A RESEARCH PRIMER FOR COMMUNICATION SCIENCES AND DISORDERS

TIMOTHY MELINE

Lamar University

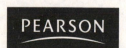

Boston   New York   San Francisco
Mexico City   Montreal   Toronto   London   Madrid   Munich   Paris
Hong Kong   Singapore   Tokyo   Cape Town   Sydney

Executive Editor and Publisher: *Stephen D. Dragin*
Editorial Assistant: *Anne Whittaker*
Vice President, Marketing and Sales Strategies: *Emily Williams Knight*
Vice President, Director of Marketing: *Quinn Perkson*
Marketing Manager: *Amanda Stedke*
Production Coordinator: *Mary Beth Finch*
Editorial Production Service: *Publishers' Design and Production Services, Inc.*
Manufacturing Buyer: *Megan Cochran*
Electronic Composition: *Publishers' Design and Production Services, Inc.*
Cover Designer: *Linda Knowles*

For related titles and support materials, visit our online catalog at
www.pearsonhighered.com.

Between the time website information is gathered and then published, it is not unusual for
some sites to have closed. Also, the transcription of URLs can result in typographical errors.
The publisher would appreciate notification where these errors occur so that they may be
corrected in subsequent editions.

Library of Congress Cataloging-in-Publication Data
Meline, Timothy J.
    Research primer for communication sciences and disorders / Timothy Meline.
        p. cm.
    Includes bibliographical references and index.
    ISBN-13: 978-0-13-701597-9 (alk. paper)
    ISBN-10: 0-13-701597-6
    1. Communicative disorders—Research. I. Title.
    RC428.M45 2010
    362.196′8550072—dc22

                                                    2009031185

Printed in the United States of America

10 9 8 7 6 5 4 3 2 1   RRD-VA   13 12 11 10 09

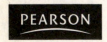

www.pearsonhighered.com

ISBN-10: 0-13-701597-6
ISBN-13: 978-0-13-701597-9

To all the animals that grace humanity

ABOUT THE AUTHOR

Dr. Timothy Meline has three children, a grandson, three dogs, and two cats. He is an accomplished writer, researcher, and sometimes artist and musician who lives in Beaumont, Texas. Dr. Meline frequently presents at state and national forums mostly on topics that are important to research in communication disorders. He also published articles in various professional journals, including those published by the American Speech–Language–Hearing Association. In addition to professional interests, he gardens, plays tennis, and reads science fiction novels.

CONTENTS

CHAPTER 2
Ethics in Communication Disorders Research   28

CHAPTER 3
Evidence-Based Practice in Communication Disorders   49

CHAPTER 4
Measurement in Communication Disorders Research   70

CHAPTER 8
Nonexperimental Research Designs in Communication Disorders   162

CHAPTER 10

Quantitative Analysis in Communication Disorders Research   **207**

CHAPTER 11

Synthesizing Research in Communication Disorders   **240**

CHAPTER 13
Writing for Research in Communication Disorders   288

PREFACE

The research enterprise is exciting and challenging—exciting in its discovery of new ideas and challenging in its demand for rigor. The importance of research for audiologists and speech-language pathologists is evident in the search for knowledge and the many contributions of research to clinical practice. In notable treatises on research, Wambaugh and Bain (2002) examined the "great need and potential for the application of research to clinical practice" (see Chapter 3 in this text), and Brobeck and Lubinsky (2003) promoted the use of single-subject research in clinical practices (see Chapter 7 in this text). Teachers of research methods regularly communicate their enthusiasm for research to students, but students benefit most from hands-on experience. Most programs in communication sciences and disorders recognize the importance of the research experience for undergraduates (Mueller & Lisko, 2003) as well as for graduate students. As Mueller and Lisko (2003) advised, "Students who design, fully execute, and disseminate a research project learn to appreciate the excitement of discovery and the reward of scholarship" (p. 124). Williams and Fagelson (2003) recounted their revision of the traditional research pedagogy as a "cooperative learning community" with journal clubs and collaborative research projects to spur learning. Many programs have adopted similar models in their curriculum, and many students have subsequently presented their research projects in state and national forums. The more research experiences invested in the undergraduate and graduate curricula, the more students appreciate how research and clinical practice are connected. Students should also see research as a legitimate career choice.

To these ends, the chapters that follow begin with the science that underpins research methods and end with an exposition on writing for presentation and publication. The intervening chapters extol many important and diverse issues in research, including evidence-based practice, ethics, group designs, single case designs, qualitative designs, survey methods, quantitative methods, research synthesis, and evaluating research for practice.

The chapters include "Technology Notes," which encourage students to appreciate and explore the technologies available for research in communication disorders. Throughout the chapters, *thought questions* follow case examples to encourage active learning. Though the chapters cover the basics and some information that is not so basic, students benefit from an introductory course in research methods, statistics, or quantitative methods in the undergraduate curriculum. As supplements, there are many excellent tutorials in the journals that address special topics in more detail. There are also many internet resources, and selected websites are referenced throughout the chapters.

The thirteen chapters are comprehensive in scope, though individual chapters may survey their topic. Chapter 1 presents the *foundation for scientific inquiry* with discussions of the basic principles of science, various types of research, variables and operational definitions, and validity issues.

Chapter 2 is an introduction to *ethics in research*. It provides a history of ethics, presents professional codes of ethics, discusses the impact of various issues in ethics, addresses human and animal research issues, and forms the relationship between evidence-based practice and ethics.

Chapter 3 is dedicated to the principles of *evidence-based practice* in communication disorders. It discusses the origins of evidence-based practice, ethics, evidence-based practice benefits and risks, and implementation issues such as clinical practice guidelines, acceptance and adherence, resistance to change, and misconceptions.

Chapter 4 addresses the *basic principles underlying scientific observations, including measurement*, data transformations, and data collection issues. In addition, it introduces descriptive statistics and the importance of visual presentation (statistical graphics) in communication disorders research.

Chapter 5 introduces the foundation for *group research* designs in communication disorders including sampling methods, subject selection procedures, and randomization issues. In addition, it introduces complex research designs and their applications in communication disorders research.

Chapter 6 surveys *qualitative research* and its applications to communication disorders research. It includes an orientation to qualitative research and a discussion of basic qualitative research designs with examples. In addition, Chapter 6 discusses credibility and transferability issues related to qualitative research outcomes as well as the combining of qualitative and quantitative approaches. Students are also introduced to qualitative analysis software applications.

Chapter 7 presents *single case designs* and their applications in communication disorders research. It explains the basic A-B-A, multiple baseline, changing criterion, and simultaneous treatment designs with case examples.

Chapter 8 presents *nonexperimental research* designs including case studies, and historical, correlational, developmental, and survey designs. In addition, replication designs including conceptual, systematic, and direct types are discussed.

Chapter 9 introduces *hypothesis testing* in communication disorders. It outlines six steps in the hypothesis-testing process and introduces the concepts of the normal distribution, standard normal distribution, distribution of test statistics, and the Central Limit Theorem. Overall, Chapter 9 forms a foundation of understanding for the discussion of quantitative methods that follows in Chapter 10.

Chapter 10 is a review of *quantitative methods* in communication disorders including tests for differences between two groups, simple analysis of variance, complex analysis of variance, and tests for analyzing categorical data. Chapter 10 also introduces effect-size statistics along with their calculation and interpretation. The availability of online resources for quantitative analysis is referenced throughout the chapter.

Chapter 11 introduces the notion of *synthesizing research* in communication disorders. It includes a review of Robey and Schultz's (1998) *Model for Clinical-Outcome Research* and presents examples of traditional narrative reviews, systematic reviews, quantitative reviews, and "best evidence" reviews. In addition, Chapter 11 discusses the epidemiology of systematic reviews, the life of a systematic review, and the importance of systematic reviews to evidence-based practice.

Chapter 12 explains the need to *evaluate research* in communication disorders for clinical practice. It includes critical questions for evaluation, case examples, and a checklist for critically evaluating research articles.

Chapter 13 discusses *writing for research* in communication disorders. The chapter includes a review of stage-process and cognitive-process models of the writing process to encourage a better understanding of the underlying process. Students are expected to acquire better writing habits as a consequence of reading Chapter 13.

A Research Primer for Communication Sciences and Disorders presents a cohesive and comprehensive introduction to research for advanced undergraduate students and graduate students in communication sciences and disorders. It was written with the philosophy that no one research design or method is the best. Each and every method and approach to research has its place, and each one contributes in its unique way, as Robey and Schultz's (1998) model explains. The characteristics that best define good research are rigorous planning and execution, not the choice of design or methodology.

The author would like to thank the following reviewers for their time and input: Janet Patterson, California State University, East Bay, and Vishakha Rawool, West Virginia University.

PART I

FOUNDATIONS OF SCIENCE AND RESEARCH IN COMMUNICATION DISORDERS

CHAPTER 1

SCIENTIFIC INQUIRY IN COMMUNICATION DISORDERS RESEARCH

> **research** (r¹-sûrch) *v.* analyze, experiment, explore, inquire, investigate, probe, scrutinize, study

Scientific inquiry aims to better understand the world and its inhabitants. This goal is achieved by accumulating a body of scientific knowledge. In daily life, information is gathered from a variety of sources including newspapers, magazines, books, and the Internet as well as from friends, coworkers, newscasters, and experts who share their professional opinions. Information is also gathered from personal experiences with the world and its inhabitants—though personal experiences are mediated by the senses and shaped through past experiences. With regard to this, Borden, Harris, and Raphael (2002) explained, "Our perceptions often match our expectations rather than what was actually said and heard" (p. 151). Borden and associates (2002) referred to this characteristic of human perception as *duality*. Most of us would agree that perceptions do not always match reality. Because perceptions are often inaccurate or subject to personal bias, scientists depend on other methods to verify their observations.

The ordinary *ways* of knowing the world are adequate for daily living but not for scientific inquiry. Science imposes a higher standard of objectivity and reliability than ordinary observations permit. The *scientific method* prescribes a set of rules and principles that guides the search for knowledge.

THE SCIENTIFIC METHOD

Scientists attempt to describe the world and logically organize the information collected into the larger body of knowledge. *Research* is the process whereby scientists attempt to understand the world and its inhabitants. Scientific research is governed by

TECHNOLOGY NOTE

Our perceptions of reality are affected by what we see and hear. Sometimes it is difficult to sort out what is real from what is fiction. Television, radio, and movies are very influential in our lives. Indeed, speech-language pathologists (SLPs) are depicted in the mass media in various ways, and the public's perception may be influenced by these depictions. SLPs are occasional characters in daytime soap operas. Actress Lela Lee depicted a speech therapist in *The Young and the Restless*. In the soap opera *All My Children* (2005), the script reads: "Lily visited Jonathan in prison … they discussed their common problems with speech troubles. Lily tried to give Jonathan hope and said that hers got better after she saw a speech therapist." A speech therapist was also depicted in *Rocket Science*, a movie about a boy who joins the high school debate team to tackle his stuttering. Why are our perceptions different from reality?

a rigid set of rules that define the scientific method. *Three important assumptions* are the underpinnings of the scientific method:

1. *Order*—Scientists believe that events occur in regular patterns, not random occurrences.
2. *Determinism*—Scientists believe that the occurrence of an event is determined by prior events.
3. *Discoverability*—Scientists expect to find answers to research questions. However, new questions arise as others are answered. In this way, scientific research is an ongoing and continuous process of discovery.

Scientific Observations

Scientists observe events to explain the relationship between two or more variables. *Variables* are properties that take on different values—as few as two or an infinite number. The scientific method imposes several conditions on observations. First, observations must be objective. *Objectivity* is the expression of reality without the intrusion of the researchers' personal beliefs, biases, or emotions. Speculation about unobserved events is expressly prohibited. Second, the events and observations of events must be *public*, because science is a social enterprise, and the research process should be open to scrutiny by all. Third, observations must be *repeatable*. A research study must be described in enough detail to allow others to replicate its methods and results. The replication process provides for a *confirmation* of results. The need to confirm or refute research results is basic to the scientific approach. Nothing is assumed to be true until it is confirmed by independent investigations.

Cause and Effect

Sometimes researchers in communication disorders observe people and events without inferring causality. For example, some studies are interested in the relationship

TECHNOLOGY NOTE

Technology is more than electronic and digital products. Its definition includes the application of science and the materials (or resources) used to achieve scientific objectives. An especially important resource for achieving scientific objectives is the brain power provided by individuals in the discipline of communication disorders. The American Speech-Language-Hearing Association's Research and Scientific Affairs Committee highlighted the need for a strong research base in the professions because of the interdependence of practitioners and researchers. The Committee recommended a reemphasis on research methods in training programs along with experiences in conducting research (American Speech-Language-Hearing Association, 1994).

between two variables such as gender and perceptions of hearing-aid use with no consideration of causality. Other studies may survey opinions about professional issues without inferring causality. Nonetheless, most research in communication disorders is interested in cause-effect relationships at some point in time.

Typically, researchers infer cause from effect by eliminating all possible causes but one. The cause–effect relationship is stated, "If A then B." There are three conditions for inferring causality: (a) the treatment occurs before the change, not after, (b) the change is observable, and (c) no other variable can account for the change. The third condition is the most difficult to satisfy because variables are not easily isolated. Thus, the relationship is more often stated as "A *implies* B." Researchers use statistics to verify implications such as $A \rightarrow B$.

Steps in the Scientific Method

Ideas for research come from a variety of sources. For example, speech-language pathology and audiology practices are rich sources of ideas for scientific study. Clinical experiences, anecdotal accounts, and case studies often inspire future investigations. Likewise, social, political, and regulatory demands for quality assurance are catalysts for studies of treatment efficacy. On the other hand, research reports, articles, editorials, letters to the editor, and textbooks are also good sources of ideas.

Once the seed of an idea exists or a problem to be solved is identified, it must be expressed in a manageable way. The scientific principle of *objectivity* requires formality throughout the research process. As a consequence, observations are usually coded so that they can be reliably recorded. In addition, *operational definitions* are written for each variable of interest. An operational definition gives meaning to a variable by specifying the activities necessary for its measurement.

The five major steps in the scientific process are as follows:

1. *Stating the problem.*   The statement of the problem should be a clear description of the problem along with a rationale for its study. Research questions are usually evident once the problem to be addressed is clear. The research questions should express the goals of the study.

2. *Formulating the research hypothesis.*   Another step in the research process is the formulation of the research hypothesis. In Friedman's words: "The construction of hypotheses is a creative act of inspiration, intuition, invention; its essence is the vision of something new in familiar material" (1953, p. 43). The hypothesis is a best guess at the answer to a research question. The research hypothesis should be supported by the existing scientific literature as well as personal experiences.

3. *Developing the research method.*   A third critical step in the research process is to develop a procedure for answering the research questions. The *research method* includes a specification of participants and a detailed plan for observing behaviors and recording data. Observations become data when they are coded in some operational form. A numerical coding is most common because numbers are easily recorded, analyzed, and stored. Numerical coding is the hallmark of quantitative research. On the other hand, qualitative research methods depend on descriptions, categories, and words for data. Whatever the nature of the data (quantitative or qualitative), a research study's success depends on the *validity* and *reliability* of its methods. Validity has to do with the meaningfulness of results, and reliability has to do with the ability to replicate results.

4. *Analyzing results.*   After collecting and recording the data, researchers analyze it. A typical analysis includes graphs, tables, and statistics. The different kinds of analysis help to accurately interpret results. If the analysis of data is faulty, the research conclusions will be faulty. For this reason, the analysis of data is an especially rigorous and demanding step in the research process. Researchers may seek advice from statisticians and other experts in data analysis because this step in the research process is highly specialized.

5. *Interpreting results.*   The interpretation of results is guided by both the research questions and hypotheses that were originally proposed. The goals for the interpretation of results are (a) to answer each research question, and (b) to support or refute the hypothesis. Sometimes, new research questions as well as methodological shortcomings are revealed when data are analyzed and interpreted. The interpretation of results is typically included in the *conclusion section* at the end of the research report.

TYPES OF RESEARCH IN COMMUNICATION DISORDERS

By convention, research is organized into various divisions; some are just dichotomous (divided into two parts). In practice, the boundaries that divide one type of research from another are artificial and often overlap. Nonetheless, these divisions are a basis for understanding the complexities of research designs.

Basic and Applied Research Types

The simplest way to distinguish between basic and applied types of research is to examine the purpose for conducting a research study. If the sole purpose is to contribute new scientific knowledge with no intention of solving a social or clinical problem or any

TECHNOLOGY NOTE

Is it science, pseudoscience, or junk science? The standards for determining whether a body of knowledge or a practice is *scientific* vary from discipline to discipline. However, scientists agree that principles such as reproducibility and verifiability are basic to all disciplines. A practice or body of knowledge is *pseudoscience* when it misuses the scientific method. Pseudoscience is identified by its; (a) use of vague, exaggerated, or untestable claims; (b) overreliance on confirmation rather than refutation; (c) lack of openness (transparency); (d) failure to progress toward confirmation of its claims; (e) personalization of issues; and (f) use of misleading language. Finn, Bothe, and Bramlett (2005) proposed 10 criteria to distinguish science from pseudoscience. They illustrated their criteria's use with several popular or controversial treatment approaches. Finally, *junk science* is a term used exclusively in political debates. The term suggests that the argument has political, ideological, or other unscientific motives.

other practical application, the research is best described as *basic research*. On the other hand, if the purpose is clearly to solve a social problem, clinical problem, or other practical application, the research is best described as *applied research*. Both types of research are highly valued in the scientific community.

Basic research is especially useful for constructing new theories and modifying existing ones. *Theories* are general explanations that attempt to explain the relationship between observable events (effects) and their origins (causes). Applied research is much narrower in scope but answers important questions of immediate social and clinical relevance. Applied research attempts to solve problems that require immediate solutions. However, basic research is often an impetus for finding solutions to practical problems. For example, Bloom's (1970) classic study of early language development was basic research but it inspired many applied research studies and contributed much to the clinical domain.

Two types of applied research with distinctly different purposes are common in communication disorders. Olswang (1990) described the two distinct purposes as follows:

> Applied research can be conducted for the purpose of better understanding the nature of communication disorders (i.e. exploring differences between normal and disordered populations), or for better understanding the clinical processes of assessment and treatment associated with communication disorders. (p. 45)

Applied research of the first type focuses on the nature of communication disorders, and any concern for immediate applications is of secondary importance. Applied research of the second type is known as *clinical research*, and its primary purpose is to study some aspect of the clinical process. Clinical research may be further divided into special areas of interest such as assessment, treatment, or clinical specialties. The demand for clinical research is increased by needs for quality assurance, best practices, and evidence-based practice. Olswang (1990) explained:

> Clinical research has been motivated in part by issues of accountability. Practitioners are asked to document the efficacy of their treatments, proving that what they do makes a difference in their clients' communicative functioning. Clinicians in school settings, health care settings, and private practice are asked to evaluate the efficacy of their services, to demonstrate that their efforts are worthwhile. (p. 45)

Laboratory and Field Studies

Another distinction in research types is between laboratory research and field research. *Field research* is conducted in everyday settings such as homes, schools, or clinics. In contrast, *laboratory research* is conducted in more or less contrived settings outside the mainstream of daily lives. Field research aims to observe behaviors as they occur in their natural environment. Field researchers may sacrifice close control over variables for closer ties to reality. In contrast, laboratory research maintains rigid control over variables but risks laboratory bias—laboratory surroundings may affect behavior in unwanted ways. For example, people who know they are being observed may change their behaviors in dramatic ways. Contemporary researchers have eliminated some of the unwanted effects of the laboratory environment to create laboratory settings that are remarkably natural.

Experimental Versus Quasi-Experimental Research Types

Experimental research is sometimes equated with laboratory research. However, many experiments are successfully conducted in field-like settings. Two requirements are central to the definition of a true experiment. First, participants are randomly assigned to two or more conditions. The random assignment of subjects to conditions is the best way

TECHNOLOGY NOTE

Scientists depend on the randomization of subjects to groups to eliminate unwanted influences. However, *simple randomization*—the method that scientists typically use— works only with large numbers. If you flip a penny 10 times, will the result always be 5 heads and 5 tails? The more times you flip the penny (assuming it's a fair penny), the more likely you are to achieve a 50/50 split. According to Lachin, Matts, and Wei (1988), 200 or more subjects are needed to guarantee a balance between groups. For a sample of 20, the chance of a 60/40 split or worse is 50 percent. We would need 100 subjects to reduce the chance of a 60/40 split to 5 percent. For experiments with small numbers of subjects, simple randomization may not work. There are alternative methods for achieving balance when experiments include small numbers of subjects (Lachin et al., 1988; Moeschberger, Williams, & Brown, 1985).

to assure equivalency, and it avoids the possibility of bias. Sometimes, researchers achieve near equivalency by *matching* subjects in condition A with those in condition B, but random assignment is the only way to assure equivalency. Second, researchers control the selection of conditions, and they can freely manipulate the conditions. If a research design does not meet these requirements, it is probably a *quasi-experimental* design. Exhibit 1.1 highlights the differences between true experiments and quasi-experiments. It also illustrates the difference between quasi-experiments and nonexperiments.

Nonexperimental designs lack any measure of comparison—no group comparison or prior measurement for comparison. They provide interesting data but do nothing to eliminate extraneous factors that might influence results. Thus, nonexperimental designs typically observe behaviors without inferring cause and effect. As an example, a speech-language pathologist (SLP) might interview patients following dysphagia treatment to assess the treatment's effects. However, without a point of comparison, the SLP cannot conclude that the outcome is due to the dysphagia therapy. It could have been the result of a number of other factors. If cause and effect are important, the SLP could interview patients who did not receive dysphagia therapy and compare their results with those who did receive therapy. Alternatively, a measurement made prior to therapy could be compared with the post-therapy outcome.

Research Designs in Communication Disorders

The majority of research designs in communication disorders are the quasi-experimental type. *Quasi* means "as if, almost or having a likeness to." Thus, quasi-experiments are almost experiments but not quite. Trochim (2004) described quasi-experimental designs as those that look like experimental designs but lack the key ingredient of

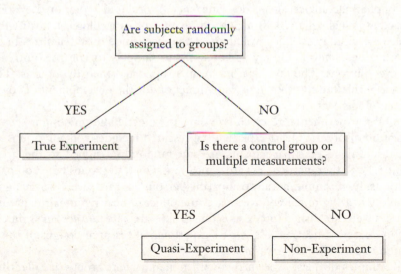

EXHIBIT 1.1
Questions for Identifying Research Types

random assignment. There are few examples of true experiments in communication disorders. In fact, Meline and Harn (2008b) identified only 16 true (randomized) experiments in American Speech-Language-Hearing Association (ASHA) journals published between 2003 and 2008. Those 16 experiments represent about 1 percent of the articles and reports published in ASHA journals during that time period. Truly randomized group experiments are somewhat underrepresented in communication disorders research. The reasons for their rarity probably include the high costs of time, money, and other resources that are typically associated with this type of research.

A case example of a true experiment is Roy, Weinrich, Gray, Tanner, Stemple, and Sapienza's (2003) study of three different treatments for teachers with voice disorders. Their research team described the experimental protocol as follows:

> This randomized clinical trial used patient-based treatment outcome measures to evaluate the effectiveness of three treatment programs. Sixty-four teachers with voice disorders were randomly assigned to 1 of 3 treatment groups: voice amplification using the ChatterVox portable amplifier (VA; n = 25), resonance therapy (RT; n = 19), and respiratory muscle training (RMT; n = 20). Before and after a 6-week treatment phase, all teachers completed (a) the Voice Handicap Index (VHI; B. H. Jacobson et al., 1997), an instrument designed to appraise the self-perceived psychosocial consequences of voice disorders, and (b) a voice severity self-rating scale. (Roy et al., 2003, p. 670)

Based on Roy et al.'s (2003) description, answer the following questions: (a) What qualifies the research design as a true experiment? (b) How many conditions were employed in the experiment? (c) In what way did the researchers control the selection of conditions?

Leydon, Fisher, and Lodewyk-Falciglia (2008) reported a randomized, controlled experimental design with tissue samples as "participants." They investigated the effect of pharmacological agents on ovine (sheep) vocal fold hydration. Leydon, Fisher, and Lodewyk-Falciglia (2008) hypothesized that pharmacological treatments to the surface of excised vocal folds would affect the magnitude of water fluxes in the vocal fold mucosae. They randomly assigned tissue samples to control (untreated) and treated conditions. The investigators' results supported their hypothesis. They concluded that the findings should provide direction for the development of voice hydration treatments.

Quasi-experimental research types are the most common designs seen in communication disorders. Quasi-experimental research includes control groups or multiple measurements, but participants are not randomly assigned to the groups (see Exhibit 1.1). Rather, participants are typically assigned to groups based on preexisting conditions. For example, a study comparing persons who are severely hearing impaired and mildly hearing impaired investigates the effect of hearing impairment after hearing loss is well established (preexists). The groups are *nonequivalent* in as much as they differ in degree of hearing loss. Quasi-experimental research designs of this sort are common in communication disorders.

Examples of quasi-experiments with nonequivalent groups are plentiful in the communication disorders literature because clinical groups are frequently compared to nonclinical groups. A case example is Hoffman and Gillam's (2004) comparison of nonequivalent groups (children with specific language impairment and children who were typically developing). They described their two groups as follows:

> The group of children with SLI contained 18 boys and 6 girls who ranged in age from 96 months to 128 months, with a mean age of 9;5 (years;months; see Table 1). All children in the SLI group had been previously diagnosed as language impaired by public school assessment teams that included, at a minimum, a speech-language pathologist, a psychological examiner, and a classroom teacher, and all were receiving speech-language services in school at the time of the study. [...] The control group also contained 18 boys and 6 girls. They ranged in age from 96 to 128 months of age, with a mean age of 9;4 (see Table 1). Participants in the control group were selected on the basis of age, grade, and gender. Like their SLI counterparts, these children demonstrated normal hearing and nonverbal intelligence. Unlike their SLI counterparts, however, these children had no prior history of speech, language, or learning disorders. (Hoffman & Gillam, 2004, pp. 117–118)

Though the children in Hoffman and Gillam's (2004) quasi-experiment were not exactly alike, the researchers took steps to establish some equivalency between the two groups. After reading Hoffman and Gillam's (2004) description of their subjects, answer the following questions: How did Hoffman and Gillam attempt to match the SLI and typically developing groups of children? In what ways were the two groups of children different?

Another case example of quasi-experimental research is Tyler, Lewis, Haskill, and Tolbert's (2003) study of phonological and morphosyntactic changes in young children. Tyler et al. (2003) described their method as follows:

> Participants included 47 preschoolers, ages 3;0 (years; months) to 5;11, with impairments in both speech and language development: 40 children in the experimental group and 7 in a control group. All children had received speech-language evaluations and were identified as potential participants through review of their evaluation results in consultation with the evaluating SLP. Children in the experimental group were enrolled in speech-language services in early childhood programs in Washoe County School District, Reno, NV. For these children, speech-language services consisted of participation in one of the four experimental interventions. The control group consisted of children who had been placed on waiting lists for speech-language services. (p. 1079)

Based on the description of Tyler et al.'s (2003) study, answer the following questions: (a) What is your opinion of their research? (b) What were the experimental conditions? (c) What features make the design quasi-experimental? (d) Could the researchers have randomly assigned subjects to conditions? (e) If you were to repeat the experiment, what would you do differently?

TYPES OF VARIABLES IN COMMUNICATION DISORDERS RESEARCH

Variables are the focus of interest for behavioral scientists. Variables are concepts that take on different quantitative or qualitative values. The opposite of a variable is known as a *constant*. Constants do not change, and they are not evident in human behavior. Examples of variables include "intelligence," which has many values, and "gender," which has two values: male and female. Thus, variables can have as few as two values or an infinite number of values. There are many different types of variables, but a critical distinction exists between those known as independent and dependent variables.

Independent and Dependent Variables

Independent and dependent variables are the focus of interest in research designs. In experimental research designs, researchers control and manipulate the independent variable however, in quasi-experimental designs, researchers cannot control or manipulate the independent variable, because it is fixed. For example, Reynolds, Callihan, and Browning (2003) chose two forms of intervention (i.e., rhyming and narrative treatments) for 16 participants. The research team purposefully manipulated the independent variable by choosing two treatment conditions and randomly assigning half of the 16 participants to each of the two conditions. Reynolds et al. (2003) actively manipulated their independent variable, but many research designs include independent variables that cannot be manipulated. A case in point is McHenry's (2003) study. McHenry (2003) included participants with varying degrees of dysarthric speech: (a) mild dysarthria, (b) moderate-to-severe dysarthria, and (c) no dysarthria (control group). In McHenry's quasi-experiment, the independent variable (dysarthric speech) was present before the study began. Therefore, it could not be manipulated by the researcher.

A second variable of central importance to research is known as the *dependent variable*. The dependent variable is the focus of observations in an experiment. It is usually a behavior that has been operationally defined. In experimental research, a relational hypothesis is typically written as a conditional statement: *If X, then Y*. In this form, *X* is the independent variable and *Y* is the dependent variable. This is true for *bivariate* research problems, which include one independent variable and one dependent variable. However, some experiments are designed to investigate *multivariate* problems—those that include more than one independent variable or more than one dependent variable. In multivariate research designs, the relational hypothesis is expressed as (a) *if X, then P and Q* or, alternatively, (b) *if P and Q, then Y*.

Active and Attribute Variables

Another important distinction made in research is one between active and attribute variables. *Active variables* are those that can be manipulated by the researcher. Examples of active variables include types of language tests, treatment procedures, noise, and other conditions that are readily changed. In contrast, *attribute variables* are measured but not manipulated. Human characteristics are attribute variables. Examples of attribute variables include language skills, intelligence, and hearing sensitivity. The assumption is that past environmental or hereditary incidents are responsible for these attributes; however, identifying exact causes is not always possible.

Continuous and Categorical Variables

A distinction between continuous and categorical variables is important for the preparation and analysis of research data. *Continuous variables* take on a range of values and possess the mathematical property known as *order*. For example, language age, chronological age, IQ, and hearing sensitivity are usually treated as continuous variables. In contrast, *categorical variables* do not have the mathematical property of order. In this case, people or objects are assigned to categories based on whether they possess some characteristic or not. Categorical variables may be dichotomous with only two values, or they may possess many values. For example, *gender* includes the categories *male* and *female*, but *hearing loss* may have five or more categories ranging from *mild* to *profound*. The number of categories depends on the classification scheme adopted by the researchers.

Artificial categories are sometimes created from continuous variables. For example, chronological age is clearly a continuous variable. However, age categories such as *young, middle-aged, old*, and *very old* are often constructed. To be meaningful, each category requires an *operational definition*. For example, the category *very old* may be operationally defined as 80 years of age and over. The important point is that categories can be created from continuous variables, and these newly created categories are treated as categorical variables. The use of variables in research designs will determine their classification as either continuous or categorical.

Extraneous Variables in Communication Disorders Research

In general, variables other than the independent variables and the dependent variables are unwanted and are often a nuisance in research. *Extraneous variables* are potential nuisance variables. In research, an extraneous variable is any variable that affects the dependent variable that is not the independent variable. If the dependent variable is affected by one or more extraneous variables, the relationship between independent and dependent variables is confounded. In this case, conclusions about the relationship between the independent and dependent variables are seriously compromised.

Extraneous variables are a regular occurrence and a persistent concern for researchers. They are particularly problematic in some research designs. However, if researchers are able to identify possible nuisance variables before a study begins, their effects may be minimized. The most troublesome extraneous variables are those that are unknown to the researchers.

OPERATIONAL DEFINITIONS IN COMMUNICATION DISORDERS RESEARCH

Research data are systematically collected and recorded according to guidelines (i.e., operational definitions) that are adopted by researchers during the early planning stages of experimentation. *Operational definitions* describe the activities necessary to measure and manipulate variables. More specifically, operational definitions are instructions for selecting subjects, measuring behaviors, and carrying out procedures.

Two Types of Operational Definitions

There are two types of operational definitions. One type specifies what behaviors will be measured. For example, a definition of stuttering lists the specific behaviors that the researcher believes represent the concept of stuttering. An operational definition is a bridge between concepts such as "stuttering" and observations such as syllable repetitions. Mizuko and Reichle (1989) adopted an operational definition for selecting participants based on specific behaviors. Their selection criteria were described as follows:

> Subjects selected for the study met the following criteria: (a) English spoken as the primary language in the home, as reported by the subject's ward; (b) no apparent secondary handicaps—either physical, sensory (auditory or visual), or emotional—as reported by the subject's ward; (c) vision within normal limits, as determined by the Child's Recognition and Near Point Test (Allen, 1957); (d) hearing within normal limits, as determined by a pure-tone audiometric screening; (e) age equivalent scores between 2 and 5 years (*M* = 3.19 years; *SD* = 0.73), as determined by the Peabody Picture Vocabulary Test (Dunn, 1981); and (f) lack of familiarity with any of the three symbol systems, as determined by parental or teacher report. (Mizuko & Reichle, 1989, p. 628)

A second type of operational definition describes the manipulation of an independent variable. The independent variable in Mizuko and Reichle's (1989) study was the *graphic symbol system*. They selected three symbol systems as the experimental conditions: (a) Blissymbols, (b) Picture Communication System, and (c) Picsyms. Mizuko and Reichle's (1989) operational definition included a description of the three symbol systems as well as reasons for choosing them:

> The rationale for selecting these symbol systems was twofold. First, these systems have been the focus of investigations with intellectually normal children (Mizuko, 1987). Second, one or more of these three symbol systems had been the focus of intervention studies with persons having moderate to severe handicaps (Goosens', 1983; Hurlbut et al., 1982; Leonhart & Maharaj, 1979). (p. 628)

The Limits of Operational Definitions

Some variables are easily measured, such as gender or social class. However, concepts like intelligence are more difficult to define. Any one or a combination of behaviors could form a definition of intelligence. In practice, researchers often rely on standardized measures of intelligence because they are reasonably objective and repeatable. Thus, a widely accepted test such as the *Stanford-Binet Intelligence Scale* is a common basis for operational definitions of intelligence. Likewise, researchers may choose a proven measure of hearing sensitivity or language ability for an operational definition. It is important that the measure chosen has been demonstrated both valid and reliable for the population of interest. Based on what you know about audiology and speech-language pathology, answer the following questions: (a) What are examples of widely accepted tests for hearing sensitivity and language ability? (b) Are they valid and reliable tests for the populations of children or adults that you treat? (c) Could these tests be used as measures for operational definitions in research?

DATA COLLECTION IN COMMUNICATION DISORDERS RESEARCH

Research data are the consequence of observing or otherwise gathering information for study. Observations become data when they are coded in some fashion. These *codings* may take the form of written records or taped recordings. If the coding is not initially in numerical form, it is usually recoded numerically to facilitate data analysis. The assignment of numerals to objects according to specified rules is known as *measurement*. The data are also known as *statistics*. The science of statistics includes four steps: (a) collection, (b) classification, (c) analysis, and (d) interpretation of numerical data. The classification, analysis, and interpretation steps are faulty if data are not gathered in a reliable fashion.

THE RELIABILITY OF COLLECTED DATA

The collection of data is a critical aspect of the scientific method and is a highly systematic process. Researchers must have a plan for gathering data that ensures both *objectivity* and *repeatability*. Care must be taken in the collection of data to avoid personal biases that may unfairly affect the data. For example, a researcher who hypothesizes improved voice quality following treatment may unwittingly rate voice quality as better than it is in reality. Procedures for ensuring the reliability and validity of data collection include (a) blinding procedures and (b) interobserver reliability measures.

Blinding Procedures

Blinding procedures are processes by which researchers, research assistants, and subjects perform the tasks prescribed by the research plan without knowledge of the research questions or hypotheses. To implement blinding procedures, researchers may recruit independent operatives to collect data and implement treatments. In the context of experimental research designs, *single blinding* is such that subjects do not know to which group they are assigned—experimental or control. In the case of *double blinding*, neither participants nor research team members know who is assigned to experimental and control groups. Blinding is an important procedure in both experimental and quasi-experimental designs. It helps to ensure the integrity of the research process.

Interobserver Reliability Measures

Interobserver reliability is established by measuring the consistency of two or more individuals who independently observe the same event. Typically, the agreement between individuals is expected to be 90 percent or more, depending on the exact nature of the observations. By convention, an *agreement index* of below 80 percent is usually unacceptable. Interobserver agreement indexes are widely used to estimate the reliability of observational data. Two common computations for interobserver agreement are (a) the total percentage agreement, also known as the *smaller/larger index*, and (b) the point-by-point agreement.

The *total percentage agreement* procedure is calculated for two sets of scores by dividing the smaller number of behaviors observed by the larger number. For example, observer A records 22 occurrences of a behavior, and observer B records 18 occurrences. To calculate the percentage of agreement, the 18 is divided by 22 to equal 0.82. The result is converted to a percentage by multiplying 0.82 by 100. The result is an 82 percent agreement between observers. This procedure assumes that the two sets of scores overlap. In other words, observer A identified the same 18 occurrences of the behavior as observer B plus 4 additional occurrences. When this assumption is not met, an alternative procedure such as the point-by-point agreement index is employed.

The *point-by-point agreement index* is a common interobserver agreement metric in communication disorders. This procedure examines targeted behaviors point by point, as shown in Exhibit 1.2. The symbol "0" represents the absence of a target behavior, and "1" represents its presence. A point-by-point inspection of the data

EXHIBIT 1.2
Example of Point-by-Point Agreement for
Interobserver Reliability

OBSERVER A	OBSERVER B
1	0 disagree
1	1 agree
0	0 agree
1	1 agree
1	1 agree
0	0 agree
1	1 agree
0	1 disagree
0	0 agree
1	1 agree

reveals 2 points of disagreement between observers A and B with a total of 8 points of agreement. Thus, 8 divided by 10 (total points of comparison) yields a coefficient of 0.80. The result is converted to a percentage by multiplying 0.80 by 100, for an 80 percent agreement between observers. The point-by-point agreement index is generally a good way to establish interobserver reliability.

INTERNAL VALIDITY IN COMMUNICATION DISORDERS RESEARCH

The concept of internal validity was first introduced by Campbell in 1957. Internal validity is the minimum requirement for meaningful interpretations of research results. *Internal validity* is defined as the degree to which the relationship between the independent variable (IV) and dependent variable (DV) is observed without the influence of extraneous variables. If there is a causal inference, the relationship is hypothesized as IV → DV.

Variables that affect the DV other than the IV are known as *confounding* (or extraneous) variables. The presence of confounding variables weakens internal validity. As a consequence, when internal validity is weak, researchers cannot imply that the IV produced the effect observed in the DV. Problems with internal validity are the most common weakness in research studies.

Nine Possible Threats to Internal Validity

Campbell and Stanley (1963) described eight common threats to internal validity, including (a) differential selection effects, (b) history effects, (c) maturation effects, (d) statistical regression effects, (e) attrition effects, (f) testing effects, (g) instrumentation effects, and (h) additive and interaction effects. These are sometimes referred to as the eight classic threats. Shadish, Cook, and Campbell (2002) added another threat, *ambiguous temporal precedence*, to the list of common threats to internal validity. Thus, nine common threats to internal validity are important considerations for researchers as they plan their investigations in communication disorders. However, the nine threats do not affect every research design. Rather, some designs are more vulnerable to certain threats—and some are less vulnerable. Exhibit 1.3 lists the common threats to internal validity, the most vulnerable research designs, and some possible remedies. The first of the nine threats to internal validity is known as ambiguous temporal precedence.

Ambiguous temporal precedence effects.   To infer causality, the treatment must occur before a change in the dependent variable is observed. However, the direction of a relationship between two variables is not always clear. When the direction of relationship between two variables is uncertain, the relationship is best described as *A ↔ B*. Correlational and longitudinal designs are especially vulnerable to ambiguous temporal precedence (ATP) effects because the temporal relationship between variables is often ambiguous.

EXHIBIT 1.3
Common Threats to Internal Validity in Communication Disorders Research, Most Vulnerable Research Designs, and Possible Remedies (Controls)

THREAT	MOST VULNERABLE DESIGN	REMEDY (CONTROL)
1. Ambiguous temporal precedences	Correlational and longitudinal designs	Choose another design if cause-effect is critical.
2. Differential selection effects	Designs with two or more groups	(a) Randomly assign subjects to groups. (b) Match subjects.
3. History effects	Observations over an extended time period	Shorten length of experimental treatment.
4. Maturation effects	(a) Lengthy experimental treatment (b) Complicated experimental task	(a) Shorten time of experimental treatment. (b) Add a control group to account for the maturation effect.
5. Statistical regression effects	Subjects selected on the basis of high or low test scores	Deselect subjects with high or low test scores.
6. Attrition effects	(a) Vulnerable subject population (b) Small sample size	Select additional subjects to offset losses.
7. Testing effects	Subjects tested more than once during an experiment	(a) Counterbalance tests. (b) Incorporate a time interval to extinguish the effect.
8. Instrument effects	Use of mechanical or electronic instruments; human observers (judges)	(a) Calibrate frequently. (b) Implement training. (c) Add perceptual anchors.
9. Additive and interactive effects	All designs are vulnerable.	Avoid vulnerabilities or minimize them whenever possible.

Controlling ATP effects. There are no specific procedures for controlling ATP effects. Rather, the only way to avoid the threat of ATP effects is to choose a research design that is not vulnerable to such effects—such as pretest-posttest designs. However, if causality is not important to the research purpose, it is known as *differential selection*.

Differential selection effects. The participants in research studies possess unique characteristics (learned and inherent), such as gender, age, intelligence, culture, and motor skills. Research designs that employ two or more groups of participants are especially vulnerable to differential selection threats. If subjects are assigned to experimental and control groups in a way that results in an unequal distribution of the subjects' unique characteristics, differential selection is a serious threat. The results from such an experiment are confounded. If there is a difference between groups, the difference may be due to the independent variable effect or possibly due to the subject-related effect.

Controlling selection effects.   In the case of research designs with one subject or one group of subjects, selection effects are not a problem. The best way to control selection effects is to randomly assign subjects to experimental and control groups. *Random assignment* of subjects to groups usually avoids differential selection effects. In research designs where two or more groups of subjects are compared, an important assumption is that the groups are homogeneous in all respects. In quasi-experimental designs, the groups are homogeneous except for the classification variable. The classification variable is the one feature that distinguishes one group from the other. For example, research in communication disorders often includes groups that are distinguished by clinical classifications—such as persons with cochlear implants. To minimize the effects of differential selection in research designs where random assignment to groups is impossible, *matching* procedures are employed. If properly implemented, matching procedures ensure that the groups are equivalent for critical features, such as intelligence, age, gender, culture, and other characteristics. The third threat to internal validity is known as *history*.

History effects.   History effects include outside events (extraneous variables) that may influence the dependent variable during the course of a study. Research designs that require observations over long periods of time are especially vulnerable to the threat of history effects. The observations in comparative studies are sometimes accomplished in a few days, so they are less vulnerable to history effects. In contrast, longitudinal designs are especially vulnerable because of the duration of time involved. Pretest-posttest designs may or may not be especially vulnerable. The degree of vulnerability will depend on the duration of time between pretest and posttest phases. If the duration of time is a few days, history effects are probably negligible. On the other hand, if the duration of time is weeks or months, history effects may threaten the validity of the experiment.

Controlling history effects.   History problems are managed by anticipating their occurrence and controlling their effect. If a research plan requires a lengthy period of treatment or observations, the opportunity for extraneous variables to interfere is high. However, a research plan that accomplishes an experimental protocol in two or three weeks will probably avoid confounding by history effects. If researchers identify an extraneous variable but are unable to avoid its effect, they may choose to eliminate its effect at the experiment's conclusion with the help of special statistical procedures. However, statistical control of an extraneous variable is only possible if the variable is measured. The fourth threat to internal validity is known as *maturation*.

Maturation effects.   Students sometimes confuse history and maturation effects. Maturation effects include changes within the organism—not outside events. Examples include changes in physical abilities and mental processes such as children's development of speech and language or motor skills. In the special case of adults with aphasia, *time post-onset* is a variable that may produce a maturation effect. Brookshire (1983) explained:

> This information is particularly important when subjects' participation in an experiment spans several days or weeks, because if short-time postonset subjects who are in a period of neurologic recovery are included, changes in their responses during the course of the experiment may reflect the effects of neurologic recovery, rather than the effects of experimental conditions. (p. 343)

In addition to longer-term maturation effects, shorter-term maturation effects such as boredom, fatigue, and inattention are risks for maturation effects. Experimental tasks that are long or complicated may produce maturation effects such as boredom and fatigue—and these factors can significantly affect the dependent variable. As a case example, Tharpe and Ashmead (2001) reported a longitudinal study of seven infants. They measured auditory sensitivity monthly from birth to 12 months of age. *Maturation* was the independent variable, as is typical in developmental research, so maturation effect was the focus of the study.

Controlling maturation effects.   Maturation effects are minimized by reducing the time required for completing observations, but shortening an experiment's length is not always possible. An alternative is the addition of a control group that is expected to mature at the same rate as the experimental group. Because the control group does not receive the experimental treatment, a difference between the groups may be attributed to the treatment effect. Short-term maturation effects may be controlled by modifying the experimental milieu in ways that minimize boredom, fatigue, and inattention. For example, planned rest periods or more comfortable surroundings may reduce fatigue and improve attention for some participants. A fifth threat to internal validity is known as *statistical regression*.

Statistical regression effects   Statistical regression predicts that participants who score very high or very low on a test tend to regress toward the mean on the next administration of the test; that is, high scores tend to move lower and low scores tend to move higher. As a case example, if participants score 10 percent on a speech discrimination test, they will probably score higher on the next administration of the test. Statistical regression effects are a threat to internal validity when subjects are assigned to groups or conditions based on extreme scores (high or low) on a test. A subsequent change in the dependent variable may be attributed to the treatment effect or statistical regression (extraneous variable).

Controlling statistical regression effects.   Statistical regression effects are minimized by not selecting subjects based on extreme test scores. For example, participants in pretest-posttest research designs can be deselected if their pretest score is extremely high or low. However, deselecting participants presents a threat of another kind known as an "attrition effect." *Attrition effects* are the sixth potential threat to internal validity.

Attrition effects.   Attrition effects (formerly known as mortality effects) involve a loss of participants due to one or more reasons. For one, participants may drop out of a study for unknown reasons, or participants may relocate to a different geographic area. Another possibility is that participants cease to meet selection criteria because of physical changes, mental changes, or extreme scores on a pretest measure. Studies that require a long period of time for completion are especially vulnerable to attrition effects. Developmental studies are especially vulnerable because they typically require many months or years for completion. Some populations are especially vulnerable to attrition effects due to chronic illnesses and other health-related characteristics.

Controlling attrition effects.   It is sometimes difficult to anticipate the loss of participants. However, researchers should plan for attrition based on the characteristics of participants and the length of the study. When attrition is expected, researchers can avoid attrition effects by selecting additional participants to offset possible losses. A seventh potential threat to internal validity is known as *multiple tests*.

Multiple-tests effects.   If participants are tested more than once during an experiment, multiple-tests effects are possible. Testing effects occur when one test affects performance on a second test. The result may be (a) a test-sensitizing effect, (b) a test-practice effect, or (c) a combination of the two effects. *Test-sensitizing effects* are changes in the subjects' anxiety levels in anticipation of test taking. Anxiety usually abates after the first test, and performance on the second test improves. However, test anxiety may increase after the first test—particularly if the subject initially perceives the test as very difficult. *Test-practice effects* are the result of acquiring specific skills that improve performance on the second test. Test-sensitizing and test-practice effects are especially troublesome in research designs with two or more administrations of the same test.

Controlling testing effects.   The method of *counterbalancing* tests is often employed to control testing effects. For example, half the participants take test A followed by test B, and the other half take test B followed by test A. In this fashion, the halves are averaged, and the adverse testing effects are minimized. An alternative is to plan an interval of time between tests to extinguish testing effects. An eighth potential threat to internal validity is *instrumentation*.

Instrumentation effects.   The threat of instrumentation effects has to do with unwanted variations in instruments used to measure human behaviors. Researchers may use mechanical or electronic devices to collect data, or they may employ human observers. Both mechanical instruments and human vary because of internal fluctuations and external influences. Mechanical and electronic equipment may change over time in response to temperature, humidity, jarring, and mechanical wear. Human observers may change over time due to distractions, inattentiveness, or physical discomforts.

Controlling instrument effects.   Mechanical and electronic instruments require frequent calibrations to ensure consistent measurements. Human observers may benefit from training to minimize the variability in their observations and judgments. For example, *perceptual anchors* usually minimize variability when rating scales are employed as observational tools. Perceptual anchors are typically auditory or visual models that serve to establish the upper and lower limits of a rating scale. In addition to training and perceptual anchors as controls, researchers may employ observers who are experts by virtue of prior training, experience, and credentials that are relevant to the study's purpose. The ninth threat to internal validity is the combined effect of two or more of the previous eight threats.

Additive and interaction effects.   Any one of the threats to internal validity may interact with one or more of the other threats. For example, selection effects often interact with maturation, history, or instrumentation effects. The direction and size of additive and interaction effects are not easily identified or measured. There are no controls for additive and interaction effects except to eliminate threats to internal validity when possible and to minimize the threats that are identified but unavoidable.

EXTERNAL VALIDITY IN COMMUNICATION DISORDERS RESEARCH

External validity refers to the generalizability of research results to other participants and settings—an especially important consideration for transferring research results to clinical practice. Threats to external validity are of two types: (a) threats to population validity and (b) threats to ecological validity. *Population validity* has to do with problems generalizing to other people. *Ecological validity* has to do with problems generalizing to other environments (Bracht & Glass, 1968). There are seven factors that may limit the ability to generalize research results to other persons and settings.

Seven Possible Threats to External Validity

To achieve some degree of validity for clinical practice, population validity and ecological validity are important considerations. The challenge for researchers is to balance the need for internal validity with a consideration for external validity. The first of seven potential threats to external validity is related to the issue of *accessible populations and target populations*.

Accessible populations and target populations.   Target populations are the entire populations that are of interest to researchers. For example, researchers may be interested in American-born, 12-year-old children with Down syndrome. The total population with these characteristics includes a large number of children distributed throughout the country and elsewhere. Accessible populations include all people who can be participants given the researchers' available resources. Many researchers are limited to recruiting participants from a restricted locale such as a city, state, or region. In this case, generalization of results is usually restricted to the accessible population.

A case example is Walden, Surr, Cord, and Dyrlund's (2004) study of hearing-aid microphone preferences in everyday listening situations. The research team recruited participants (16 males, 1 female) from the accessible population of hearing-impaired adults with hearing aids fitted at the Walter Reed Army Medical Center. Based on this short description of the Walden et al. (2004) study, answer the following question: Should we generalize Walden and colleagues' results to other persons and other settings? Another possible threat to external validity involves the *description of the independent variable*.

Describing the independent variable explicitly.   The procedures followed by researchers must be described in sufficient detail to be duplicated in other settings. Detailed descriptions of procedures are especially important if results are to be generalized to clinical practice settings. Another threat is the possibility of multiple-treatment interference.

Multiple-treatment interference effects.   If participants receive more than one treatment consecutively, the external validity of subsequent treatments is uncertain because the subsequent treatment may have reacted to the initial treatment. Thus, the effects of subsequent treatments may not be generalizable to situations without the benefit of a preceding treatment. Another possible threat to external validity is known as *novelty and disruption*.

Novelty and disruption effects.   "A new and unusual experimental treatment, e.g. a [teaching] innovation, may be superior to a traditional treatment primarily because it is novel" (Bracht & Glass, 1968, p. 443). In other words, the difference between treatments may disappear when the novelty is gone. A different kind of effect is known as a *disruption effect*. The treatment effect is disrupted because researchers are less skillful in their administration of a new and unfamiliar treatment. Thus, the new treatment may be less effective than the traditional treatment. A familiarization routine before a study begins may reduce the novelty effect, and practice will minimize the disruption effect. Another threat is the possibility of experimenters unknowingly influencing subjects.

Experimenter effects.   Researchers may unintentionally affect the behaviors of participants. Experimenter effects are typically associated with (a) differences in the researchers' behavior, such as mannerisms or verbal reinforcements; (b) the researchers' appearances, such as clothing, gender, or age; and (c) bias in the researchers' observations and recording of data. Experimenter effects are minimized by ensuring that researchers interact with participants in a uniform manner. A better solution is for researchers to employ assistants who are blind to the study's purpose, and then have only the assistants interact with participants. Biases in observations as well as in recording data are minimized by employing independent observers and utilizing blinding procedures. Another possible threat to external validity involves pretest/posttest research designs.

Pretest and posttest sensitization effects.   The experimental effect may be confounded by the presence of pretest or posttest administrations. Pretest and posttest sensitization effects limit the generalization of results to those situations where the pretest or posttest is also present. The use of unobtrusive measures minimizes the effect of pretests and posttests. A final threat that may affect external validity is the measurement of the dependent variable.

Measurement of the dependent variable.   The operational definition of the dependent variable may limit generalization and transferability of results to clinical practice settings. For example, if a dependent variable such as cognitive development is operationally defined by a series of Piagetian tasks, the research results may not generalize to cognitive development that is measured in other ways.

CONCLUSION

The *literature* (body of research reports) in communication sciences and disorders is rich with examples of scientific inquiry including a wide range of designs, methods, and topics of interest. The published articles provide opportunities to evaluate methods and to acquire ideas for research and clinical practice. A case in point is Stewart, Pankiw, Lehman, and Simpson's (2002) report of hearing in users of recreational firearms. Their purpose was to determine hearing loss and hearing handicap for shooters. To recruit participants, Stewart et al. (2002) approached customers as they entered a sporting goods store the weekend before deer-hunting season. The research team asked customers to participate in the study. The 232 volunteers (45 females, 187 males) were also given a $5 gift certificate for the purchase of any item in the sporting goods store as an incentive. The participants completed short questionnaires to collect demographic data and information about firearm use. The research team subsequently obtained hearing thresholds in a mobile hearing unit with sound booths. Participants who were identified with hearing loss > 25 dB (n = 177) completed the *Hearing Handicap Inventory for Adults* (Newman et al., 1990).

Stewart et al. (2002) found that males, older individuals, and blue-collar workers exhibited more high-frequency hearing loss and a greater hearing handicap than others. Based on what you know about Stewart and colleagues' (2002) study, answer the following questions:

1. What is your evaluation of their method for recruiting participants?
2. What threats to internal validity may have been present in their study?
3. What is your evaluation of their study's external validity?
4. Who was their target population?
5. Who was their accessible population?
6. If you were to repeat their study, in what ways might you change their method?
7. How are their results useful for clinical practice?

For students, teachers, and clinicians who have a special interest in research, plentiful examples of research are found in the scholarly journals, including those published by the American Speech-Language-Hearing Association (ASHA), the American Academy of Audiology (AAA), and the National Student Speech Language Hearing

Association (NSSLHA). These professional associations publish a number of scholarly, peer-reviewed journals:

1. The *Journal of Speech, Language, and Hearing Research (JSLHR)* pertains broadly to studies of the processes and disorders of speech, language, and hearing, and to the diagnosis and treatment of such disorders (ASHA, 2008).

2. The *American Journal of Audiology: A Journal of Clinical Practice (AJA)* pertains to all aspects of clinical practice in audiology (ASHA, 2008).

3. The *American Journal of Speech-Language Pathology: A Journal of Clinical Practice (AJSLP)* pertains to all aspects of clinical practice in speech-language pathology (ASHA, 2008).

4. *Language, Speech, and Hearing Services in Schools (LSHSS)* pertains to speech, hearing, and language services for children and adolescents, particularly in schools (ASHA, 2008).

5. *Contemporary Issues in Communication Science and Disorders (CICSD)* publishes papers pertaining to the processes and disorders of speech, language, and hearing, and to the diagnosis and treatment of such disorders, as well as articles on educational and professional issues in the discipline (NSSLHA, 2008).

6. The *Journal of the American Academy of Audiology (JAAA)* publishes articles and clinical reports in all areas of audiology, including audiological assessment, amplification, aural habilitation and rehabilitation, auditory electrophysiology, vestibular assessment, and hearing science (AAA, 2008).

The American Speech-Language-Hearing Association archives journals from 1980 to the most current issues. A search engine on ASHA's website permits students, audiologists, and speech-language pathologists (ASHA members) to search the journals by topic, key word, and author's name. The American Academy of Audiology provides a search engine on its website for members to search *JAAA* from 1990 to the current issue. These periodicals are also indexed in searchable databases such as ComDisDome, PubMed, PsychInfo, and Ebscohost.

CASE STUDIES
Scientific Inquiry in Communication Disorders Research

Case 1.1: Snooping for Unusual Data
You collected the following pretest data for 12 participants. Is there a problem with the data? How should you proceed?

54	49
13	50
61	60
67	60
44	50
89	46

Case 1.2: Nuisance Variables for Professor Ross?
Professor Ross and you are planning a follow-up study to determine the speech outcomes for 20 students that you treated for pervasive /s/ problems when they were in elementary school. The former students are between 13 and 21 years of age. What internal validity problems do you anticipate?

Case 1.3: A Question of Time
You begin an investigation of treatment outcomes for 10 adults with aphasia, but the participants' post-onset times are varied. Is there a threat to internal validity? How should you proceed with the study?

Post-Onset Time (weeks)	
8	20
52	24
12	48
50	51
58	60

Case 1.4: Solving the Conflict Between Internal Validity and External Validity
In planning your thesis proposal with Professor Mark, you make the point that the study should have good external validity because you want the results to be transferable to clinical practice. However, he says that is not possible because you will jeopardize the study's internal validity. He asks you to write a brief explanation of how you will maintain internal validity and make the results useful for clinical practice at the same time. What is your plan?

Case 1.5: Is Replication a Legitimate Scientific Pursuit?
As a doctoral student, you are expected to propose an original research study for completion of requirements. You have searched the literature and found one good experiment on the topic that you have chosen. You attempt to convince your advisor that there is a need for a replication of that experiment, but she says that is not original research. What argument will you use to convince your advisor that a replication research design is appropriate for your thesis?

STUDENT EXERCISES

1. Physical dimensions are easily measured because there are natural units of measurement such as inches or pounds. However, psychological variables are not easily measured because they lack natural units of measurement. This is a problem for *construct validity*. What is your operational definition for the construct known as *language development*?

2. Review one issue from a contemporary journal in communication disorders. How many research articles in the issue include one or more research questions? How many statements of hypotheses can you find?

3. Locate a research report on a topic of interest in communication disorders. What *participant selection criteria* were specified by the researchers? What is the population of interest that the sample represents? What is the level of generalization for the research results?

4. Examine the methods section of a research article in communication disorders. What are the procedures and what instruments were used by the researchers? Did the researchers employ *blinding procedures*?

5. Locate a research article on communication disorders. What operational definitions were included in the methods section of the report? Evaluate the researchers' operational definitions. Are the definitions valid ones?

6. The principle of randomization is quite important in scientific research, especially for ensuring internal validity in research designs. Search and locate a study in communication sciences and disorders that utilizes randomization to assign subjects to experimental and control groups. How many subjects did it include? Did the researchers use a simple randomization method? Simple randomization uses random numbers, drawing names from a hat, or a similar procedure for assigning subjects to groups. What is the likelihood that the researchers controlled the influence of unknown variables with their randomization procedure?

CHAPTER 2

ETHICS IN COMMUNICATION DISORDERS RESEARCH

ethics (ĕth′ ĭks) *n.* beliefs, conduct, conscience, conventions, decency, goodness, honesty, honor, ideals, imperatives, integrity, morality, practices, principles, standards, values

Research ethics are rules of conduct that are based on a history of sound and logical research practices. Ethical standards are not intended to slow the progress of science. Instead, they should encourage honesty in reporting data, accuracy in describing procedures, and fairness in the treatment of research participants. Matters of ethical conduct are inseparable from matters of research design, because some designs are more likely to cause discomfort or harm to participants. Thus, ethical decision making in research is accomplished during the initial planning process.

A SHORT HISTORY OF HUMAN RIGHTS

The impetus for formalizing rules of conduct in experimentation and research comes from a long history of human rights abuses. Accounts of human rights abuses for the sake of experimentation are present in the earliest recorded history. A watchdog group, the Alliance for Human Research Protection, provides a chronology of human research that dates back to the sixth century BCE. The chronology includes major milestones for the advancement of good ethics in research as well as accounts of the worse abuses.

A nineteenth-century example of human rights abuse is Dr. Arthur Wentworth's spinal taps of 29 children for no therapeutic purpose. He hypothesized that the procedure was harmless. At the experiment's conclusion, Dr. Wentworth pronounced the surgical procedure painful but harmless. The experiment may have provided some new information for medical science, but its participants suffered intolerable abuse. Dr. Wentworth was subsequently reprimanded by his colleagues and widely criticized by others.

An atrocity of human rights abuse with official sanctions began around 1932. At that time, the U. S. Public Health Service (PHS) began a longitudinal study of untreated syphilis in more than 400 African American men in Tuskegee, Alabama. The study continued for 40 years. The participants were not told they had syphilis, and when a cure (penicillin) became available in 1943, it was not offered to them. The project ended in 1972 when the story appeared on the front pages of newspapers. A PHS employee had revealed the shocking facts to an Associated Press reporter.

In remarks at the White House in 1997, President Bill Clinton apologized to survivors and relatives, saying, "The people who ran the study at Tuskegee diminished the stature of man by abandoning the most basic ethical precepts" (The White House OPS, 1997). The discipline of speech-language pathology has suffered lapses in research ethics as well.

The Monster Study

In 1939, Professor Wendell Johnson and a graduate student, Mary Tudor, sought to increase disfluencies in children who stuttered and children who were normally fluent. According to Silverman (1988), a primary objective of the study was to determine whether labeling a person as a "stutterer" would have any effect on his or her speech fluency.

The participants in Tudor's study were children living in a state-supported orphanage. Johnson and Tudor deceived the children and misled the orphanage's staff. At the study's outset, Tudor told the children:

> The staff has come to the conclusion that you have a great deal of trouble with your speech. The types of interruptions which you have are very undesirable. These interruptions indicate stuttering. You have many of the symptoms of a child who is beginning to stutter. (Tudor, 1939, p. 10)

The caretakers were told that the children showed definite symptoms of stuttering. Tudor further advised the caretakers to watch the children's speech all the time and stop them when they had interruptions. At the end of the study, she reported that "every subject reacted to his speech interruptions in some manner. Some hung their heads; others laughed with embarrassment. In every case the children's behavior changed noticeably" (Tudor, 1939, p. 147). When the study concluded, Tudor made no attempt to debrief the children or the children's caretakers.

In 2002, Ambrose and Yairi reexamined Tudor's methods and results. They suggested that the experiment caused an unpleasant reaction in some of the children but no lasting affect. However, Silverman (1988) examined the same data and concluded, "the implications of the findings seem clear—asking a child to monitor his speech fluency and attempt to be more fluent can lead to increased disfluency and possibly stuttering" (pp. 230–231). Thus, there remains some controversy over the real impact of Johnson and Tudor's (1939) methods. What is your opinion?

What Is Moral Conduct?

The basis for moral conduct has been disputed for centuries. Since Plato's time, philosophers have asked: Should we judge an action only in relation to certain conditions, or should we judge it as right or wrong independent of any conditions? *Relativism* holds that rules of conduct vary with individual needs, customs, and historical evolution, while *absolutism* maintains that the rules of conduct are always the same (Abelson & Friquegnon, 1991).

Johnson and Tudor planned their study at a time when moral neutrality was an accepted practice in the scientific community. Rosnow and Rosenthal (1997) described the period as the "see no evil, hear no evil" era of positivistic science. From a relativistic point of view, Johnson and Tudor did what others were doing at the time. However, from an absolutist perspective, what they did was surely wrong. In any case, by today's standards, Johnson and Tudor's (1939) study was clearly indefensible in its methods and procedures.

What Are the Rights of Research Participants?

The rights of individuals have been debated since the earliest annals of recorded history. The ethical principle *primum non nocere* (first, do no harm) was inspired by the Hippocrates, a Greek physician who lived in the fifth century BCE. In 1865, Claude Bernard, a French physiologist, published a book about human experimentation and admonished researchers, "never perform an experiment which might be harmful to [the patient] even though the result might be highly advantageous to science, i.e., or the health of others" (1957, p. 101).

TECHNOLOGY NOTE

The emergence of new technologies is a challenge for ethics in research as well as clinical practice. Technological advancements raise new questions about what is acceptable conduct in experimentation and other professional endeavors. For example, Meline and Mata-Pistokache (2003) addressed the hazards inherent in email technology. Technological innovations such as email are useful tools for research, but their emergence requires a reexamination of codes of ethical conduct. A related issue is the use of technology to extend audiology and speech-language pathology services across state boundaries (cf. Frazik, 2003). The Digital Era Copyright Enhancement Act (1999) addressed new legal issues stemming from advances in technology. Likewise, the American Speech-Language-Hearing Association's Board of Ethics published new guidelines to address the plagiarism dilemmas created by advances in technology (ASHA Ethics Board, 2002).

In 1947, in the aftermath of World War II, the Nuremberg Code was adopted (The Nuremberg Code, 1947). It addressed the importance of free choice in experimentation as follows: "The voluntary consent of the human subject is absolutely essential." In 1966, the National Institutes of Health's Office for Protection of Research Subjects issued a policy statement establishing independent research review bodies— to be known as institutional review boards (IRBs). Their purpose was to ensure the rights and welfare of people in clinical trials both before and during their participation.

What are institutional review boards (IRBs)?   Typically, institutional review boards are composed of no less than five experts and laypeople with varying backgrounds to ensure a complete and adequate review of research proposals (U.S. Food and Drug Administration, 2008).

Institutional review boards evaluate the potential risks to participants, assess the safeguards, and recommend modifications as needed. Since the 1970s, institutional review boards have expanded their responsibilities to the evaluation of the designs and statistical features of research proposals. IRBs are sometimes criticized for not being consistent when evaluating risks (Rosnow & Rosenthal, 1997). Indeed, Kimmel (1991) reported that gender, specialty area, and work setting all influenced estimates of risk. Exhibit 2.1 lists the basic principles for evaluating research risks. The first two principles are to be followed by researchers, and the last six principles are to be followed by institutional review board members.

EXHIBIT 2.1
Principles for the Evaluation of Research Risks by Researchers and Institutional Review Boards

---

RESEARCHERS
1. Provide information on potential risks and benefits.
2. Provide information on probability, magnitude, and harm associated with each risk.

INSTITUTIONAL REVIEW BOARDS
1. Evaluate validity of the researcher's assessment of risks and benefits.
2. Determine if the proposed study meets the standard for minimal risk—i.e., the probability and magnitude of harm or discomfort anticipated in the research are not greater in and of themselves than those ordinarily encountered in daily life.
3. If more than minimal risk is involved, consider alternative procedures with lesser risks.
4. Evaluate risks against benefits.
5. Consider potential long-term consequences for individual participants.
6. Recognize difficulties and biases when estimating risks.

Labott & Johnson, 2004.

The Belmont Report.   The publicity from the Tuskegee Study caused the U.S. Congress to pass the National Research Act in 1974. The National Research Act created the National Commission for the Protection of Human Subjects of Biomedical and Behavioral Research. The Commission was charged with identifying the basic ethical principles that should underlie the conduct of biomedical and behavioral research involving human subjects and to develop guidelines that should be followed to assure that such research is conducted in accordance with those principles.

In 1979, the National Commission for the Protection of Human Subjects of Biomedical and Behavioral Research published *Ethical Principles and Guidelines for Research Involving Human Subjects* (*The Belmont Report*) (National Institutes of Health, 1979). The *Belmont Report* was so named because the National Commission convened in the Smithsonian Institution's Belmont Conference Center. The Commission accomplished three goals:

1. Distinguished between research and practice
2. Identified three basic ethical principles
3. Described applications for the three basic principles

In regard to the third goal, the applications for the three basic principles described in the *Belmont Report* were (a) informed consent, (b) risk-benefit assessment, and (c) selection of research participants. The *Belmont Report* is important because it is the framework for contemporary codes of professional conduct in research.

ANIMALS IN RESEARCH

What Separates Animals from Humans?

Many scientists have adopted the attitude that the use of laboratory animals in research raises no serious moral questions (Hoff, 2003). This attitude is similar to the moral neutrality for human research participants that existed before the demands for reform in the 1960s. The moral neutrality in animal research is rooted in the unique features that separate humans from animals. Hoff (2003) cited a number of features that are proposed to distinguish humans from animals. They include (a) rationality, (b) the ability to communicate meaningfully with others, (c) the human capacity for suffering, (d) Cicero's humanistic principle, and (e) humans' dominant position in the animal world.

The first feature that is proposed to distinguish humans from animals is *rationality*, the human capacity to reason and acquire intellectual knowledge. However, Hoff (2003) pointed out that not all humans are rational. Nonetheless, most humans possess intellectual abilities far beyond the abilities of nonhuman animals. The second feature is the *ability to communicate meaningfully with others*. However, some animals such as the great apes have shown a capacity to communicate meaningfully with humans. The third feature that is proposed to distinguish humans from animals is the *human capacity for suffering*. According to Hoff (2003), it is sometimes assumed that the subjective experience of pain is quite different for humans and animals. Although humans can suffer in ways that animals cannot, animals experience physical pain in much the same way as humans (Hoff, 2003). According to Hoff (2003), pet owners, naturalists, and zoo patrons know that animals can suffer from feelings of loneliness, jealousy, boredom, frustration, rage, and terror.

The fourth feature is the *humanistic principle* proposed by Cicero (106–46 BCE). The humanistic principle asserted that "just being human" is a sufficient basis for the special moral status of humans. However, the humanistic principle is an arbitrary principle with no rational basis.

The fifth argument for distinguishing humans from animals is the *natural superiority of humans* over all other animals. However, the "natural order of things" does not provide a sufficient basis for special moral status for humans (Hoff, 2003). "It is fair to say that no one has yet given good reasons to accept a moral perspective that grants a privileged moral status to all and only human beings" (Hoff, 2003, p. 474).

Does the use of laboratory animals in research raise serious moral questions? Many argue that moral neutrality is unacceptable in animal research. What is your opinion?

Why Are Animals Used in Research?

The primary use of animals in research is in the domain of biomedical research. Inasmuch as humans are morally protected from invasive and possibly harmful procedures, the alternative is to experiment with other species. About 17 million animals are used for biomedical research each year (North Carolina Association for Biomedical Research, 2007). The main benefits of using animals for experimentation are (a) to aid medical advances and (b) as teaching tools for learning about body and function and perfecting surgical skills. The main arguments against the use of animals in experimentation involve (a) the moral issue of animal rights and (b) the validity of *animal models*.

Animal models are prototypes for the human body and its functions. The value of an animal model depends on the similarity between the animal's organs and systems and the human equivalent. The use of animal models is controversial. Animals are very different from humans, but some animals have organs and systems that are remarkably

TECHNOLOGY NOTE

The Humane Society of the United States (HSUS) advocates an end to the use of animals in research and testing that is harmful to the animals. The HSUS promotes research methods that may potentially replace or reduce animal use or refine animal use so that the animals experience less suffering or physical harm. Their website includes a map of the United States with the numbers of animal research facilities in each state. For example, there are 85 facilities in Texas, 29 in Florida, 176 in California, and 86 in New York. How many animal research facilities are in your home state? You can access the HSUS home page at www.hsus.org.

similar to those of humans. The animals frequently used in speech and hearing experiments include cats, dogs, rabbits, guinea pigs, chinchillas, monkeys, rats, and mice.

How Are Animals Used in Research?

Some animal species have biological similarities to humans that qualify them as good models for specific human diseases or other human afflictions. For example, rats provide a model for cancer, rabbits for atherosclerosis, and monkeys for polio. In addition to the prospective benefits for humans, animal research may provide some benefit for other animals. Typically, veterinarians are able to use results from animal research for treating domestic, farm, and zoo animals.

Animals are surrogates for humans in research because of the similarities in structure and the function of their biological systems. Animals with short life spans, such as rats, enable researchers to study the effects of aging or the progress of a disease within an abbreviated time frame.

As a case in point, cats have well-developed mechanisms for hearing similar to those of humans. Like humans, cats acquire noise-induced hearing loss as well as other hearing problems. Cats and dogs are common subjects in hearing experiments. Wilson and Mills (2005) reviewed the many experiments of brainstem auditory-evoked response in dogs. In these studies, the researchers typically employed chemical restraint, earphones, and needle electrodes inserted in the scalps of dogs.

Another model for hearing experiments has included chinchillas as subjects. Davis, Qiu, and Hamernik (2005) adopted the chinchilla model to study the effects of noise on hearing. Reportedly, the chinchilla's sensitivity and frequency responses for sounds are similar to those of humans. Davis et al. (2005) exposed chinchillas to 90–110 dB SPL continuous noise for five days. After five days, the chinchillas were euthanized, and their cochleae were studied.

A third model for hearing experiments used cats as subjects. Ryugo, Cahill, Rose, Rosenbaum, Schroeder, and Wright (2003) included white cats with congenitally rapid onset of deafness and pigmented cats as controls in their experiment. The cats were bred and born at the Johns Hopkins University farm. Ryugo et al. (2003) tested the hypothesis that white cats would exhibit progressive cochlear degeneration and hearing loss. The researchers performed repeated ABR tests up until the time of sacrifice (i.e., euthanasia). According to Ryugo et al. (2003), cats were sacrificed at various ages

TECHNOLOGY NOTE

The North Carolina Association for Biomedical Research (NCABR) promotes public understanding and support for bioscience research. Its website includes informational links for educators, students, organizations, and the general public. In addition, the NCABR's home page at www.ncabr.org includes online video and educational materials. It provides answers to questions about the care and use of animals in research. For example, how are animals used in biomedical research cared for?

ranging from birth to 1 year. After sacrifice, the cochleae and brains were harvested for histologic analysis.

The preceding cases illustrate some common uses for animals in hearing research. However, the details regarding purpose, methods, and results are omitted. To judge the merits of an individual study, the published report should be examined in detail. In addition to animal models to study hearing, scientists use animal models to study the larynx and trachea.

Rousseau, Hirano, Chan, Welham, Thibeault, Ford, et al. (2004) used 18 rabbits as subjects. Their purpose was to assess the mechanical properties of scarred vocal folds. The researchers created a scar on one vocal fold, while the other vocal fold served as a control. After six months, the larynges were excised for histologic examination.

To study laryngeal transplantation and nerve re-innervation, several animal models have been used. The animal models have included dogs, cats, rats, and pigs. The first studies of laryngeal transplantation in the 1960s used dogs as subjects. In 1995, experimenters performed 11 canine laryngeal transplants to study laryngeal transplant viability and immunosuppression (Anthony, Allen, Trabulsy, Mahdavian, & Mathes, 1995). This experiment and others led to the first true human laryngeal transplant in 1998.

The first laryngeal transplant patient was a 40-year-old man who had suffered severe trauma to the throat 20 years earlier (Birchall, Lorenz, Berke, Genden, Haughey, Siemionow, et al., 2006). Reportedly, the patient regained limited voice and normal swallow function. However, the procedure has not been repeated.

Animal models are also used to improve tracheal reconstruction following laryngectomy (ten Hallers, Rakhorst, Marres, Jansen, van Kooten, Schutte, et al., 2004). Improved tracheal reconstruction methods may lead to better prosthetic voice for patients.

Protections for Animals in Research

The first protections for animals in research came in 1966 with the enactment of the Animal Welfare Act (7 U.S.C. et seq.). The Animal Welfare Act has been amended by the United States Congress several times, most recently in 1991. The Act applies to all public and private animal research facilities in the United States.

The United States Department of Agriculture (USDA) determines which animal species will be included under the Animal Welfare Act. The USDA currently includes guinea pigs, hamsters, gerbils, rabbits, dogs, cats, primates, marine mammals, farm animals, and warm-blooded wild animals. The animals not included are rats, mice, and birds.

In 1984, the federal agencies that use or fund biomedical research developed the *United States Principles for the Utilization and Care of Vertebrate Animals Used in Testing, Research and Training* (Office of Laboratory Animal Welfare, 1984). The federal agencies that use or fund animal research are the Food and Drug Administration (FDA), the Environmental Protection Agency (EPA), the Consumer Product Safety Commission (CPSC), and the Occupational Safety and Health Administration (OSHA).

The FDA requires animal trials before prescription and over-the-counter medications can be tested with humans. The other federal agencies use data from animal studies to regulate the environment, to minimize risks to consumers from household products, and to protect workers. The 1984 principles included the following requirements:

1. The procedures involving animals must be relevant to human or animal health.
2. The researchers must use the minimum number of animals to obtain valid results.
3. The researchers must consider alternatives to using animals.
4. The living conditions for animals must be appropriate for their species.
5. The researchers and caretakers must be properly trained and qualified.

In 1985, the Public Health Service (PHS) published their *Policy on Animal Care and Use of Lab Animals* (Health Research Extension Act, P.L. 99–158). Its requirements are similar to those in the Animal Welfare Act. It extended the requirements to all PHS research initiatives involving vertebrate animals, including rats, mice, and birds. The PHS agencies include the National Institutes of Health, FDA, Centers for Disease Control and Prevention, the Agency for Healthcare Research and Quality, Indian Health Service, and others. The National Institutes of Health (NIH) published the *Guide for the Care and Use of Laboratory Animals*. The NIH Office of Laboratory Animal Welfare's webpage includes links to the *Guide*, public laws, and other resources concerning animal research. The URL for its webpage is http://grants.nih.gov/grants/olaw/olaw.htm.

In addition to the statutory acts that regulate animal use in research, there are voluntary professional standards for laboratory animal care. The American Association for Accreditation of Laboratory Animal Care (AAALAC) was established in 1965. The Association is an independent, peer-review accreditation program for animal research facilities. More than 730 organizations, institutions, and companies are currently accredited. The AAALAC lists currently accredited facilities at www.aaalac.org/accreditedorgs/index.cfm. However, some facilities choose not to be listed.

Abuse and Misuse of Animals in Research

Though the experimentation and the care of animals used in research are regulated, the protections are not sufficient to avoid abuse and misuse. Many of the 17 million animals used in research each year either are not protected, or current protections fail to protect them. There are many cases of animal abuse in government, the military, universities, and companies. The news media sometimes publicize cases of animal abuse, but most cases are not publicized.

In a case that did become public, the Associated Press reported a controversial experiment that was conducted at the University of New Mexico (Associated Press, 2007). Officials at the University of New Mexico defended the experiment saying there was nothing wrong with the research, but an animal protection group called it a perversion of science. According to the Associated Press story, mice were hung by their tails with adhesive tape, electrically shocked, and forced to swim until nearly drowning. The experiment was designed to study hopelessness and depression for a science fair project. The news of the experiment prompted New Mexico governor Bill Richardson to issue an official statement, which said, "I am disappointed that this abuse was allowed to happen under any circumstances" (State of New Mexico, Office of the Governor, 2007).

The immoral and moral uses of animals in research continue to be debated. The current regulations and oversight may not be sufficient to protect animals from abuse and misuse. For example, researchers can adopt new animal models for research that include animals not protected by the USDA. Alternatively, they can choose to ignore the current regulations. In any case, "animals should not be used in painful experiments when substantial benefits are not expected to result" (Hoff, 2003, p. 477). The use of animals in research is likely to remain a controversial topic for researchers, students, and animal rights advocates.

PROFESSIONAL CODES OF ETHICS IN RESEARCH

Today, most researchers agree on a set of moral principles to guide the conduct of experimentation. However, new and changing technologies are a challenge for professional associations and state license boards that are responsible for establishing standards for ethical conduct. The speech-language pathology and audiology professions are likely to adopt new technologies for their practices and research endeavors as they become available. The *California Occupation Guide* described audiology and speech-language pathology as *high-tech* professions:

> Future speech-language pathologists (SLPs) and audiologists will routinely use computers to screen the speech and language skills of students and adults with communication disabilities and to provide further diagnostic testing when needed. Clients in therapy can use programs between sessions that not only present stimuli, but evaluate responses and give immediate feedback automatically. (California Employment Development Department, 1995)

Technology affects methods for experimentation as well as those for clinical interventions. Researchers are increasingly using the Internet for online experimentation and chat rooms and email for collecting research data. These uses raise new concerns for privacy, confidentiality, and informed consent. The increased dependence on high-tech resources such as networked computers and the Internet will probably require further examination of existing codes of conduct for researchers and clinicians.

The set of principles that guide the conduct of experimentation is formalized and written as a *code of ethics*. Organizations of physicians, psychologists, audiologists, speech-language pathologists, and others have adopted codes of ethics that address standards for acceptable behaviors (*prescriptions*) and unacceptable behaviors (*proscriptions*). Because members of professional organizations may engage in research activities in addition to clinical practice, codes of ethics usually address standards for research along with standards for clinical practice.

The *Belmont Report* recognized practice and research as distinctly different activities, though the two activities may overlap, such as in research that aims to discover more effective therapy techniques. *Practice* refers to interventions with the sole purpose of improving the well-being of an individual client or patient. On the other hand, *research* tests hypotheses, makes conclusions, and extends results to the population of interest. For research, the benefit to society as a whole may outweigh the well-being of individual participants. The *Belmont Report* identified three basic ethical principles: (a) respect for persons, (b) beneficence, and (c) justice.

Ethical Principle One: Respect for Persons

The principle of *respect for persons* requires researchers to recognize participants in experiments as persons of worth who participate by free choice. An application of this principle is called *informed consent*. The basic elements of an informed consent document are listed in Exhibit 2.2.

Informed consent is the knowing consent of an individual or legally authorized representative who is able to exercise free choice without undue inducement, force, fraud, deceit, duress, constraint, or coercion (Korchin & Cowan, 1982). To meet the standard of respect, researchers must ensure that participants are provided complete information about the experiment, participants understand the information, and participants are willing volunteers.

Ethical Principle Two: Beneficence

A second ethical principle that is identified in the *Belmont Report* is *beneficence*. Researchers should make every effort to ensure the well-being of research participants. Researchers are expected to (a) do no harm to participants and (b) maximize benefits and minimize risks to participants. *Benefit* refers to something of positive value to participants, and *risk* refers to the possibility of harm to participants. Inhumane treatment of participants is never acceptable, and risks should never exceed the minimum necessary to achieve the research goals. Benefits should always outweigh risks in an analysis of risks and benefits.

Ethical Principle Three: Justice

A third ethical principle that is identified in the *Belmont Report* is *justice*. This principle is concerned with the equal treatment of people in society. It concerns the fair and equitable distribution of burdens and benefits. The Tuskegee study is an example of injustice, because the burden was on African American men but syphilis affects people of all races, genders, and classes. The choice of research participants should be evaluated for possible selection biases. For example, participants may be selected because they are readily available (convenience sampling) or selected because of inherent vulnerabilities. In the latter case, institutionalized persons, students, patients, immigrants, and the poor are especially vulnerable. The selection of participants should correspond closely to the purpose of the research.

EXHIBIT 2.2
Basic Elements of a Consent Form

1. *Explanation of the Procedures*   The purpose of the study and a description of the procedures should be included. The activity should be identified as research.

2. *Risks or Discomforts*   Any foreseeable risks and discomforts to the participant should be described. Risks should be quantified if possible.

3. *Benefits*   Expected benefits from the research to the participant or others should be described.

4. *Alternative Procedures*   Alternative procedures or treatments that might be beneficial to the participant should be disclosed.

5. *Confidentiality*   The degree of confidentiality should be described, including who will have access to the participant's records.

6. *Termination of Participation*   Individuals should be informed that they are free to withdraw consent and discontinue participation in the research at any time without prejudice. In addition, circumstances under which the investigator may terminate their participation without their consent should be disclosed.

7. *Costs to Participants*   Costs to individuals from participation in the study should be disclosed including no costs.

8. *Payment for Participation*   Any amount or other payment to be paid to the subject for participation should be specified.

9. *Questions*   An offer to answer any questions concerning the procedures along with a name and phone number of a person to contact should be included.

10. *Legal Rights*   A statement indicating that the individual is not waiving any legal rights by signing the form should be included.

11. *Patient Initials*   If the consent form has more than one page, a provision for initialing the first pages should be included.

12. *Signatures*   A place for signatures of the participant, a witness, and dates of receipt should be included.

13. *Copy for Participant*   A copy should be provided to the participant.

14. *Additional Elements for Research with Children*   Children should be given an opportunity to consent to or refuse participation. Their expression of consent or refusal should be indicated on the form. Signatures are expected for older children. Younger children may demonstrate consent in a variety of ways.

NOTE: A *waiver* may be appropriate if a child is not capable of indicating consent because of the child's mental state or chronological age. In every case, consent of at least one parent or legal guardian is required. If more than minimal risk is involved, both parents (legal guardians) should signify consent. Special provisions may be made for children who are wards of the state, an agency, or institution.

Statements of Ethics in Research

The rules of conduct found in codes of ethics written by professional organizations are obligatory for their members. For example, the American Psychological Association (APA) addressed the issues of respect for persons, beneficence, and justice in *Ethical Principles of Psychologists and Code of Conduct* (American Psychological Association, 2002).

The American Speech-Language-Hearing Association (ASHA) addressed the issues of respect for persons, beneficence, and justice in its *Code of Ethics* (2003). The preamble to ASHA's *Code of Ethics* included "speech, language, and hearing scientists" as a group of individuals who are governed by the *Code*. The members of the American Speech-Language-Hearing Association are obliged to abide by the following rules of conduct regarding research.

1. *Principle of Ethics I. (Preface)*   Individuals shall honor their responsibility to hold paramount the welfare of persons they serve professionally or participants in research and scholarly activities and shall treat animals involved in research in a humane manner. [*beneficence*]
2. *Principle of Ethics I. (Rules of Ethics C)*   Individuals shall not discriminate in the delivery of professional services or the conduct of research and scholarly activities on the basis of race or ethnicity, gender, age, religion, national origin, sexual orientation, or disability. [*justice*]
3. *Principle of Ethics I. (Rules of Ethics F)*   Individuals shall [...] inform participants in research about the possible effects of their participation in research conducted. [*respect for persons*]
4. *Principle of Ethics I. (Rules of Ethics N)*   Individuals shall use persons in research or as subjects of teaching demonstrations only with their informed consent. [*respect for persons*] (ASHA, 2003)

In 2007, ASHA's Committee on Research Integrity and Publication Practices published *Guidelines for the Responsible Conduct of Research: Ethics and the Publication Process*. The *Guidelines* outlined expectations for ethical conduct to include protections for humans and animals and publication issues, such as authorship and potential conflicts of interest.

The American Academy of Audiology (AAA) addressed issues of privacy, informed consent, and freedom of choice in the *Code of Ethics* of the American Academy of Audiology:

> Principle 5, Rule 5d: Individuals shall not carry out teaching or research activities in a manner that constitutes an invasion of privacy, or that fails to inform persons fully about the nature and possible effects of these activities, affording all persons informed free choice of participation. [*respect for persons*] (American Academy of Audiology, 2007)

In addition, the AAA's *Code of Ethics* (2007) addressed the *confidentiality* of information and records in research (Principle 3); *informed consent* in research (Principle 4, Rule 4d); and *beneficence*: "Individuals shall exercise all reasonable precautions to avoid injury to persons in the delivery of professional services or execution of research" (Principle 2, Rule 2c).

State license laws and regulations for audiologists and speech-language pathologists may incorporate statements of ethics that specifically address research endeavors. For example, Illinois's *Professional Conduct Standards* specify the following behaviors as unethical or unprofessional conduct:

> Failing to inform prospective research subjects or their authorized representative fully of potentially serious after effects of the research or failing to remove the after effects as soon as the design of the research permits. (State of Illinois Division of Professional Regulations, 2004)

ISSUES IN RESEARCH ETHICS

Research Participants

Research plans typically include human subjects in their procedures. However, the term *subject* is not sufficient to include all the people who may participate in an experiment. The term *participant* is a better choice to describe individuals who have an active role in a research study. A research participant should be viewed as a partner or collaborator, not simply a cooperative subject (Korchin & Cowan, 1982). Research participants are not only those who receive a treatment, but they may be those individuals who assume supportive roles. For example, research studies sometimes include observers who are employed to judge a behavior or other event. These *judges* are considered to be participants in a study and are entitled to the same rights as other participants, such as informed consent.

Researchers choose participants for their studies based on their purpose and methodology. For example, a research report in the journal *Language, Speech, and Hearing Services in Schools* sought to investigate language-impaired children's social pretend play and conversational behaviors (Dekroon, Kyle, & Johnson, 2002). The researchers selected seven boys as participants. Three participants were language impaired and four were not. As a general principle, the choice of participants is expected to match the purpose of the study. In this case, it was not clear why the researchers selected only boys as participants. On the other hand, a research report in the *American Journal of Audiology* included 191 women (no men) as participants (Erler & Garstecki, 2002). The Erler and Garstecki (2002) study's stated purpose was to determine whether women vary by age in the degree of stigma they attach to hearing loss and hearing-aid use. In this case, the selection of women as participants closely matched the stated purpose of the research.

Distributive justice has to do with the inclusion or exclusion of research participants based on genuine needs and not based on social, racial, sexual, or cultural bias. An injustice occurs when researchers purposely exclude a class of people who may benefit from research or when researchers purposely include a class of people because of convenience or based on their vulnerabilities. There are classes of people, such as women and ethnic minorities, who may be excluded from research that could otherwise be beneficial to them. Likewise, there are classes of people, such as disadvantaged individuals, who may be disproportionately included in research studies that contain significant risks. Researchers are encouraged to select participants carefully to avoid social injustices and to ensure the benefits of research are distributed fairly.

Informed Consent

There are many potential barriers to informed consent. Achieving the goal of informed consent is confounded when participants are especially vulnerable or unable to fully comprehend the information. This is a special problem for children, as well as adults with diminished cognitive abilities. For example, adults who are unable to make informed decisions, such as some individuals with aphasia or with Alzheimer's disease, are especially vulnerable.

Individuals who reside in institutions are sometimes recruited for participation in research studies. For example, a study reported in the *Journal of Speech and Hearing Disorders* included 272 prison inmates as participants (Walton, McCardle, Crowe, & Wilson, 1990). Though the participants signed an informed consent form prior to their participation in the study, they may or may not have been willing volunteers. Institutionalized persons, such as nursing home residents and prisoners, are especially vulnerable because of their dependency on others.

To ensure voluntary and informed consent with special populations, proxy consents may be sought from parents, custodians, or other responsible persons. However, parental consent or consent from others, no matter how well informed, is not sufficient to place a child or any vulnerable person in a potentially harmful experiment (Court of Appeals of Maryland, 2001).

Another barrier to informed consent is *comprehension*—or the lack of it. Nearly half the population in the Unites States reads at or below the eighth-grade level, and some Americans have little or no reading skills. In 1982, Korchin and Cowan reported that some consent documents require college-level reading ability. Today, readability remains an important issue because the language in consent forms is sometimes two or three grade levels above recommended reading levels (Paashe-Orlow, Taylor, & Brancati, 2003). The reading level for informed consent documents should be between the sixth- and eighth-grade levels, which is the reading level found in newspapers. However, the reading level should be adjusted accordingly for special populations. To ensure readability, researchers can test their consent documents with several prospective participants from the target population before the experiment begins.

The following description was included in the informed consent form for a study of the effects of vocal training on respiration, phonation, and articulation. The participants ranged in age from 18 to 35 years.

> You are invited to participate in this research study. The purpose of this form is to give you a written description of the research study and to have you sign this informed written consent. Speaking and singing are sophisticated ways of communication. We are interested in recording samples of your speaking and singing voice during this and subsequent semesters so we can gain a better understanding of the changes in the articulatory, vocal and respiratory systems and effectiveness of vocal training. In order to

TECHNOLOGY NOTE

The readability level of a passage can be checked by using a tool that is built into Microsoft Word. On the *Tools* menu, click *Options*, click the *Spelling & Grammar* tab, and check the box labeled *Show readability statistics*. Highlight the text to be analyzed and click on the *Spelling and Grammar* tab on the *Tools* menu to begin the readability analysis. The result is a list of readability statistics that includes the Flesch Reading Ease score and the Flesch-Kincaid Grade Level. The Flesch scores are based on the average number of syllables per word and words per sentence. The Flesch-Kincaid Grade Level score rates text based on the U.S. grade-level system, and the Flesch Reading Ease score is based on a 100-point scale—the higher the score, the easier the passage is to read.

accomplish this we will ask you to speak and sing. You will stand through the entire experiment. Your speech and singing will be recorded as well as the movements of your rib cage and abdomen, and the activities of respiratory muscles. The respiratory measures will evaluate how far the rib cage and the abdomen move during speaking and singing activities. The activity of your muscles will be recorded using electromyographic techniques to determine which muscles are contracting during your speech and singing. (Mendes, 2000)

The Flesch-Kincaid Grade Level for the passage from the Mendes (2000) informed consent form is 12.0—meaning that a 12th grader should be able to understand the text. What factors should be considered when evaluating the readability of an informed consent form? How could the Mendes (2000) description be made more readable?

In practice, informed consent is traditionally provided to participants in written form with an opportunity for questions and answers. However, some participants require special considerations to ensure their understanding of informed consent. For example, special care is needed for participants from different ethnic, cultural, and socioeconomic groups to avoid misunderstandings based on different values and beliefs. Special accommodations are necessary for individuals who are hard of hearing, deaf, or blind to ensure their comprehension for informed consent.

Researchers have an obligation to openly communicate with participants before, during, and after the study. Before a study begins, individuals should consent or decline to participate based on a full disclosure of information about the study. As a research study progresses, participants should be kept informed and given opportunities to ask questions, express concerns, or withdraw from the study. This is especially important in studies of long duration.

Though full and honest disclosure is the general rule of conduct, *deception* is necessary in planning some experiments. However, deception should only be used in exceptional cases where the truth would make the experiment impossible. For example, an experiment by Collins and Blood (1990) used a "cover story" to disguise the true purpose of their study. The real purpose was to observe nonstutterers' perceptions of stutterers who acknowledged their stuttering and their perceptions of stutterers who did not acknowledge their stuttering. However, participants were informed as follows:

> [Participants were told that] they would be working on a class project examining the effects of working with a stutterer. They were told that they would be working with one of two men and that because their schedules were unpredictable, they would observe videotapes of the two men ahead of time to indicate their preference. They would return a week later to complete the working task with the individual. (Collins & Blood, 1990, p. 77)

After completing the experiment, the true purpose of the experiment and the need for a cover story were explained to participants. If deception is deemed necessary, ethics require that participants are debriefed as soon as possible when a study concludes.

Privacy and Confidentiality

The data collected during the course of a study are privileged information. Information gathered about participants is confidential unless otherwise agreed on before hand. Data should be used for the present research purpose, not for other purposes. To ensure confidentiality, the anonymity of participants should be established from the start. For example, secret codes can be assigned to participants to protect their true identities. The American Speech-Language-Hearing Association's *Code of Ethics*, Principle of Ethics I (Rules of Ethics K, L) requires that researchers adequately maintain and appropriately secure research records, and researchers shall not reveal, without authorization, any personal information about research participants (ASHA, 2003).

Withholding Treatments

Experimental research designs require the random assignment of subjects to two or more conditions. One condition is an experimental treatment, and the other condition is a control condition without treatment. Control groups are also known as comparison groups. A control group is needed to confirm the effect of a treatment on an experimental group. The decision to withhold treatment from persons who may otherwise benefit from the treatment is difficult. However, Hersen and Barlow (1976) challenged the traditional viewpoint that withholding treatment is problematic:

> An oft-cited issue, usually voiced by clinicians, is the ethical problem in withholding treatment from a no-treatment control group. This notion, of course, is based on the assumption that the therapeutic intervention, in fact, works, in which case there would be little need to test it at all. Despite the seeming illogic of this ethical objection, in practice many clinicians and other professional personnel react with distaste at withholding treatment, however inadequate, from a group of clients who are undergoing significant human suffering. (p. 14)

To minimize risk to participants and maximize benefits, researchers should do a risk-benefit analysis when planning their study. Factors such as length of the study and the potential for harm to participants are important considerations. Researchers should weigh potential benefits against potential risks. *Benefit* is a product of the scientific worth of the study and the value to individual participants. *Risk* is any potential harm to the welfare of a participant. For example, if research procedures may cause physical discomfort, emotional stress, or loss of income, these are risks to welfare. However, the possible risks to participants are many and varied, as described by Metz and Folkins (1985):

> They might include physical risks from exposure to radiation, electric shock, vocal abuse, and so on. A risk from experimental therapy must be less than the optimal clinical result. There are also emotional risks, such as a potential for embarrassment, invasion of privacy, or undue stress. There may be a risk of adverse financial effects on subjects. There is a risk of misleading subjects (and their families) about their health or abilities. Also, risks which are acceptable with some populations may not be allowed with other groups, such as children. (p. 27)

Special safeguards are needed to protect children, individuals with physical disabilities, students, patients, and other vulnerable populations when they participate in experiments.

Collecting Data, Describing Procedures, and Reporting Results

Before presenting data to the scientific community, a researcher should be certain that observations are accurate. In addition, details of research procedures should be honestly described. A researcher should also describe mishaps that occurred during the course of the study if they might have influenced results. For example, loss of subjects (*attrition*) or breakdown of equipment are significant mishaps and should be reported.

Matters of honesty are addressed in ASHA's *Code of Ethics*, Principle of Ethics I (Rules of Ethics M): "Individuals shall not ... misrepresent services rendered, products dispensed, or research and scholarly activities conducted (ASHA, 2003). A commitment to honesty is essential for the advancement of science. Dishonesty hinders science and denies the possible benefits to society (cf. Bok, 1999). For example, researchers must replicate experiments in new settings with different participants to confirm results. If the details of studies are not reported accurately and honestly, attempts to replicate results may be fruitless.

When a research study is completed, researchers typically disseminate their results to colleagues by way of professional meetings and scientific journals. In fact, researchers are obliged to share their results with others. If researchers choose not to report publishable results, they are engaging in self-censorship (McGue, 2000). Self-censorship is a disservice to society and the research community because it can have a negative affect on the accumulated record of research. It is important that all publishable research results are made available to colleagues and other interested parties.

Scientific research is often the product of collaboration by two or more investigators. When planning a study, researchers should discuss matters of authorship early to avoid misunderstandings later. Authorship is reserved for those persons who conceive, design, perform, or write for publication or presentation. Authorship includes a responsibility for the content of a research report. Typically, the first author of a research report is the person who contributed most to the study.

Conflicts of Interest in Research

Researchers sometimes face conflicts of interest because of the dual roles that they assume. For example, researchers are often teachers or clinicians, and they move from one role to the other role on a regular basis. As teachers, researchers may unfairly induce students to participate in research. For this reason, teacher-researchers should recruit students from outside their own classrooms. As clinicians, researchers may unfairly recruit patients for their own research endeavors. For this reason, clinician-researchers should recruit research participants from outside their practice or take other precautions to ensure that human rights are fully respected.

Honoring Promises and Commitments to Participants

The research investigator should ensure that any and all promises and commitments made to participants are fulfilled. These may include promises such as providing a summary of research results to participants, continuing therapy, or paying for their participation.

EVIDENCE-BASED PRACTICE AND ETHICS IN RESEARCH

The accumulation of research is important to clinical practice because research is the source of evidence for best practices in audiology and speech-language pathology. ASHA's *Code of Ethics*, Principle of Ethics I (Rules of Ethics B) states: "Individuals shall use every resource, including referral when appropriate, to ensure that high-quality service is provided" (ASHA, 2003). Evaluating research for its application to clinical practice is one of the most important resources available for ensuring that high-quality clinical services are provided. To meet this obligation, clinicians must be able to evaluate the credibility of results and the transferability of research outcomes to their clinical settings.

Scientists prescribe a set of rules and standards to ensure that research is a systematic and ethical endeavor. These rules and standards are collectively known as the *scientific method*. Meline and Paradiso (2003) wrote, "To establish [evidence-based practice], the scientific method must be adopted by clinicians as well as researchers" (p. 274). Herbert, Sherrington, Maher, & Moseley (2001) defined *evidence-based practice* as the systematic use of best evidence, typically high-quality clinical research, to solve clinical problems.

CONCLUSION

Research is an honorable endeavor, but disregard for ethics can seriously diminish the effort and may have ill effects on science's legitimate pursuit of the truth. A thoughtful research plan that prospectively addresses ethical concerns is important, but diligence throughout the research endeavor is needed to ensure a high standard of ethics. People and animals deserve the greatest care and consideration when they participate in research studies. The present-day ethical standards for scientific research are good, but they require the good-faith efforts of students and scientists to ensure they are adopted in practice. Chapter 3 addresses scientific research and its importance to audiology and speech-language pathology evidence-based practices.

CASE STUDIES

Case 2.1: Mrs. Toller's Dilemma
As a speech-language pathologist, your patient, Mrs. Toller, is recruited for an experiment planned by you and Professor Stanford. Mrs. Toller is being treated for swallowing problems. The research plan includes experimental and control groups, and assignment to one or the other group is random. Mrs. Toller has a 50 percent chance of being selected for the experimental (treated) group and a 50 percent chance of being selected for the control (untreated) group. What are the potential ethical issues? What should you do?

Case 2.2: Authorship for Professor Baker
You are completing a thesis with your advisor, Professor Stangerson. You and Professor Stangerson agreed during the initial planning that you would be the first author and Professor Stangerson would be the second author on any presentation or publications of the results. However, Professor Stangerson received statistical advice from Professor Baker who is the clinical audiologist, and Professor Stangerson wants to include Professor Baker's name on a presentation of the results. What are the potential ethical issues? What should you do?

Case 2.3: Deception in the Classroom
You and Professor Gregson are planning a research study in several fourth-grade classrooms to investigate teachers' perceptions of students with speech and hearing impairments. You plan to tell teachers that the study is about nutrition and its affect on classroom behavior. What are the potential issues? How should you proceed?

Case 2.4: Students for Ethics in Animal Research
Three students, Jacob, Tamatha, and Katherine, are preparing an hour-long PowerPoint presentation for their final project in research class. Topics were randomly assigned to students. Their team's topic is to support the value and ethics of animal research. What main points should they emphasize to support the value of animal research? How should they support ethics in research?

Case 2.5: Appointment to the Institutional Review Board
You are nominated to be appointed to the Institutional Review Board as an expert member. As a part of the nomination process, you have to list your qualifications. Appointment to the IRB is very important, so you want to do your best. What are your qualifications?

STUDENT EXERCISES

1. In her classic book about lying in public and private life, Sissela Bok (1999) examined the reasons why debriefing subjects after deception may not succeed. What did Bok say about deception in experimentation?

2. In 1939, Tudor and Johnson studied 22 children in an Iowa orphanage (Tudor, 1939). The *Tudor Study* received much attention when a report in the *San Jose Mercury News* characterized it as the "Monster Study." How did Ambrose and Yairi's (2002) report and the *Mercury News* report differ?

3. Informed consent documents may be difficult to read according to Paasche-Orlow, Taylor, and Brancati (2003). They gathered research data from templates of informed consent forms at 114 medical schools. Institutional review boards often post models (templates) for informed consent on their local websites. If your school or a school nearby posts a template for informed consent, what is its readability level?

4. The National Institute on Deafness and Other Communication Disorders (2004) offers guidelines for communicating informed consent to individuals who are deaf or hard of hearing. What are its recommendations for facilitating communication with special populations?

5. The National Institutes of Health's Office of Human Subjects Research (2004) recommends additional safeguards when research participants have impaired decision-making capacity. What additional safeguards do they recommend?

6. The *Cedar Rapids Gazette* (Iowa) reported a settlement in the lawsuit over the 1939 University of Iowa "Monster Study." Several of the children who participated in the study and descendants of others (some of the children were deceased) shared a $925,000 award for their suffering. Try searching with the key words "monster study" online to retrieve additional news regarding Johnson and Tudor's study. The *Cedar Rapids Gazette* Online is found at www.gazetteonline.com.

7. Search online or whatever sources you choose to find two or three research studies that include animals as subjects. Once you locate the reports, answer the following questions. What were the animal species? What did the researcher(s) say about the care of the animals? What did they say about the benefit of the research? In your opinion, was the research justified? Explain your rationale for your last answer.

CHAPTER 3

EVIDENCE-BASED PRACTICE IN COMMUNICATION DISORDERS

> **evidence** (′ ɛ v ɪ dəns) *n.* Information that helps form a conclusion, grounds for belief, data in proof of the facts, something that makes plain or clear, a clue, confirmation, corroboration

WHAT IS EVIDENCE-BASED PRACTICE?

Evidence-based practice (EBP) is a process that aims to provide clients and practitioners with the information needed to choose the best procedure for a client's benefit. At its best, clinical decisions should be based on the most up-to-date scientific and clinical evidence relevant to a particular condition, whether the condition is deafness, stuttering, dysarthria, or any other condition within the scope of audiology or speech-language pathology practices.

Because the individual client's benefit is paramount, practitioners and clients collaborate to make the best decision given the available choices. The available choices are derived from the scientific research, the practitioner's clinical experience, and the client's unique attributes. Clearly, research plays an important role (perhaps a primary role) in EBP, but research alone should not prescribe best practices for every client. Rather, research evidence is considered within the context of the clinician and client relationship. Exhibit 3.1 illustrates the interplay between research, practitioner experience, and client preferences/attributes. Though Exhibit 3.1 depicts each variable as equal in its influence, the exact contribution of each variable will depend on the specific case. For example, if there is little scientific evidence to support one or another treatment as the best practice for a particular condition, the clinical decision may depend more on the clinician's expertise and client preferences and less on scientific research.

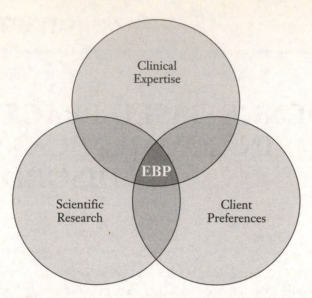

EXHIBIT 3.1
Three Variables That Interact to Influence Clinical Decisions

Evidence-based practice is an ideal model for best practices, but its implementation is sometimes troublesome. The history of its origins helps one to appreciate EBP's place in the practices of audiology and speech-language pathology. Its history began in the early days of medicine.

A Short History of Evidence-Based Practice

Perhaps Hippocrates (c. 460–370 BCE) should be credited with planting the first seeds for evidence-based practice. Hippocrates was a Greek physician who is credited with making medicine a profession apart from theurgy and philosophy. Hippocrates greatly advanced the systematic study of clinical medicine. He prescribed practices for physicians based on his objective observations and written records, which included environmental consequences as well as family histories. Clearly, Hippocrates' ideas are the precursors of modern medical practices.

The earliest systematic clinical trial.   The experimental design known as the *systematic clinical trial* is the mainstay of modern-day research. Systematic clinical trials are important because they are often the best source of information for evidence-based practice. An important 18th century figure in the history of evidence-based practice is James Lind. Lind was the first doctor to conduct a systematic clinical trial (Bartholomew, 2002).

In the year 1747, James Lind was commissioned as a naval doctor aboard the HMS *Salisbury*. A common infirmity among sailors at that time was scurvy. Scurvy is a disease with symptoms that include liver spots on the skin and bleeding gums. In 1747, the cause of scurvy was unknown to Lind or his medical colleagues. Today, it's known that the cause of scurvy is a deficiency in ascorbic acid (vitamin C). In Lind's era, scurvy was untreated and left many sailors with open wounds, lost teeth, and impaired mobility.

Lind speculated that the cause of scurvy was faulty digestion. With this theory in mind, he set out to test a myriad of possible remedies that included vinegar, mustard and garlic purges, oranges, lemons, and an elixir of vitriol. To test his theory, Lind divided sailors with scurvy into six pairs with each pair receiving a different treatment. The sailors who received the oranges and lemons were quickly cured.

Lind's experiment was successful, but his story has an unfortunate epilogue. Though the experiment's results were convincing, Lind and his medical colleagues failed to grasp its importance. According to Bartholomew (2002), Lind's theory and imperfect knowledge of bodily functions led him to the wrong conclusions. In as much as vitamins and their effect were unknown in Lind's time, that line of reasoning was not considered. Lind published the results of his clinical trial in 1753, but 42 years passed before sailors were prescribed regular doses of citrus juice to prevent scurvy. Lind's story teaches a valuable lesson for contemporary scientists and practitioners. The connections between causes (treatments) and effects (clinical outcomes) are easily misinterpreted and often misunderstood (Meline, 2007b).

The evidence-based practice movement.   Historical figures like Hippocrates and Lind set the stage for the evidence-based practice movement of the 20th century. By the early 1900s, the scientific method was recognized as the best means to discover evidence in the form of cures, treatments, evaluations, and other practices. According to Levant (2005), the use of "control groups" was a common practice in experimental research as early as 1912. This was an important milestone for research because the inclusion of control groups in experiments provides a comparison between treated and untreated participants. For example, pharmaceutical researchers typically give a real pill to participants in an experimental group and administer a placebo (inert look-alike pill) to participants in a control group. In this fashion, they are able to compare placebo effects and drug effects to judge the drug's efficacy accordingly. Thus, control groups are an important if not critical feature in group research designs. Research results that support a particular approach, treatment, or device without a control group for comparison are of questionable validity.

The term "evidence-based medicine" (EBM) first appeared in print in Guyatt's 1991 article in the *ACP Journal Club*. The original model for EBM appeared in the Evidence-Based Medicine Working Group's 1992 article in the *Journal of the American Medical Association* (Steinberg & Luce, 2005). According to White (2004), the original EBM model was soundly criticized as impractical. White (2004) described the original model as follows:

> The original model of evidence-based medicine presented in 1992 in the *Journal of the American Medical Association* went something like this: A clinical question would arise at the point of care and the physician would conduct a literature search yielding multiple

(sometimes hundreds of) articles. The physician would then select the best article from the results, evaluate the research, determine its validity and decide what to do—all while the patient waited in the exam room (p. 51).

Clearly, the original model of evidence-based practice was difficult or nearly impossible to implement in real-world medical practices. Nonetheless, the driving forces were strong enough to continue the movement and ultimately reshape the model into something more practical. The driving forces in evidence-based decision making included (a) the recognition that there was substantial geographic variation in practices that could not be explained simply by cultural differences or individual attributes, (b) strong evidence that many clinical practices were providing no benefit or doing more harm than good, (c) indications that many patients were not receiving beneficial services, and (d) rising health care costs (Steinberg & Luce, 2005).

An additional driving force for EBP was the rise of the Internet in the 1990s. The phenomenon of networking (connecting computers around the globe) gave rise to the *Information Age*. At no previous time in history, with the exception of Gutenberg's printing press (c. 1450), had access to information taken such a dramatic leap. The expanding Internet allowed vast amounts of information to be accessed and updated with relative ease. Clearly, the Internet provided unparalleled access to information and made evidence-based practice an achievable goal (Meline, 2006a).

An important figure leading up to the 1990s, and whose ideas have significantly impacted evidence-based practice, was Archie Cochrane (1909-1988). Cochrane was an untiring advocate for better evidence in medical and nonmedical practices. He also advocated for randomized controlled clinical trials and the development of systematic reviews of clinical trials (Chalmers, 2007). Systematic reviews are collections of clinical trials on a particular topic that are gathered, synthesized, and evaluated by experts. The use of systematic reviews significantly shortens the time needed for practitioners to access evidence for clinical practice.

Not surprisingly, Cochrane embraced James Lind as his hero. In 1979, Cochrane wrote a critical review of the medical profession and challenged medicine to provide better evidence for its diagnoses and treatments. Cochrane's challenge was the catalyst for establishing the Cochrane Database of Systematic Reviews. Today, the Cochrane Collaboration is a leader in developing evidence-based health care and is a repository for systematic reviews. The Cochrane Collaboration's homepage (www.cochrane.org) includes a menu of general topics such as Ear, Nose, and Throat Disorders, Developmental Learning Problems, Neuromuscular Diseases, and others. Individual topics lead to lists of systematic reviews that describe what is known about conditions and treatments such as swallowing difficulties, autism spectrum disorders, auditory integration training, and more. The systematic reviews in the Cochrane Database and in similar databases are important sources of information for audiologists and speech-language pathologists.

Evidence-based practice first appeared in journals of the American Speech-Language-Hearing Association (ASHA) in 1995. Wiley, Stoppenbach, Feldhake, Moss, and Thordardottir's (1995) article titled "Audiologic Practices: What Is Popular Versus What Is Supported by Evidence" set out to illustrate disparities between published scientific evidence and common clinical practices. Shortly thereafter, Bess (1995) wrote an editorial that strongly supported evidence-based audiology. A series of letters to the editor followed (Bloom, 1995; Deutsch, 1995; Fitzgibbon, 1995; Menzel, 1995). The commentary was mixed. Some supported the idea of evidence-based audiology, and others were highly critical. In any case, this spirited exchange appeared to mark the birth of evidence-based practice in audiology.

Discussions of evidence-based practice for speech-language pathology first appeared in ASHA journals in 1999–2000. In 1999, Thorpe espoused EBP principles and cautioned against the adoption of auditory integration training (AIT) as a clinical practice without scientific evaluation of its merit. The following year, Logemann and O'Toole (2000) introduced a clinical forum on dysphagia in the schools with the declaration, "In this era of evidence-based practice, it is critical that we use diagnostic and treatment techniques that have data that support their efficacy" (p. 26). Shortly thereafter, Silliman's (2000) editorial extolled the virtues of adopting evidence-based practice for teaching language and literacy in the schools.

Speech-language pathologists increasingly recognized the importance of evidence-based practice in the period from 2000 to 2005. The American Speech-Language-Hearing Association's convention abstracts identified only 3 presentations on the topic of EBP in 2002, 9 presentations in 2003, and 10 presentations in 2004 (Meline, 2006a). The 2005 ASHA convention theme was "Using Evidence to Support Clinical Practice." Given the theme, it is not surprising that "evidence-based practice" appeared more than 50 times in the convention program.

Several important initiatives followed EBP's acceptance as the standard for professional practice. In 1997, ASHA established the National Center for Evidence-Based Practice in Communication Disorders (N-CEP). The N-CEP is a resource for education, training, and assistance to audiologists and SLPs. The N-CEP manages the National Outcomes Measurement System (NOMS), which collects data on the effectiveness of speech-language pathology services. A few years later, in 2000, the Learning Disabilities Initiative (responsiveness to intervention) sought to establish a research base to identify students with learning disabilities. These initiatives were important steps for implementing evidence-based practice into local schools, clinics, hospitals, and other service delivery centers.

WHAT ARE THE ETHICS OF EVIDENCE-BASED PRACTICE?

Professional codes of ethics typically include statements such as "Individuals shall use every resource, including referral when appropriate, to ensure that high-quality service is provided" (ASHA, 2003). In an era of evidence-based practice, this statement implies that practitioners are obligated to use the best evidence available in their practices. Indeed, the strongest arguments in support of evidence-based practice are (a) EBP identifies the best evaluated procedures as well as useless and harmful procedures, and (b) EBP enables audiologists and speech-language pathologists to make better-informed decisions (Kerridge, Lowe, & Henry, 1998). However, it is not always clear which procedures are beneficial and which are useless or harmful.

Evidence-Based Practice Benefits

Practitioners are expected to do no harm to their clients and are expected to maximize benefits. At its best, evidence-based practice helps practitioners avoid harmful interventions, and it maximizes benefits by identifying best practices. Nonetheless, clinical decision making is difficult at times.

Clinical decision making is relatively easy when procedures, treatments, assessments, and devices are supported as beneficial by a preponderance of scientists and clinicians. Alternatively, clinical decision making is easy when interventions are clearly useless. However, researchers and clinicians frequently question the effectiveness of interventions, and the research outcomes for many interventions are mixed (Meline, 2007b). Interventions with mixed results are referred to as *controversial interventions* (Pannbacker & Hayes, 2007). They usually remain controversial until a preponderance of scientific evidence either supports or refutes their usefulness.

In the special case of therapies with no apparent evidence either supporting or refuting them, Bernstein Ratner (2006) encouraged practitioners to keep an open mind. According to Bernstein Ratner (2006), "no evidence that something works YET is not the same as evidence that it does not work" (p. 262). However, when the clinician's choice is between an intervention that is proven to work and one that is untested, evidence-based practice favors the proven intervention.

The ethics of evidence-based practice begin with the client. Loewy (2007) argued that evidence-based practice must be aimed at the client's best interests and not competing interests. The American Psychological Association's Presidential Task Force on Evidence-Based Practice recommended that "clinical decisions should be made in collaboration with the patient, based on the best clinically relevant evidence, and with consideration for the probable costs, benefits, and available resources and options" (Levant, 2005, p. 18). In any case, evidence-based practice begins with the client, and the client's welfare is most important.

Clearly, evidence-based practice is beneficial for clients. EBP helps to ensure that the best resources are available for assessing and treating clients' conditions. The best resources include a consideration of client values, clinician experience, and scientific evidence.

Evidence-Based Practice Risks

Though the core values of evidence-based practice are clearly beneficial to clients, EBP's implementation is troublesome. Implementation is typically accomplished through practice guidelines or standards that may be shaped by costs, political considerations, and other factors that are unrelated to beneficence. The criticisms of evidence-based practice most often voiced as possible threats are (a) individual client autonomy and (b) social justice.

Threats to individual client autonomy are realized when patient choices are unnecessarily limited. For example, if practitioners blindly adopt clinical practice guidelines without considering alternatives, some clients—especially those who are "outliers" in the research on which the guidelines are based—may be denied a legitimate choice (Beach & Faden, 2005).

Beach and Faden (2005) warned: "At its extreme, patients could face only one choice, the approved course of treatment or no treatment." Thus, limiting a client's choice when reasonable alternatives are available violates the ethical principle of *respect for persons*. To adhere to this principle, practitioners must ensure that clients are provided complete information regarding alternative courses of treatment.

Another potential problem with implementing evidence-based practice is *social justice*. The ethical principle of justice concerns the equal treatment of people in a society. Justice requires that benefits are equally and fairly distributed. The impact of evidence-based practice on justice in health care is a concern (Beach & Faden, 2005). One aspect of this problem is that racial/ethnic minorities and women are often underrepresented in clinical trials. Thus, there is less scientific research to substantiate or deny the use of interventions with these populations. Another aspect of the problem concerns vulnerable populations, such as those disadvantaged by poverty, advanced age, or mental illness. Though these groups of people have greater need for services, they may be disenfranchised because of lack of relevant research or poor access to health care (Rogers, 2004). Practitioners should be sensitive to these issues and take steps to ensure that individual social and cultural factors are considered along with scientific evidence when making clinical decisions.

A SIMPLE MODEL FOR EVIDENCE-BASED PRACTICE

Straus, Richardson, Glasziou, and Haynes (2005) described a five-step model for evidence-based practice. It is superior to other models in its simplicity and clarity of purpose. In short, the Straus et al. (2005) EBP model contained the following five steps:

1. Formulate an answerable question about prevention, diagnosis, prognosis, or therapy. Clinicians ask, What information is needed?
2. Locate the best evidence to answer the question. Clinicians ask, Where is the evidence?
3. Evaluate the evidence for *validity* (i.e., being true, somewhat true, or not true), *impact* (size of the effect), and *utility*. Clinicians ask, How useful is the evidence likely to be in my practice?
4. Integrate the critical evaluation from step 3 with clinician's clinical experience and client's unique biology, values, and circumstances.
5. Implement and evaluate effectiveness and efficiency—seek ways to improve them. Clinicians ask, Does it work as expected?

The Straus et al. (2005) model includes five distinct steps, but audiologists and speech-language pathologists do not have to engage in all five steps all of the time. Rather, there are different modes for practicing evidence-based decision making. Some audiologists and SLPs may choose to become expert in all five steps, while others prefer to be "end-users." End-users focus mostly on steps 4 and 5. It is also possible for audiologists and SLPs to switch between modes of EBP depending on their clinical needs. Most practitioners are probably end-users most of the time, rather than engaged in all five steps (Meline, 2006a).

Audiologists and speech-language pathologists frequently rely on others to identify the scientific evidence and evaluate it for validity, impact, and applicability for clinical practice. When feasible, this practice is cost effective in terms of time and effort. However, practitioners will have to engage in all five steps when systematic reviews or clinical practice guidelines are not available.

IMPLEMENTATION ISSUES FOR EVIDENCE-BASED PRACTICE

What Are Clinical Practice Guidelines?

The Institute of Medicine's (1990) *Clinical Practice Guidelines* paper is the authority for definitions, attributes, implementation, and evaluation. The Institute of Medicine (IOM, 1990) defined clinical practice guidelines as "systematically developed statements to assist practitioners and patient decisions about appropriate health care for specific clinical circumstances"(p. 38).

Clinical practice guidelines are developed in accordance with the Institute of Medicine's eight attributes for good practice guidelines. The eight attributes for practice guidelines are (a) validity, (b) reliability/reproducibility, (c) clinical applicability, (d) clinical flexibility, (e) clarity, (f) multidisciplinary process, (g) scheduled review, and (h) documentation (Institute of Medicine, 1990, p. 59). IOM provided a discussion of each attribute as it relates to the development of good guidelines. For example, as regards *clarity* as an attribute, the IOM (1990) proposed that "practice guidelines should use unambiguous language, define terms precisely, and use logical, easy-to-follow modes of presentation" (p. 59). The other attributes are discussed with equal specificity.

The American Academy of Audiology and the American Speech-Language-Hearing Association are among the professional groups that are developing clinical practice guidelines. According to the AAA, "clinical practice guidelines (CPG) advance the mission of the American Academy of Audiology (Academy) by providing a framework of clinical recommendations to audiologists for the express purpose of providing state-of-the-art care for individuals with hearing and balance disorders" (July 2006). The Academy of Neurologic Communication Disorders and Sciences is developing clinical practice guidelines for medical conditions such as dysarthria, acquired apraxia of speech, aphasia, dementia, and spasmodic dysphonia (Golper, Wertz, Fratalli, Yonkston, Myens, Katz, et al., 2001). Though adherence to guidelines is a matter of individual choice, adherence is likely to strengthen the practices of audiology and speech-language pathology in the eyes of the public, clients, and colleagues.

What Are the Acceptance and Adherence Issues?

Clinical practice guidelines are typically developed by professional bodies and made public for the benefit of consumers. The consumers include service providers (audiologists and SLPs) and their clients. Clinical practice guidelines are disseminated in various ways, but their acceptance is not automatic.

Dissemination involves getting the clinical practice guidelines to the intended users. To disseminate clinical practice guidelines, professional bodies such as ASHA and AAA typically publish guidelines online, distribute printed materials, or provide informational seminars to their members and the public. However, passive dissemination alone is unlikely to change practice behaviors (Centre for Reviews and Dissemination, 1999).

Activities aimed at disseminating clinical practice guidelines serve to (a) raise awareness of research findings, (b) facilitate readiness for change, and (c) encourage consideration of practice alternatives (Centre for Reviews and Dissemination, 2001). Though dissemination is critically important, activities that promote implementation are equally important. *Implementation* refers to the concrete activities and interventions undertaken to turn policy objectives into desired outcomes (Pressman & Wildavsky, 1973). Implementation activities serve to (a) increase the adoption of research findings, (b) facilitate changes in practice, and (c) reinforce and support changes in practice (Centre for Reviews and Dissemination, 2001).

Once clinical practice guidelines are developed, their dissemination to constituents is relatively easy, but the guidelines are unlikely to be adopted without strategic interventions. The reasons for resistance to change in professional practices are numerous. The most prevalent reasons are (a) persistence of the status quo, (b) high stress levels, and (c) reluctance of individuals to work together for change.

Persistence of the status quo is a serious obstacle to change. There is a natural tendency to return to previous practice patterns without strong motivation to change and regular reminders. Furthermore, health care providers may be resistant to change in their practices because of high stress levels. Stress levels are typically high in health care professionals, and heightened stress can reduce the ability to change practice behaviors. A third obstacle to change is getting the right groups and individuals together to implement change in local practices. The difficulty getting people together for change may be due to withdrawal because of stress, limited time and resources, or geographic separation. Given the numerous obstacles, implementing new practice guidelines is a difficult task.

TECHNOLOGY NOTE

The National Guideline Clearinghouse (NGC) is a public resource for evidence-based clinical practice guidelines. NGC was created by the Agency for Healthcare Research and Quality, U. S. Department of Health and Human Services. It is a repository for clinical practice guidelines. NGC's home page on the Internet is accessed at http://www.guideline.gov. Users search the NGC database by typing keywords into the search box on the home page. The *What's New This Week* section announces new and updated guidelines.

Resistance to Change in Clinical Practices

Resistance to change in clinical practices has been documented in some areas of medicine. A recent example is the treatment of asthma. Asthma in children is a serious public health concern, and current guidelines for its treatment are well known to pediatricians. Nonetheless, a national survey of pediatrician's attitudes, beliefs, and practices reported that 88 percent were familiar with the guidelines, but only 35 percent of pediatricians followed them (Flores, Lee, Bauchner, & Kastner, 2000).

In another case of resistance to change, Smeele et al. (1999) related that a hospital adopted asthma guidelines, tested them for six months to eliminate barriers, and educated the staff. However, following the hospital's six-month campaign, adherence to the guidelines was only 68 percent. The case examples presented here suggest that clinical practice guidelines are easily disseminated, but their acceptance and adoption are likely to present a challenge.

An interesting case in speech-language pathology is the use of nonspeech oral motor exercises to change speech sound productions. Nonspeech oral motor exercises include blowing, tongue push-ups, pucker-smile, cheek puffing, and tongue curling (Lof, 2007). According to Lof, there is no scientific evidence that supports the use of nonspeech oral motor exercises to benefit speech. Based on the current scientific evidence, nonspeech oral motor exercises are not harmful to clients but are useless for promoting better speech. Nonetheless, clinicians are likely to persist in using nonspeech oral motor exercises in their practices for the reasons previously discussed. Exhibit 3.2

EXHIBIT 3.2
Best Practices for Behavioral Change

1. Passive dissemination alone is unlikely to change practice behaviors.
2. Compliance is lower for practice recommendations that are complex and less easily implemented.
3. Multifaceted interventions are more effective than single interventions.
4. Focused approaches are most effective.
5. Mailed educational materials are not effective.
6. Ongoing feedback with reminders is effective.
7. Feedback with specific recommendations is more likely to change practice behaviors than general feedback on current behaviors.
8. Disseminating educational materials such as clinical practice guidelines, audiovisual materials, and electronic publication is not effective.
9. Educational outreach visits are effective.
10. No "magic bullet" exists that can reliably be expected to change practice behaviors in all circumstances and settings.

Timmerman & Mauck, 2005.

lists 10 best practices for behavioral change based on Timmerman and Mauck's (2005) review of the literature.

COMMON MISCONCEPTIONS ABOUT EVIDENCE-BASED PRACTICE

Misconception: EBP Is a Cookbook Approach to Clinical Practice

Evidence-based practice is sometimes criticized as a "cookbook" approach to the delivery of clinical services. To the contrary, EBP incorporates the best scientific evidence, but the best scientific evidence is not always transferable to clinical practice. There are many factors that hinder the transfer of scientific evidence to practice. First, scientific research is typically conducted in ideal surroundings, which may be quite dissimilar from those in local practices. "There is a huge difference between efficacy (how well something works in the laboratory or the controlled environment of the clinical research trial) and effectiveness (how well it works in the 'real world' of the hospital ward, the clinic, the home and the community)" (Greenhalgh, 1998, p. 1716). Those treatments that are shown to be useful in clinical trials are more easily transferred to clinical practices if they are flexible and can be fit to the client's particular needs. Those with rigid protocols are least likely to be successfully transferred.

Second, the majority of the scientific evidence comes from group research designs such as randomized clinical trials. Typically, researchers report group statistics such as averages and standard deviations and neglect individual participants' performances. However, the performances of individual participants are important for clinical practice considerations. Inasmuch as a client may be unlike the "average participant" in a study, he or she may not respond to the treatment in the same way as participants in the study.

Third, there may be a strong "therapist effect" when transferring scientific evidence into clinical practices (Bernstein Ratner, 2006). For sure, there are differences in clinical expertise. *Clinical expertise* refers to competencies attained through education, training, and experience. The traits associated with clinical expertise include (a) recognizing meaningful patterns, (b) disregarding irrelevant information, (c) acquiring and organizing extensive knowledge, (d) adapting to new situations, (e) self-monitoring one's knowledge and performance, and (f) continuing to learn. Clinicians who possess these traits are likely to be more effective in transferring scientific evidence to practice.

Clinical practice guidelines provide a framework but are not the sole source of information for making clinical decisions. For example, the American Academy of Family Physicians (AAFP, 2004) published clinical practice guidelines for the diagnosis and management of acute otitis media (AOM). However, AAFP cautioned that the guidelines are not intended to replace clinical judgment or establish a protocol for all children with this condition. Furthermore, the guidelines may not provide the only appropriate approach to the management of AOM.

It is clear that clinical practice guidelines are not applicable in the same way to every client. Clinical judgment must be used in deciding how to apply scientific evidence to individual children and adults. In other words, EBP informs but does not replace the clinician's judgment (Meline, 2006a, 2007a).

Misconception: EBP Is Solely a Matter of Science

Scientific evidence is one component of evidence-based practice. The American Speech-Language-Hearing Association's (2005) position statement specifies that audiologists and speech-language pathologists "recognize the needs, abilities, values, preferences, and interests of individuals and families to whom they provide clinical services, and integrate those factors along with best current research evidence and their clinical experience in making clinical decisions."

A case example is Gillon's (2000) study of $5\frac{1}{2}$- and $7\frac{1}{2}$-year-old children in New Zealand. Gillon's research participants were delayed in phonological skills but typical in other respects. She compared pre- and posttest performances of experimental and control groups after 20 hours of treatment. The experimental group was given a phonological awareness program while the control group was given a traditional treatment. The experimental group gained 34% but the control group gained only 1%. Gillon's (2000) outcome represents strong evidence in favor of her phonological awareness program, but evidence alone is not enough for clinical decisions. To make an informed decision, clinicians must appraise the validity, impact, and applicability of the evidence. The following questions are relevant to Gillon's (2000) study.

1. Is my client similar enough to the population studied?
2. Does the program's benefit outweigh its potential harm?
3. Does the program fit with my client's values and preferences?
4. Does the program's benefit outweigh its cost?
5. How does my clinical experience mesh with the current evidence?

The *Critical Appraisal of Research Studies* (CARS) is presented in Exhibit 3.3. The CARS helps to identify inconsistent reporting, possible biases, weakness in methods, validity of conclusions, and clinical applications for results. It is an initial appraisal tool that serves to identify relevant research studies for transfer to practice.

However, the final decision regarding clinical intervention will consider the client's individual needs and incorporate the clinician's expertise (Meline, 2006a, 2007a).

Misconception: Textbooks Are Good Sources for Answering Specific Clinical Questions

There are two types of clinical questions: (a) questions that ask for general information about a condition and (b) questions that ask for specific information to support clinical decision making. *General questions* contain two essential elements: (a) a question root

EXHIBIT 3.3
Ten Questions for the Critical Appraisal of Research Studies (CARS)

DIRECTIONS

A critical appraisal of a study for evidence-based practice aims to identify inconsistent reporting, possible biases, weakness in methods, validity of conclusions, and clinical applications for results. The 10 questions for the critical appraisal of research studies (CARS) help to identify strengths and weaknesses in core values common to good clinical research. Strengths are identified as *Yes* answers to questions 1–9 and *No* to question 10. The Guidelines for Appraisal may help form general conclusions. However, appraisers should weigh each question according to its relevance in their clinical practice.

GUIDELINES FOR APPRAISAL

10 strengths	Likely to be of use in my clinical practice.
8–9 strengths	May or may not be relevant depending on the weakness.
1–7 strengths	Probably not relevant for my clinical practice.

INTRODUCTORY SECTION

1. Are the purpose and goals clearly stated? *Yes   No*

METHODS SECTION

2. Is the sample size adequate/justified? *Yes   No*
3. Are subjects similar enough to my client(s) to transfer outcomes? *Yes   No*
4. Were the measurements valid and reliable? *Yes   No*

RESULTS SECTION

5. Was a significant change reported between pre-/posttests, different treatments, or participant groups? *Yes   No*
6. Was the change interpreted for clinical importance? (effect size, criterion-based standard, or subject self-evaluation) *Yes   No*

CONCLUSIONS SECTION

7. Were the research questions answered? *Yes   No*
8. Were conclusions consistent with the results? *Yes   No*
9. Were study limitations discussed? *Yes   No*
10. Is there an alternative explanation for study outcomes? *Yes   No*

(*who, what, where, when, how* or *why*) and (b) a verb. A few examples: (a) Why do children stutter? (b) When is sensory integration appropriate? (c) How are targets for conversational recasts chosen?

In contrast, *specific questions* contain four essential elements: (a) a problem of interest, (b) an intervention, (c) a comparison, and (d) a clinical outcome. An example of a specific question: In clients with phonological delay, does a phonological awareness program compared to traditional intervention result in larger gains?

Some textbooks (e.g., Kamhi, Masterson, & Apel, 2007; Reilly, Douglas, & Oates, 2004; Rosenfeld & Bluestone, 2003) are repositories of clinical evidence, but they usually require frequent updates to be current. Textbooks are best for answering general questions but not the best for answering specific clinical questions.

Exhibit 3.4 illustrates an approach to evidence-based information access for answering specific clinical questions (Straus et al., 2005). The time needed to access information increases from the pyramid's top to its base. At the pyramid's apex, "Computerized Decision Support Systems" represents the ideal means for accessing EBP information. In theory, computerized decision support systems link client electronic clinical records to relevant information about the problem and integrate the two. Many hospitals and clinics track patient health data via electronic medical records (EMRs), but EMRs are not yet integrated with evidence-based information for assisting clinical decision making.

A step lower on the pyramid are synopses of individual research studies. Synopses are abstracts of the best new clinical research that are relevant to clinical practice. Examples of online medical synopses that are regularly updated are (a) EBM Online, (b) ACP (American College of Physicians) Journal Club, (c) UpToDate, and (d) Best-Treatments (NHS Direct).

A step below synopses on the pyramid is "Systematic Reviews." If synopses are not available or more detailed information is needed, systematic reviews of relevant scientific research are an excellent source of information. Examples are (a) the systematic

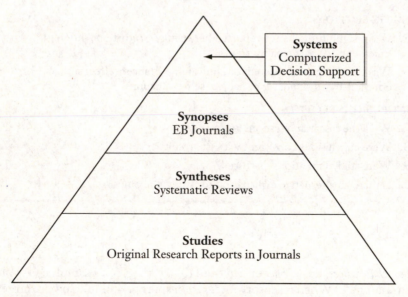

EXHIBIT 3.4
The 4S Approach to Evidence-Based Information Access
Adapted from Straus et al., 2005, Figure 2.1, p. 34.

reviews published in peer-reviewed journals or those developed by special interest groups and (b) the Cochrane Library's collection of health care reviews.

At the pyramid's base, the most time-consuming source of EBP information is original research reports in peer-reviewed journals. Practitioners can locate original research reports and systematic reviews via searchable electronic databases such as MEDLINE or PubMed. In addition, professional organizations such as the American Academy of Audiologists and the American Speech-Language-Hearing Association provide members access to their current publications as well as their collections of archived journals. If a global search is desired, search engines such as Google and 360 Search enable users to search multiple resources simultaneously from a single interface (Meline, 2006a, 2007a).

Misconception: Reading Journals and Attending Conferences Are Sufficient for EBP

Are reading journals and attending conferences enough for evidence-based practice? The answer is *no*, because it is impossible to prospectively acquire all the information needed to treat all future clients. The prospective learning acquired from reading journals and attending conferences is important but not sufficient for evidence-based practice. Rather, EBP requires ongoing day-to-day monitoring for new evidence (Meline, 2006a, 2007a).

Misconception: EBP Is Useless When There Is No Good Evidence

An important consideration when gathering information from research studies is known as *evidence grading*. Evidence grading is premised on the idea that research designs vary in their ability to measure and predict the usefulness of clinical interventions. In other words, higher grades of evidence are more likely to correctly predict outcomes than lower grades of evidence. This hierarchy of research evidence from high to low is displayed in Exhibit 3.5.

Exhibit 3.5 pictures the evolution of the scientific evidence from ideas at the base to the accumulation of scientific evidence via systematic reviews at the top. The pyramidal shape signifies the availability of more evidence at the bottom and less at the top. Presumably, the relevance of the information increases from bottom to top. Though it is a useful concept, evidence grading has some serious flaws.

First, evidence grading is based on the strength of research designs, so randomized clinical trials (RCTs) are high on the pyramid. However, studies of the same general design may dramatically differ in their quality. Thus, consumers cannot assume that all RCTs are relevant. Neither can consumers assume that all systematic reviews are done with the same care. Second, the highest levels of evidence do not exist for all clinical problems. Therefore, a specific clinical question, such as how to best manage the needs of clients with Asperger syndrome, may not be answered by research evidence in the upper levels of the pyramid.

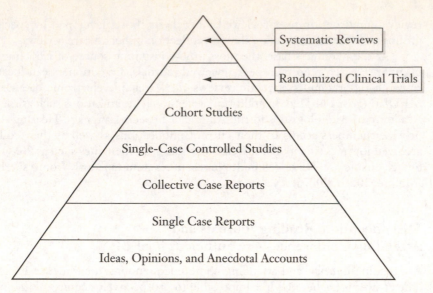

EXHIBIT 3.5
Grading Evidence for Evidence-Based Practice

An important goal for evidence-based practice is to identify the need for more scientific evidence. When none or only a few studies exist that address a particular clinical problem, it simply means that there is a need to investigate the problem. Thus, EBP is useful for identifying research needs as well as recommending best practices (Meline, 2006a, 2007a).

Misconception: EBP Is Just Numbers and Statistics

Clearly, evidence-based practice is more than just numbers and statistics. The relevant information gleaned from scientific evidence must be individualized for each client, and clinical decisions are based on clinical expertise and client preferences as well as numbers and statistics (Meline, 2006a, 2007a).

Misconception: EBP Is Ineffective Without Randomized Controlled Trials

Although randomized controlled clinical trials (RCTs) are the "gold standard" for judging clinical efficacy, RCTs are often not available or may not be appropriate for answering some research questions. For example, qualitative research (see Chapter 6) is better suited for answering questions about clients' experiences, attitudes, and beliefs. Furthermore, RCTs are sometimes seriously flawed, and flawed studies do not provide good evidence for clinical practice. For example, there are good reasons for discarding clinical pharmaceutical trials with adults who stutter when they fail to wash out (i.e., eliminate residual) drug effects before testing (Meline & Harn, 2008a).

EVALUATING RESEARCH FOR EVIDENCE-BASED PRACTICE

The challenges for audiologists and speech-language pathologists are (a) to identify the highest level of evidence that is available for answering their clinical questions and (b) to evaluate its appropriateness for their clinical setting. Exhibit 3.6 recommends 10 steps to achieve an evidence-based practice. These steps may ease the burden of incorporating EBP principles into local practices. Following examination of the various approaches to research in succeeding chapters, Chapter 12 provides further methods and techniques for evaluating research for audiology and speech-language pathology practices.

EXHIBIT 3.6
Ten Steps to Evidence-Based Practice

1. Organize an EBP team in your workplace.
2. Prioritize clients for EBP needs. For example, if you have students who are not progressing in the way you want, focus on locating the best available evidence for their needs.
3. Don't try to establish EBP in all practice areas at once. Try targeting the weakest area or the clinical area of greatest need.
4. If you utilize a controversial intervention in your practice, watch for new information to either support or reject the practice.
5. Establish contacts (consultation) with experts in other work settings.
6. Work to establish local norms when regional and national norms do not represent your clients.
7. Convince your boss that an extra block of time each week (no matter how small) for EBP initiatives will pay off in client satisfaction, outcomes, and cost benefits.
8. Get a good pocket guide to help evaluate new evidence as it becomes available. The *Pocket Guide to Critical Appraisal* by I. K. Crombie (1990, BMJ Books) is a good one.
9. Don't forget that EBP is meant to be client centered. Resist sales pitches for branded products that are more product centered than client centered.
10. Under no circumstance should you give up. The search for evidence-based practice is unending, but in the process you will become more expert, others will value your added expertise, and you will gain substantial self-esteem.

Meline, 2007a.

TECHNOLOGY NOTE

An important initiative that aims to improve the quality of research used in decision making in health care is the *CONSORT Statement. CONSORT* is short for Consolidated Standards of Reporting Trials. It specifies 22 criteria that are a standard way for authors to report the results of randomized clinical trials (RCTs). The CONSORT also facilitates complete and transparent reporting, which aids in the critical appraisal and interpretation of RCTs. The companion for the reporting of nonrandomized research designs is the *TREND Statement. TREND* is short for Transparent Reporting of Evaluations with Nonrandomized Designs. Further information about CONSORT is found online at www.consort-statement.org.

WHAT IS THE FUTURE OF EVIDENCE-BASED PRACTICE?

To a large degree, evidence-based practices in audiology and speech-language pathology will follow the course set by evidence-based medicine. In that regard, electronic journals dedicated to EBP in audiology and speech-language pathology will emerge. Similarly, clinical textbooks in audiology and speech-language pathology will address current needs via frequent electronic updates. Surely, the American Academy of Audiology, the American Speech-Language-Hearing Association, and other professional entities will develop clinical practice guidelines much as the American Academy of Physicians has done.

Scientists and clinicians will increasingly recognize the value of a variety of research paradigms including qualitative methods, single-participant designs, replication designs, and research integration (topics for later chapters). Regarding research integration, Glass (2000) has envisioned a time when researchers will be able to combine the raw data from many experiments without meta-analytical techniques.

New possibilities for evidence-based practice will follow advances in technology, but technological evolution sometimes has unintended consequences (Dewar, 1998; Meline & Mata-Pistokache, 2003). The exact future for evidence-based practice is unclear, though its future promises to be exciting (Meline, 2006a, 2007a).

CONCLUSION

Evidence-based practice is a powerful concept with obvious benefits for clients, audiologists, and speech-language pathologists. On the other hand, EBP is a challenge to implement and possibly a burden for practitioners who are already overworked. The growing availability of good systematic reviews as well as the advent of clinical practice guidelines promises to ease the burden. Once clinical practice guidelines are developed, the professional bodies will face the challenge of finding ways to encourage their acceptance and use. In addition, audiologists and speech-language pathologists are challenged to sort out the good practices from potentially bad clinical practices. In that regard, Exhibit 3.7 offers some cautions for consumers to observe.

Exhibit 3.8 displays a decision tree. It highlights the critical steps in the process of choosing research outcomes that are relevant for clinical practice. The decision tree begins

EXHIBIT 3.7
Some Cautions to Observe in Evidence-Based Practice

1. Some authority figures in audiology and speech-language pathology advocate strongly for their programs, products, and interventions to be the accepted standard in the professions. Be alert for authority figures with potential for personal gain that may bias their opinions.

2. Don't believe any claims you read until you (and others) have critically evaluated their validity. Lof (2007) warned about exaggerated claims for products in catalogs, at CEU events, and in non peer-reviewed periodicals. Huff's (1982) *How to Lie with Statistics* is an informative exposé of advertisers' use of statistics to deceive consumers.

3. Be alert for third parties, organizations, governmental bodies, and the like that impose specific procedures as the standard of care to the exclusion of others. Some standards are justified, but others may unnecessarily limit care.

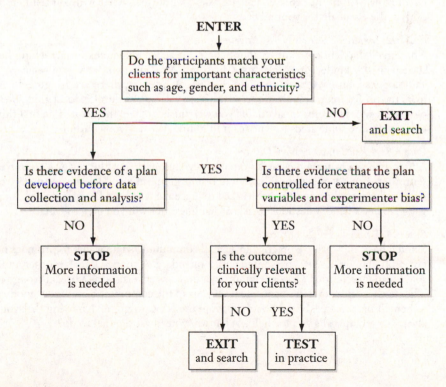

EXHIBIT 3.8
Decision Tree for Research to Evidence-Based Practice

with the question, Are participants in the study similar enough to the individuals in your practice to justify further analysis? If the answer is *yes*, an evaluation of the research method is warranted. However, if the answer is *no*, it is best to exit and search for more relevant studies. If the study's outcome is relevant to your practice, the procedure (test or treatment) is assessed with clients. Decision trees like the one in Exhibit 3.8 are helpful tools for understanding the decision-making process from research outcomes to practice.

CASE STUDIES

Case 3.1: Should I Change Interventions?

Debbie is a speech-language pathologist with three years of experience in a school. Her caseload includes three adolescents with pervasive /r/ problems. Their speech articulation is improving slowly with traditional interventions. However, Debbie is considering a new intervention that she read about in a magazine article. It is a device that when fitted to the mouth has shown dramatic improvements in similar students with pervasive /r/ problems. To back up their claim, the inventors presented a pretest/posttest study with 10 participants who had pervasive /r/ problems but no other participants. All 10 participants were treated with the device for four weeks, and they averaged a 50% improvement in speech productions. Because the device is expensive, Debbie is reluctant to propose this new intervention to the parents. As a fellow SLP in the schools, you are asked for advice. What will you tell her? Be sure to explain the rationale for your advice.

Case 3.2: Smallville Schools Need Guidelines

The Smallville Schools want to adopt clinical practice guidelines for screening hearing and speech in the kindergarten classes. Chris and Amy are members of a team of SLPs and audiologists who have been assigned the task. At present, there are no guidelines available from the professional organizations, so the team will have to develop local guidelines. As a recognized leader in professional affairs, you were hired to help the team. The first thing for you to do is outline some steps for the team to follow. What is your outline?

Case 3.3: A Revolutionary New Device?

A new assistive hearing device is touted as revolutionary, but the reviews are mixed. At present, there are several studies, but some results are positive and some are negative. Julia is a new graduate student and has been asked to present a report on the new device. As a help, you will give her a list of questions to ask. What questions will you give to Julia?

Case 3.4: Samuel's Private Practice

Samuel has a new private practice in a small community, so he wants to promote his practice favorably. However, he is presented with a quandary. A young client's mother and father are sold on an intervention (XYZ program) that they saw advertised as a breakthrough for autism. The mother and father are prominent citizens in the community, and their goodwill is likely to benefit his practice. Should Samuel adopt the XYZ program? Knowing that your advice is always sound, he calls you for help. What will you advise Samuel to do?

STUDENT EXERCISES

1. You've been assigned the role of team leader in your workplace. Your first assignment is to plan a strategy to achieve a 90% compliance rate for adoption of the new clinical practice guidelines for infection control. What is your plan?

2. Search the National Guidelines Clearinghouse (NGC) for EBP clinical practice guidelines related to speech, language, hearing, or swallow disorders. What is your result?

3. Locate three advertisements in magazines, journals, or on the Internet that market products, devices, programs, or interventions for speech, language, hearing, swallow, reading, or any other disorder in the audiology or speech-language pathology scopes of practice. Once you've found them, evaluate each advertisement for its accuracy and fairness.

4. Social justice is an important issue in discussions of evidence-based practice. To evaluate social justice criticisms, randomly select five abstracts or full-text articles from print journals or online. Once you have the five articles in hand, tabulate the numbers of participants in each study and their characteristics: male/female, ethnicity, race, and age. Given your results, would you say that social justice is a problem?

5. Locate a clinical research study in your area of interest. Use the CARS instrument to evaluate its strengths and weaknesses. Based on your evaluation, would you use the intervention in your practice?

6. What is one clinical recommendation that has been developed by the AAA or the Academy of Neurologic Communication Disorders and Sciences? Does this clinical recommendation reflect the IOM's attributes for good guidelines?

CHAPTER 4

MEASUREMENT IN COMMUNICATION DISORDERS RESEARCH

measurement (′me-zhər-mənt) *n.* a calculation, amount, computation, degree, estimation, evaluation, frequency, quantity, range, size, or time

Measurement is the process of systematically assigning numbers to objects, persons, or events according to some prescribed rules. For example, height and weight are measured according to the rules governing linear space and mass. The construct of intelligence is measured according to rules that govern the psychometric properties of human intelligence. The values that result from measurements (e.g., 6 feet tall, 100 IQ) are understood because their meanings are shared in society.

The purpose of measurement is to specify differences in the degree to which objects, persons, and events possess the characteristic being measured. Thus, we can say that a test score of 90 is different from a score of 80. In this case, the characteristic presumed to be measured is knowledge of the subject matter.

In order to handle, store, and utilize measurements, researchers collect and organize them in the form of *data*. The singular of *data* is "datum," but researchers almost always refer to data in the collective sense. Once their observations are gathered, researchers transform them into data that are permanently recorded on paper, magnetic tape, flash memory, or other media. Data are usually expressed numerically because numbers are easy to organize, analyze, and interpret, but data can also be recorded as words, photographs, videos, and other representations. When collection and storage are complete, researchers employ statistics to analyze and interpret the data.

Statistics is the branch of mathematics that analyzes and interprets data. Depending on the measurement, data can have very different properties. For this reason, Stevens (1946) proposed four distinct scales of measurement: *ordinal, interval, ratio*, and *nominal*. He also classified statistical procedures (e.g., mean, median, *t* test) according to the *scales* for which they were permissible. Stevens used the term *permissible* to describe the set of transformations that preserve a scale's mathematical properties. Thus, each of Stevens' scales was defined by a unique set of permissible transformations. For example, any monotone transformation—one that preserves inequalities of its arguments—is permissible for *ordinal scale data*. Thus, log, square root (if the data are not negative), and linear transformations (e.g., adding constants) were permissible transformations for ordinal data. However, if the data were *ratio scale*, the data could be multiplied by a constant, but adding constants or taking logs was not permitted. Stevens' (1946) taxonomy is used today, but the use of scale types to select or specify statistical methods is controversial. The most prominent criticisms of Stevens' (1946) taxonomy are the following:

1. Stevens' types do not exhaust the possibilities even for simple data.
2. Stevens' categories do not describe the attributes of real data that are essential to good statistical analysis.
3. Stevens' scales can often be wrong. (Velleman & Wilkinson, 1993)

The criticisms not withstanding, Stevens' (1946) classification system is a starting point for students of measurement theory. For sure, Stevens' taxonomy is not as precise or useful as first proposed. However, it can be helpful when its practical limitations are understood.

CHARACTERISTICS OF DATA

Measurement theory is important to the interpretation of statistical analyses. The data that researchers gather from observations of physical events and human behaviors must be organized, analyzed, and interpreted to make rational conclusions. The analysis depends to some degree on the characteristics of the data. However, doing statistics is not simply a matter of declaring the scale type of the data and picking a model (Velleman & Wilkinson, 1993). Mathematicians recognize the practical limitations inherent in Stevens' taxonomy, which separates data into ordinal, interval, ratio, and nominal categories.

Ordinal-Level Data

According to Stevens (1946), ordinal-level data have the mathematical property of inequality but lack other arithmetic properties. Thus, ordinal-level data can be ordered from high to low, best to worst, or least to greatest. If a group of people were lined up from shortest to tallest, we could tell who was shorter and who was taller, but we would not know the actual height of any person. These are characteristics that are common to ordinal-level data. A real-life example of ordinal-level data includes grading scales (e.g., A, B, C). In this case, the grades reflect order, but other properties are lacking. Therefore, we can say that an A is better than a B but not how much better. Ordinal-level data are not very precise in their measurement.

An ordinal-level measurement frequently used in communication disorders is the *rating scale*. A rating scale usually consists of a set of integers designed to elicit judgments about some feature or attribute. In psychometrics, rating scales typically refer to a statement that expresses an attitude or perception toward some person, place, or thing.

The Likert scale is one type of rating scale (Likert, 1932). Respondents are asked to indicate their degree of agreement with one or more statements. Traditionally, Likert scales have five response categories, with numbers assigned to each category. For example:

Statement: *I am satisfied with my hearing aid.*

Response choices:
1. Strongly disagree
2. Disagree
3. Undecided
4. Agree
5. Strongly agree

Other types of rating scales may have more or fewer than five response categories. For example, the *GRABS Voice Rating Scale* contains four response categories (Kent, 1997). GRABS rates voice quality by grade (i.e., hoarseness), roughness (i.e., jitter and shimmer), aesthetic (i.e., weakness), breath (i.e., air leakage), and strain (i.e., hyperfunction). The GRABS response categories are labeled as follows:

0	1	2	3
Normal	Slight	Moderate	Extreme

According to Stevens' (1946) definition, we can reliably conclude that a rating of 3 on the GRABS scale is worse than a rating of 1, but we cannot say that the rating of 3 is three times worse than the rating of 1. In other words, ordinal-level data possess the property of inequality but do not have equal intervals. For this reason, ordinal data in their raw form may not be suitable for statistical analysis. However, mathematical transformations of the data sometimes remedy this problem.

Interval-Level Data

Interval-level data possess the arithmetic properties of inequality and equal intervals. Thus, it is appropriate to compute differences but not to multiply or divide. For example, the difference between intelligence scores of 100 and 50 is 50—but it is not fair to say that the person with a score of 100 is twice as intelligent as the person with 50, because interval-level data have an artificial origin and no true zero point. A *true zero point* indicates the absence of whatever property is being measured. Is it possible to score zero on an intelligence test, a standardized speech-language test, or any other psychometric instrument? The answer is no, because psychometric instruments do not measure the absence of the concept being tested. In fact, they assume that the construct

TECHNOLOGY NOTE

Likert scales are subject to bias from several sources: (a) Respondents may avoid extreme points (i.e., *central tendency bias*), (b) respondents may tend to agree with all the statements (i.e., *acquiescence bias*), or (c) respondents may try to portray themselves or their organization more favorably (i.e., *social desirability bias*). Furthermore, Friedman, Herskowitz, and Pollack (1993) reported a "left-side-of-scale" bias. They asked 208 students to rate their college on 10 statements with five response categories, but half the scales were ordered from left to right—*strongly agree, agree, undecided, disagree, strongly disagree*. The other half were ordered in reverse, with *strongly disagree* on the far left. The scale with the *strongly agree* category on the left resulted in a greater degree of agreement than the scale with *strongly disagree* on the left. Friedman et al. (1993) proposed a left-side-of-scale bias. If responses were presented top-to-bottom, would you expect a similar bias?

is always present to some degree. Real-life examples of interval-level data include temperature in degrees (Celsius or Fahrenheit) and calendar dates. Calendar dates have no zero, but thermometers do have a zero point. Does zero on a thermometer mean there is no temperature? Obviously, there is temperature, and it is chilling when the thermometer reads zero.

Ratio-Level Data

Stevens (1946) described the ratio level of measurement as having all the properties of interval-level data plus a true zero point. Ratio-level data are sometimes referred to as *continuous* data. Because ratio-level data have all the mathematical properties, operations such as [20 ÷ 10] are possible. Examples of ratio-level data include common measurements such as length in centimeters, weight in pounds, height in inches, and time in seconds. Ratio-level data also include familiar units of measurement for sound intensity (decibels) and sound velocity (meters per second).

Nominal-Level Data

Nominal level does not measure anything. Rather, it is used to label people, objects, behaviors, events, or other entities. The numbers on football jerseys are often cited as a real-life example of nominal-level data. However, NFL players are assigned numerals by playing position—quarterbacks, punters, and place kickers, 1–19; running backs and defensive backs, 20–49; and so on—so the numbers on football jerseys are not entirely arbitrary.

In science, researchers sometimes include gender (male, female) or socioeconomic status (low, middle, high) as variables of interest. These categories are qualitative variables, but numbers are often assigned to them. In this case, the numbers are arbitrarily assigned to the categories without numerical meaning. For example, socioeconomic categories could be assigned the numbers 1 (high), 2 (middle), and 3 (low) without meaning. The numbers are no more than labels for the several categories. Arithmetic operations are not possible, so we cannot do much statistically with nominal data.

THE LIMITATIONS OF STEVENS TAXONOMY

Modern statisticians have argued that the Stevens (1946) classification scheme was overly simple (Velleman & Wilkinson, 1993). As a general rule, the more we can manipulate the data, the more powerful the statistical analysis. In this regard, nominal-level data are very weak, and ratio-level data are very strong. One problem with Stevens' taxonomy is that, in real life, a scale of measurement may not correspond precisely to any of his categories: "A careful data analyst should not assume that the scale type of a variable is what it appears to be even when clear assurances are made about the data" (Velleman & Wilkinson, 1993 p. 68). Sometimes, data are mistakenly assigned to the wrong level of measurement. For example, SPSS (statistical software) 16.0's help for Variable Measurement Level cited *zip codes* as an example of a nominal variable, but zip codes are not arbitrary. SPSS's help for Variable Measurement Level advised the following.

> You can specify the level of measurement as scale (numerical data on an interval or ratio scale), ordinal, or nominal. Nominal and ordinal data can be either string (alphanumeric) or numeric.
>
> **Nominal**. A variable can be treated as nominal when its values represent categories with no intrinsic ranking (for example, the department of the company in which an employee works). Examples of nominal variables include region, *zip code*, [emphasis added] and religious affiliation. (SPSS, 2008)

In fact, zip codes are numbered so that the first digit represents a certain group of states, the second and third digits represent a region in that group, and the fourth and fifth digits represent a group of delivery addresses within that region. This is an example of data that do not easily fit into Stevens' (1946) categories.

Perhaps most controversial was Stevens' (1951) proposal that statistics should be prescribed or proscribed according to his typology. According to Stevens' (1951) reasoning, analyses on nominal data should be restricted to summary statistics such as the number of cases and the mode. Permissible statistics for ordinal data included these plus the median and percentiles. Interval and ratio data allowed all of these plus means and standard deviations. Modern statisticians agree that the choice of statistical methods should not be restricted to the scale type at hand (Velleman & Wilkinson, 1993). In this regard, Guttman (1977) wrote:

> There is widespread folklore concerning mythical statistical "rules" that forbid or permit calculations involving "scales," these "rules" being independent of context. [...] Permission is not required in data analysis. What is required is a loss function to be minimized. Practitioners like to ask about *a priori* rules as to what is "permitted" to be done with their unordered or numerical observations, without any reference to any

overall loss function for their problem. Instead, they should say to the mathematician: "here is my loss function: how do I go about minimizing it?" Minimization may require treating unordered data in numerical fashion and numerical data in unordered fashion. (p. 105)

In statistics, a *loss function* represents the loss (a real cost in some sense) associated with an estimate (such as a parameter) being wrong as a function of the degree of wrongness. Loss function measures the distance between what is estimated and the true value. For example, the mean (average) is the statistic for estimating location that minimizes the expected loss experienced under the squared-error loss function, while the median is the statistic for estimating location that minimizes expected loss under the absolute-difference loss function. However, other statistics would be optimal under different (atypical) circumstances. Loss functions in economics are usually expressed as [cost in dollars = loss/time period]. In medicine, cost is sometimes expressed as lives lost (i.e., mortality).

Clearly, the choice of statistical methods is more complicated than the Stevens (1946) classification scheme implied. Prior to analyzing data, researchers should seek a statistician's advice. A case in point is when researchers collect data that are not ideally suited for statistical analysis, such as percentages, fractions, or other non-normal data. However, data can often be modified to better conform to the requirements of statistical tests. Simple transformations can often make data more amenable to good data analysis (Velleman & Wilkinson, 1993).

DATA TRANSFORMATION IN COMMUNICATION DISORDERS

Data transformations are modifications of the data values that simplify their structure, such as making the distribution of the data more symmetrical. Transformations can also make variability more nearly constant across variables and relationships more nearly linear (Velleman & Wilkinson, 1993). The most powerful statistical methods assume the data are normally distributed, but most raw data are not. Data transformations can usually improve the normality of variables. Mathematicians have also developed methods that convert ordinal-level measurements to interval and ratio scales (Guttman, 1968; Hoaglin, 1988).

The first step in evaluating the data is to determine whether a variable is substantially non-normal. The subjective approach is to visually inspect the distribution of data. However, many researchers prefer an objective approach such as an examination of skew and kurtosis or inferential tests of normality (e.g., Kolmorogov-Smirnov). The best practice is to combine both visual inspection and objective tests to evaluate normality. Researchers should also inspect their data to ensure there are no mistakes in data entry or extreme values (i.e., outliers) in the distribution. Both of these conditions can contribute to non-normality.

If data are substantially non-normal, the next step is to choose a transformation that will improve normality. The most useful data transformations include logarithms and simple powers and roots that are monotone but nonlinear transformations. Square

TECHNOLOGY NOTE

The data collected in experiments are sometimes in the form of fractions or percentages. These are ordered data, but the relative distances between the raw scores are variable. This is problematic because scores in the middle are typically biased against scores at the ends of the range. Before statistical analysis, it is usually desirable to transform fractions and percentages into odds ratios and compute the natural logs of the odds ratios. This procedure transforms the fractions and percentages into mathematically more useful interval-level data. The raw data can be transformed in most popular statistical packages and with many pocket calculators. An alternative is the Chang Bioscience webpage, which includes a log-odds ratio calculator: www.changbioscience. com/stat/logr.html. The user simply enters the odds ratio, and the log-odds ratio is calculated.

root, log, and inverse operations are commonly used transformations in communication disorders. All of these transformations reduce non-normality by reducing the relative spacing of scores on the right side more than on the left side of the distribution. If done correctly, the data remain in the same relative order as prior to the transformation.

The *square root transformation* takes the square root of every value. If the data include negative values, a constant must be added to move the minimum value in the distribution above 0. It is best to move the minimum value to 1.00, because numbers of 1.00 and above behave differently than values between 0.00 and 0.99. The square root of values between 0.00 and 0.99 always becomes larger, whereas the square root of values above 1.00 is always smaller. Thus, the square root of 8 is 2.83, and the square root of 0.80 is 0.89.

Logarithms are another class of transformations that improve normality. A logarithm is the power a base number must be raised in order to get the original number. For example, if we choose base 10, $1 = 10^0$, $100 = 10^2$, and so on. Another option is the *natural log*, where the constant e (2.7182818) is the base. In this case, the natural log of $10 = 2.303$, $100 = 4.605$, and so on. If the data include negative values, a constant must be added to move the minimum value to 1.00.

The *inverse transformation* simply computes $1/x$ to find the inverse of a number (x). This has the effect of making very small values large and very large values small. For example, the inverse of 0.50 is 2 and the inverse of 100 is 0.01. The inverse transformation reverses the order of scores, so it is best to reverse the distribution prior to applying the inverse transformation. To reverse the distribution, the variable is multiplied by –1, and a constant is added to raise the minimum value above 1.00. Following the transformation, the values are restored to their original order.

MULTIPLE MEASURES IN COMMUNICATION DISORDERS

Diener and Eid (2006) are strong advocates for the use of multiple measures in the behavioral sciences. Multiple measurement methods include more than one and sometimes several different measures to estimate the underlying constructs in experiments. Diener and Eid (2006) argued that no single behavior ever represents the influence of a single construct. They reasoned that "every measurement method, even the best ones, possesses substantial shortcomings and limitations (p. 457)." It follows that "by using different methods, researchers can eliminate specific artifacts from their conclusions because the artifacts are unlikely to influence all the diverse measures they use" (Diener & Eid, 2006).

The construct that typically underlies clinical research is an important change (for better or worse) in the client's life. Kazdin (2001) described three methods for evaluating the clinical significance of change in intervention studies. The methods are (a) comparison, (b) subjective evaluation, and (c) social impact. The *comparison method* evaluates clinical outcomes relative to the performance of others (e.g., a normative sample or a preset criterion). *Subjective evaluation* includes the opinions and judgments of the client, friends, and family that a change makes a difference. Finally, *social impact* has to do with change on a measure that is considered to be important in everyday life, e.g., attendance at school, social avoidance, or communication success.

A case example of subjective evaluation in communication disorders is research with persons who stutter (PWS). Multiple measures are typically included in these experiments. In experiments with PWS, the comparison is often a 5% disfluency rate, the subjective evaluation is the opinion of the client, and social impact is reflected in change in social behaviors. The combination of these methods is a better indicator of clinically significant change than any single measure (Meline & Harn, 2008a).

DESCRIPTIVE STATISTICS IN COMMUNICATION DISORDERS

After the dependent variable is measured, researchers arrange the data in a meaningful way. Such an arrangement of data is called a *data summary*. Data summaries most often appear in *tabular form* (i.e., tables). If the total number of observations is small, the individual data can be presented in a frequency table. Exhibit 4.1 depicts a

EXHIBIT 4.1
Frequency Table Organized Across 5 Categories for 5 Participants

	CATEGORIES				
	A	B	C	D	E
Participant 1	5	8	2	3	0
Participant 2	12	12	7	13	30
Participant 3	6	0	3	2	7
Participant 4	9	11	26	8	9
Participant 5	22	10	12	9	11

frequency table with five categories and five participants. As an alternative to frequency data, the results could be presented as simple count data (i.e., the number of occurrences of the behavior). The presentation of data in one form or another usually depends on the authors' preference, but transparency and clear reporting are guiding principles. Results should be fully disclosed in the clearest possible way to avoid misinterpretation.

Frequency distributions are informative; however, shorthand methods for describing the specific features of data are also useful methods. The most common shorthand methods employed by researchers are known as descriptive statistics. A descriptive statistic is a measure of a specific feature or characteristic of a set of data. Descriptive statistics are routinely used to summarize data. Common types of descriptive statistics are (a) measures of location, (b) measures of variability, and (c) measures of individual location. All are regularly used in communication disorders research.

Measures of Location

Measures of location are single values that describe an entire set of data. The value chosen depends on the particular characteristic to be described as well as the measurement level of the dependent variable. Measures of location include two broad categories: (a) central location and (b) fractiles. Several statistical measures describe central location—the center or middle of a set of data. There are three common measures of central location: (a) mean, (b) median, and (c) mode.

A common measure of central location is the arithmetic mean or average. The mean of n numbers is their sum divided by n. For example:

$$8 + 11 + 15 + 6 + 3 = 43$$
$$n = 5$$
$$\text{mean} = 43/5 = 8.6$$

The number (n) of values in a sample is known as the *sample size*. By convention, the mean is assigned the symbol $\bar{x}$, which is read as "x bar." The symbol Σ is uppercase *sigma*, the Greek letter. Sigma is the conventional notation for summation. The symbol x is assigned to the individual values in a set of data. Thus, the formula for computing the mean is:

$$\text{mean} = \frac{\Sigma x}{n}$$

The formula reads: "the mean equals the sum of xs divided by n." The mean is a valid indicator of central location if the data are normally distributed (or nearly so). If the data include extreme scores at the top or bottom, the mean may be a poor indicator of central location.

Another measure of central location is known as the *median* (mdn). The median for a set of numbers is the midpoint or center of the data. Computing the median requires ordinal-level data or a higher level of measurement. Ranked scores and rating scales are common examples of ordinal-level data. If interval or ratio level data are not normally distributed, the median may be preferred over the mean as a measure of central location. A better solution is to transform the data if possible.

Computing the median is simple for some sets of data but complicated for others. In all cases, the first step is to arrange the scores in order from low to high. When the sample size is odd and no two values are alike, the median is the middle value. Thus, for the set of data [3, 6, 8, 11, 15] the middle value and the median is 8. When the sample size is even and no two values are alike, the median is the average of the two middle values. Thus, for the set of data [3, 6, 8, 11, 15, 20] the median is [8 + 11 / 2 = 9.5]. Computing the median is more complex when there are data with the same values. For example, the data set [3, 6, 8, 8, 8, 11, 15] contains a three-way tie [8, 8, 8]. However, if the tie is *balanced* (equally distributed) the median is the average of the tied values. Thus, the median for the data set [3, 6, 8, 8, 8, 11, 15] is 8 because the center is balanced with values of 8 on both sides. A second example [3, 6, 8, 8, 11, 15] includes an even number of values with a two-way tie. Because the tie is balanced, the median is the average of the two center values [8 + 8 / 2 = 8].

In the previous example, the median was found by *inspection*. However, unbalanced ties require estimation of the median. For example, median by inspection is not possible in the data set [2, 4, 5, 5, 5, 7] because the tied value [5] is unbalanced. Therefore, the estimated median is computed in 10 steps:

Step 1. Order the data from low to high.
2, 4, 5, 5, 5, 7

Step 2. Divide the scores into halves.
2, 4, 5 | 5, 5, 7

Step 3. Identify an interval a half-unit below and a half-unit above the middle value(s).
middle value = 5
interval = 4.5 to 5.5

Step 4. Identify the lower limit (L) of the interval.
lower limit (L) = 4.5

Step 5. Compute the sample size (n).
sample size (n) = 6

Step 6. Count the frequency of observations below the lower limit.
frequency below (Fb) = 2 [2, 4]

Step 7. Count the frequency of observations within the interval.
frequency within (Fw) = 3 [5, 5, 5]

Step 8. Divide n by 2 (constant) and subtract the frequency below.
(6 / 2) − 2 = 1

Step 9. Divide the above value by the frequency within the interval.
$$1 / 3 = 0.33$$

Step 10. Add the value above to the lower limit of the interval.
$$5 + 0.33 = 4.88 = \text{est. median}$$

The computations described in steps 1–10 are expressed in a single formula:

$$\text{est. median} = L + \left[\frac{(n/2) - \Sigma Fb}{\Sigma Fw} \right]$$

The 10 steps are appropriate to estimate the median when using actual observed scores. However, there are situations when data are grouped for analysis. In these cases, the interval is typically greater than one, and special procedures are needed to estimate the median (cf. Hinkle, Wiersma, & Jurs, 1988).

A third measure of central location is known as the *mode*. The mode is used almost exclusively with nominal data. If the researchers' dependent variable consists of numbers assigned to categories with no arithmetic meaning, the mode is the only valid measure of central tendency. The mode is defined as the value that occurs most frequently in a set of data. For example, in the data set [2, 7, 3, 2, 2, 1], the mode is 2. The mode is a relatively uninformative statistic for centrality, but it is the only index of central location for the nominal-level data.

There are two general categories for statistical measures of location in a set of data: (a) measures of central tendency and (b) fractiles. Statistical procedures are called *fractiles* when they divide a set of data into two or more nearly equal parts. Fractiles identify the proportion of observations above and below them. For example, the median is a fractile that divides data into two equal parts: 50% above and 50% below the median. Other fractiles include quartiles, quintiles, deciles, and percentiles. *Quartiles* are statistical boundaries that divide the data into 4 nearly equal parts. They are referred to as the first, second, third, and fourth quartiles. The second quartile is also known as the median. *Quintiles* divide the data into 5 nearly equal parts. *Deciles* divide the data into 10 parts, and *percentiles* divide the data into 100 parts. Computing quartiles and other fractiles is similar to computation of the median. The constant in the numerator of the formula is changed according to number of divisions, such as 4 for quartiles:

$$\text{est. quartile} = L + \left[\frac{(n/4) - \Sigma Fb}{\Sigma Fw} \right]$$

The 4 in the numerator would be replaced by 5 for computing quintiles or 100 for computing percentiles.

Measures of Individual Location

Measures of individual location are used to specify the location of one participant in relationship to a group of participants. They include (a) ranks, (b) percentile ranks, and

(c) standard scores. The simplest procedure—known as *ranks*—orders a group of participants in terms of their performances on some measure from low to high or high to low. For example, in the data set [66, 80, 91, 94, 99] the participant with a score of 94 is ranked second when the scores are ranked from high to low. Another measure of individual location is known as *percentile ranks*.

Percentiles are fractiles that divide the data into 100 equal parts. The relative position for an individual within a group of participants is given by the individual's percentile rank. For example, an individual whose score places him or her at the 80th percentile for the group performed above 80% and below 20% of the group. A third measure of individual location is known as the *standard score*.

Standard scores (also known as z scores) are raw scores that are converted to standard deviation units. They are useful as indicators of individual location when data are normally distributed. A standard score is calculated as follows (the x signifies one subject's score):

$$z = x - \text{mean/standard deviation}$$

The standard score gives an individual's location relative to the average or mean for the group of individuals. For example, if the mean and standard deviation are 100 and 15 respectively, an individual who achieves a score of 130 is two standard scores (z scores) above the mean for the group. An individual who scores 85 is one standard score below the mean for the group. Based on what you know about standard scores, answer the following question: How would you evaluate a score of 115 on a standardized test with a mean of 100 and a standard deviation of 10?

Measures of Variability

Unequal values are a typical trait of the data that is collected in experiments. The degree of dispersion in a set of data is known as variability (or spread). The degree of variability is important in research and clinical practice. For example, suppose a child scores 90 on a test that has a mean of 100. The child's score is 10 points below the mean, but what does that mean? Is the child's performance delayed? These questions are answered by knowing the normal variability associated with a test instrument. Measures of central location are not very meaningful without measures of variability. There are many measures of variability, including (a) number of different categories, (b) range, (c) variance, and (d) standard deviation.

Counting numbers of different categories.   Counting numbers of different categories is a simple measure of variability for use with nominal data. For example, if 60 percent of participants are categorized as low socioeconomic status (SES), it is useful to know whether socioeconomic status is divided into two categories or seven.

The range.   Another index of variability is known as the *range*. The range is the largest observed value minus the smallest observed value. In practice, researchers usually report the two extreme values, such as [range = 11–123]. The range is useful when comparing variations between two sets of data. For example, consider the following data:

Sample A: Range = 45 to 90
Sample B: Range = 12 to 99

Sample B appears to be more variable than sample A. However, knowing the range of scores tells us nothing about the variability of scores falling between the two extremes. An examination of the individual values in samples A and B ordered from low to high is revealing. The scores in sample B are fairly distributed from top to bottom.

Sample A: 45, 49, 89, 89, 90, 90
Sample B: 12, 22, 49, 65, 79, 99

However, the scores in sample A are grouped together at the extremes. Thus, range alone is a poor indicator of variablity. However, the range is the usual measure of variability for *ordinal data*. It is sometimes reported as an indicator of variability for interval and ratio-level data, though other measures of variability are more informative.

The variance.   *Variance* can be calculated for either interval- or ratio-level data. Variance considers the dispersion of individual values around the mean. Exhibit 4.2 duplicates the values from samples A and B. In addition, the mean for each sample and the variability of each score in relation to the mean are reported. The differences displayed in Exhibit 4.2 are used for calculating variation in the two samples. The variances are calculated in three steps:

Step 1. Square each difference to eliminate + or – signs.

Step 2. Sum the squared differences.
          Sample A = 2417.34
          Sample B = 5583.34
Step 3. Divide the sum by the number of values minus 1.

The number 1 is a constant subtracted from n because the data are a sample of the population. The sample variability is expected to underestimate the population variability. The denominator $[n - 1]$ compensates for the error in estimation.

Sample A = 2417.34 / (6 – 1) = 483.47
Sample B = 5583.34 / (6 – 1) = 1116.67

The values computed in step 3 are the variances for samples A and B. The variance (i.e., dispersion of scores around the mean) is greater in sample B than in sample A. In other words, individual scores are spread out in sample B but grouped closer together in sample A. Variance has a major shortcoming as a descriptive measure because its value is not expressed in the same unit of measurement as the sample scores. For this reason, variance is not easily interpreted. However, this fault is overcome by transforming the variance into what is known as a *standard deviation*. The term "stan-

EXHIBIT 4.2
Computing Variances from Raw Scores and Their Differences from the Mean for Two Samples

	SAMPLE A		SAMPLE B	
SCORE	DIFFERENCE	SCORE	DIFFERENCE	
45	−30.3	12	−42.3	
49	−26.3	22	−32.3	
89	−13.7	49	−05.3	
89	−13.7	65	10.7	
90	14.7	79	24.7	
90	14.7	99	44.7	
Mean = 75.3		Mean = 54.3		

dard deviation" was first used in 1893 by Karl Pearson, who was a founder of the discipline of study known as *statistics*.

Standard deviation.   The standard deviation (SD) is derived from the variation. To express variation in the same unit of measurement as the original data, the square root of the variation is calculated. The square root of the variation in sample A = 21.99, and the square root of the variation in sample B = 33.42.

$$SD = \sqrt{\text{variation}}$$

The standard deviation is easily interpreted. If the SD for a set of data is small, it means the values are spread closely around the mean. If the SD for a set of data is large, the values are spread further away from the mean. Descriptives such as *standard deviation, mean, variance*, and *range* are routinely included in statistical software (see Exhibit 4.3, SPSS 16.0 descriptives menu).

The Coefficient of Variation

The *coefficient of variation* is a measure of relative variation. In some situations, it may be more meaningful to express standard deviation as a percentage of what is being measured. This is particularly true when making comparisons between two or more sets of data. The coefficient of variation (CV) is expressed as [CV (%) = (SD / mean) (100)].

As an example, assume researchers want to compare variations in age between two groups of participants with the following characteristics:

Group A: Mean = 30 years, SD = 2.4
Group B: Mean = 26 years, SD = 3.9
$CV_{GROUP A}$ = (2.4 / 30) (100) = 8%
$CV_{GROUP B}$ = (3.9 / 26) (100) = 15%

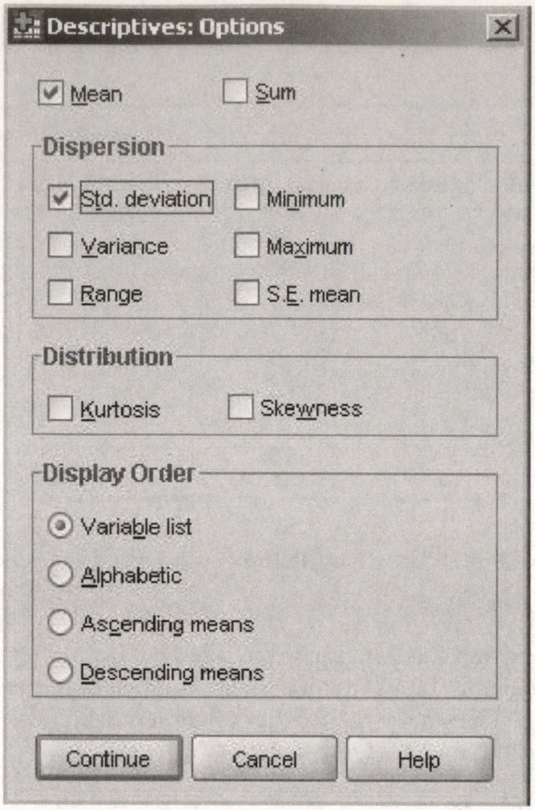

EXHIBIT 4.3
SPSS 16.0 Descriptives Options Menu
SPSS for Windows, Rel. 16.0. (2008).

TECHNOLOGY NOTE

Though best remembered as a nurse, Florence Nightingale (1820–1910) enlisted tutors to learn mathematics when she was 20 years old. She learned arithmetic, geometry, and algebra years before she became interested in nursing. Florence Nightingale applied her skills with mathematics to medical statistics and invented colorful diagrams to dramatize medical data and to persuade authorities in England to accept her proposals for hospital reform. She is recognized as a pioneer in the graphic presentation of data. Florence Nightingale's work with medical statistics earned her membership in the Statistical Society of England.

Thus, age is less variable in group A, with a coefficient of variation of 8%, than in group B, with a coefficient of variation of 15%.

STATISTICAL GRAPHICS IN COMMUNICATION DISORDERS

The method of *statistical graphics* is defined as "graphical methods for analyzing data" in Chambers, Cleveland, Kleiner, and Tukey's (1983) classic textbook. The goals of statistical graphics are to (a) visually communicate information to others, (b) record data compactly, and (c) visually analyze data to learn more about its structure (Chambers et al., 1983). Statistical graphics techniques aim to organize data in ways that facilitate the recognition of patterns in the set of data. They provide information about the distribution and shape of the set of data. For example, statistical graphics techniques display the distribution of data so that symmetry and asymmetry are recognizable. Statistical graphics techniques are useful for analyzing data from one variable (univariate data) as well as two variables (bivariate data).

Univariate Statistical Graphics

To examine the characteristics of data from one sample, a variety of statistical graphics techniques are available. The most common and useful techniques are (a) histograms, (b) bar graphs, (c) stem-and-leaf plots, and (d) box plots.

Histograms are constructed from frequency tables. The intervals chosen for analysis are displayed on the horizontal axis, and the measurement in each interval is represented by the height of a rectangle on the vertical axis (see Exhibit 4.4.1). Histograms are like bar graphs except that the columns in bar graphs are separated by a small distance (see Exhibit 4.4.2). Histograms are an aid to visualize patterns for quantitative variables, whereas bar graphs are used to graph qualitative variables. Histograms provide information about (a) central tendency, (b) variability, (c) skewness, (d) presence of outliers, and (e) the presence of multiple modes in the data.

A second statistical graphics technique is known as the stem-and-leaf display. Stem-and-leaf displays are analogous to histograms. They provide the same information about the data but in a different way. Exhibit 4.5 shows a typical stem-and-leaf display for 25 test scores. The numbers to the left of the vertical lines are *stems* (tens digits). The numbers to the right are *leaves* (unit digits). For example, [5 | 2 7] represents the test scores 52 and 57. Like histograms, stem-and-leaf plots display the shape and distribution of a set of data. Another statistical graphics technique is known as the *box plot*.

Box-and-whiskers plots (also known as box plots) display the shape and distribution for a set of data with (a) a box, (b) whiskers, and (c) outliers. Exhibit 4.6 shows the typical features of the box-and-whiskers plot.

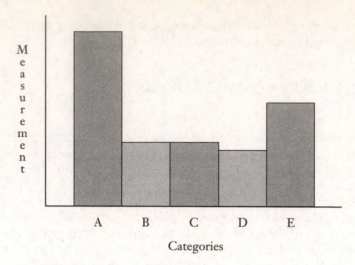

EXHIBIT 4.4.1
A Typical Histogram Display

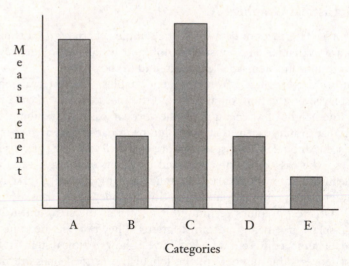

EXHIBIT 4.4.2
A Typical Bar Graph Display

The median is displayed as a horizontal line inside the box. The upper and lower boundaries of the box are the third (Q_3) and first (Q_1) quartiles respectively. The distance between Q_1 and Q_3 is the interquartile range, which contains 50% of the data. The whiskers extend from the box to the highest value within the upper limit and the lowest value within the lower limit. Values falling outside the upper or lower limits are designated as *outliers*. Outliers are extreme values that may be misfits in a set of data.

```
5 | 2 7

6 | 7 8 9

7 | 1 3 3 5 6 6 7 8 9

8 | 2 3 4 4 5 9

9 | 1 4 5 5 7
```

EXHIBIT 4.5
Typical Stem-and-Leaf Display

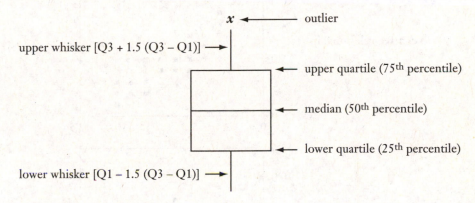

EXHIBIT 4.6
Features of the Box-and-Whiskers Plot

Bivariate Statistical Graphics

Bivariate data consist of the values of two variables, such as height and weight, from one participant. For a group of participants, the values are recorded as (X_1, Y_1) (X_2, Y_2) (X_3, Y_3) and so on. *Scatterplots* are the statistical graphics method of choice for displaying bivariate data. Exhibit 4.7 is a series of three scatterplots with coordinates X (abscissa) and Y (ordinate). X is the horizontal plane, and Y is the vertical plane. In a scatterplot, the X coordinate records values for one variable, and the Y coordinate records the values for the second variable. The purpose is to display the relationship between two variables in terms of the direction of the relationship (i.e., positive or negative) and the shape of the relationship (i.e., linear or curvilinear). Researchers visually inspect the data in scatterplots to identify extreme or suspicious values. Exhibit 4.7 displays three possible relationships (i.e., positive, negative, and none) between X and Y variables. The graphics modules in statistical software packages such as SPSS 16.0's chart builder (see Exhibit 4.8) include scatterplot, bar graph, histogram, and boxplot functions.

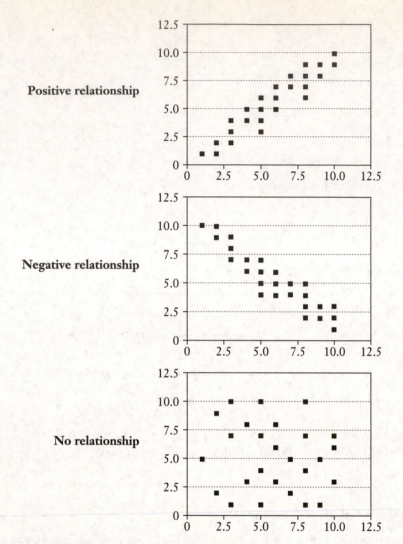

EXHIBIT 4.7
Bivariate Relationships in Scatterplots

Comparing Two or More Samples

Mean plots, standard deviation plots, and box plots can be used to compare the observations from two or more samples. For example, mean plots and standard deviation plots can be used to graph values across time for one subject (i.e., time series) or to compare two groups of subjects such as experimental and control groups. Box plots are useful for comparing central tendencies, spreads, and outliers.

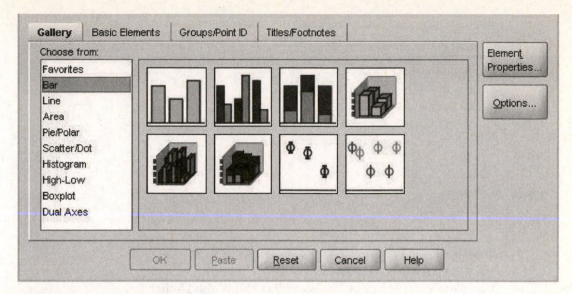

EXHIBIT 4.8
SPSS 16.0 Chart Builder Menu
SPSS for Windows, Rel.16.0. (2008).

TECHNOLOGY NOTE

Microsoft Excel's Tool Menu includes a *Data Analysis* submenu with histogram and descriptive statistics functions. *Excel's Chart Wizard* includes bar chart, scatterplot, and line graph options—but it lacks a box plot function. Though *Microsoft Excel* does not have a built in box and whisker plot function, researchers can create box plots using stacked bar or column charts and error bars in combination with line or *XY* scatter charts. *Peltier's Excel Page* is a source for *Microsoft Excel Tips and Tricks*: http://peltiertech.com/Excel/index.html. Alternatively, researchers can utilize add-ins or macros that supplement *Excel's* usual functions.

Exhibit 4.9 compares two box plots labeled A and B. Based on your understanding of box plots, answer the following questions: In what ways do the two box plots in Exhibit 4.9 differ? What else can you say about the box plots in Exhibit 4.9?

Graphing Individual Observations

In addition to statistical summaries for group data, summaries for individual participants may provide additional information. For example, group means may indicate positive increases for a targeted behavior, but individual performances may provide additional information. Information about individual outcomes is especially important

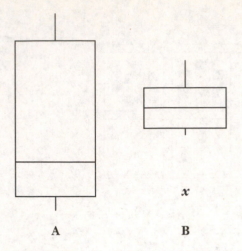

x

A   B

EXHIBIT 4.9
Comparison Between Box Plot A and Box Plot B with Outlier x

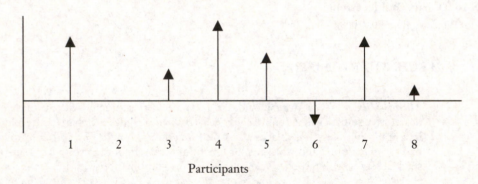

Participants

EXHIBIT 4.10
Example of Individual Participant Performances Graphed

for clinical practice. Exhibit 4.10 displays clinical outcomes for 10 participants. The outcome is positive for the group as a whole, but an examination of individual results shows that participant 2 made no gain (or loss), and participant 6 regressed.

CONCLUSION

Researchers must collect, organize, and interpret their quantitative and qualitative data. They recognize that their data possess unique characteristics that may affect the precision of measurements as well as the choice of statistical methods. Therefore, researchers inspect their data and sometimes modify it before analysis is done. The "garbage in, garbage out" (GIGO) analogy calls attention to the reality that it is difficult to produce a good result with bad input. In research, the quality of the data determines the validity of results. If data are inappropriately handled, the results will be of questionable value.

Researchers strive to persuade consumers that their interpretation is the best fit for the data. To this end, a clear and logical presentation of the data in summary and graphical forms meets the objective. Statistical software packages such as SPSS, Minitab, and S-Plus include a variety of tools for organizing data in graphical form. Statistical graphics are a means to explain results to consumers in a convincing fashion.

CASE STUDIES

Case 4.1: Collaboration and Consultation
Professor Longworth and a research assistant completed a preliminary of data collected from a comparison of two treatment approaches for facilitating language. The average improvement for group A is 20%, and the average improvement for group B is 10%. As a consultant, what additional analyses of the data do you suggest to the two researchers?

Case 4.2: Challenge for Clinician-Researchers in Schools
Two clinician-researchers are planning an experiment to test the effectiveness of a new reading fluency program. Because the experiment will be conducted during school hours in second-grade classrooms, the researchers are concerned about possible nuisance variables. What nuisance variables should they anticipate?

Case 4.3: Controlled Experimentation at General Hospital
Researchers at General Hospital collected data from a randomized-controlled experiment in which 20 dysphagic patients were divided into two groups: One group received the experimental treatment and the other group received a placebo. The statistical summaries included the following results:

Experimental group:	mean = 14	SD = 12
Control group:	mean = 8	SD = 2

Based on the preliminary results given, what are your conclusions? Is the experimental treatment an effective one?

Case 4.4: Zach and Britney's Dilemma
Zach and Britney are student researchers who have completed their data collection. However, a visual inspection reveals several extreme values to the far right of the distribution, and an objective test indicates that the data are not normally distributed. What steps should Zach and Britney take before attempting to analyze their results?

Case 4.5: Sarah's Argument
Sarah is co-investigator for a study of swallow function that employed ordinal-level measurement of the dependent variable. Because the measurement is ordinal, the principal investigator wants to use weaker nonparametric statistics to analyze the data, but Sarah objects. She believes that the stronger parametric statistics can be used. What points should Sarah make to convince her co-investigator that parametric statistics are appropriate?

■ ■ ■ ■ ■

STUDENT EXERCISES

1. Select a research report from a professional journal and answer the following questions: What kinds of data are included? What are the levels of measurement? What summary statistics are reported? What statistical graph methods are used—if none, what methods could have been used?

2. Select a research report from a professional journal. What nuisance variables, if any, are discussed, and what nuisance variables might they have encountered?

3. What is an acceptable operational definition for an experiment in which dysphonic patients are the participants? Write an operational definition for selecting dysphonic participants. Repeat the exercise for cochlear implant patients.

4. For a set of data, the median is 50 and the mean is 50. What do these results indicate?

5. A scatterplot shows a negative and curvilinear distribution for the research team's data set. What do these results indicate?

6. Identify an experiment that reports transformations of the data. What kind of transformation did the researchers utilize? What was their rationale for transforming the data?

PART II

RESEARCH DESIGNS FOR SCIENTISTS/PRACTITIONERS IN COMMUNICATION DISORDERS

CHAPTER 5

GROUP DESIGNS IN COMMUNICATION DISORDERS RESEARCH

> **design** (dĭ-zīn') *v.* to conceive or fashion in the mind, to formulate a plan, to create or execute in a highly skilled manner

A *research design* is a plan that includes protocols for selecting participants, controlling extraneous variables, implementing treatments, observing variables, and ensuring ethical procedures. Kerlinger (1973) characterized research designs as the blueprints of the research architect and engineer. Indeed, the value of a research design depends on its quality. A poor design leads to faulty conclusions, whereas a good design leads to meaningful conclusions. However, a good design alone does not ensure the scientific merit of a research study. A well-thought-out hypothesis is also important. The *hypothesis* is a tentative explanation for an observation, phenomenon, or clinical problem that can be investigated. Formulating hypotheses is a prerequisite to developing sound research designs. A good design with a poorly conceived hypothesis is unlikely to achieve scientific recognition.

WHAT IS A GOOD HYPOTHESIS?

The hypothesis is the building block on which a research design rests. It guides the choice of methods, procedures, and choice of participants as well as interpretation of results. The statement of the hypothesis should be clearly and concisely stated. To evaluate the hypothesis, we should ask: (a) Does it link the two or more variables thought to be related? (b) Is the hypothesis testable? (c) Does the theory or logic of the proposed relationship make sense? If the answers are affirmative, the hypothesis is probably well conceived.

WHAT DETERMINES THE QUALITY OF A RESEARCH DESIGN?

The quality of a research design is judged by its ability to (a) answer the research questions and (b) control extraneous variables. Some research designs are inherently better than others because they are less vulnerable to extraneous variables and threats to internal validity. A high level of internal validity ensures that the relationship between independent and dependent variables can be clearly interpreted. Because weaker designs have poorer mechanisms to control extraneous variables, the risk of reaching faulty conclusions is greater. Though it is important to choose the best research design available, the strongest designs are not appropriate for answering many research questions. As Kerlinger (1973) said:

> The most important social scientific and educational research problems do not lend themselves to experimentation although many of them do lend themselves to controlled inquiry of the ex post facto [quasi-experimental] kind. (p. 392)

For the reasons Kerlinger (1973) cited, scientists utilize a variety of research designs, both experimental and quasi-experimental. Though there are many different research designs, most are simply variations of a small number of basic designs. A research plan requires several steps: (a) identify the population of interest, (b) develop a sampling protocol, (c) select a design that answers the research questions, and (d) choose an appropriate statistical test.

SAMPLING PROTOCOLS IN COMMUNICATION DISORDERS

A first step in developing a research design is to identify the population of interest. The *population of interest* (i.e., target population) consists of all possible individuals who have at least one characteristic in common. For example, the population of adults with aphasia includes every individual who is adult and manifests aphasia. Because the population of adults with aphasia is very large and includes many subgroups, the population of interest is usually limited to subpopulations by specifying additional characteristics. For example, a study of persons with aphasia might be limited to those individuals with recent strokes and left brain lesions.

It is usually not possible to observe every individual in a population, so a sample of individuals is extracted from the target population. A *sample* is a set of data that represents only a part of the population. The goal for sampling is to extract a relatively small number of observations from a population. The resulting sample serves as a basis for generalizations about the population as a whole. For example, a sample size of 50 might be chosen to represent a population of 10,000 persons.

Sampling Methods in Communication Disorders

Sampling methods are protocols for gathering a sample from the target population. The sampling method known as *simple random sampling* ensures that each individual in the population has an equal chance of being selected for the sample. To carry out simple random sampling, each individual is selected by a chance process such as drawing numbers from a hat. This kind of random selection is important to ensure that results and conclusions can be generalized to the larger target population.

Due to practical constraints, *convenience sampling* (also known as "accidental sampling") is sometimes substituted for simple random sampling. The convenience sampling process selects participants from the pool of individuals that are available because of their close geographic proximity or other reasons of convenience. The problem with convenience sampling is that it severely limits the researchers' ability to generalize results to the larger population.

A practical alternative to simple random sampling is *stratified sampling*. The stratified sampling approach divides the target population into a number of non-overlapping subpopulations, also known as *strata*. Examples of strata are geographic regions and chronological age groupings (e.g., young, middle-aged, old). Once strata are chosen, the researchers select random samples from each of the subpopulations.

Selecting Participants for Research Studies

Selecting participants for research studies is a critical aspect for all experiments. Decisions regarding the characteristics of research participants are important for validity as well as the transferability of results. It is important that researchers establish appropriate selection criteria as a part of their overall plan of study. A case example is Gelfand, Schwander, and Silman's (1990) study of ears. They adopted a list of 11 selection criteria for their investigation of normal ears and cochlear-impaired ears and described their selection criteria as follows:

> [The selection criteria] included (a) measurable auditory thresholds ≤ 110 dB HL (ANSI-1969) at 500, 1000, and 2000 Hz for both ears; (b) no significant changes from prior pure tone thresholds (± 5dB) and speech recognition scores (Raffin & Schafer, 1980); (c) no significant air-bone gaps (Studebaker, 1962); (d) middle ear pressure within ± 50 daPa of atmospheric pressure; (e) static acoustic immittance not exceeding 3000 ohms; (f) no reflex delay (Olsen, Stach, & Kurdziel, 1981); (g) no abnormal threshold adaptation (Olsen & Noffsinger, 1974); (h) no evidence of ear disease; (i) no history or complaints of neurological involvement; (j) normal radiological findings when these tests were done; (k) no evidence of functional overlay; and (l) complaints and history consistent with cochlear involvement. Therefore, the subjects had normal hearing or sensorineural hearing losses attributable to cochlear involvement. (Gelfand et al., 1990, p. 199)

Why did Gelfand and co-investigators (1990) choose these particular criteria? They supported their choice of selection criteria by referencing authoritative sources.

Participant selection criteria should be based on sound principles, and the adoption of established standards from authoritative sources is one way to achieve a valid set of criteria.

The criteria for participant selection are often discussed and debated in professional forums. For example, Logemann (1987) suggested that research participants in studies of dysphagia should be homogeneous. According to Logemann (1987), the homogeneity should be based on (a) the nature of the physiologic or anatomic swallowing disorder, (b) the nature of the underlying disease or dysfunction causing dysphagia, and (c) the stage of the disease or recovery process.

Also concerned about participant selection criteria were Yairi, Watkins, Ambrose, and Paden (2001), who proposed a definition for stuttering, and Plante (1998), who recommended selection criteria for participants with specific-language impairment. Typically, discussions relevant to participant selection issues in communication disorders are found in published sources, including journal articles, research notes, and letters to journal editors.

Participant selection criteria are critically important to the quality of designs because they affect internal validity, the ability to generalize results, and the ability of others to confirm results through replication.

What Is a Representative Sample?

Clinical research is most beneficial when participants represent all persons at risk for the behavior or disease being studied. For example, conclusions from samples that include only males limit transferability of results to the general population of males. In 1990, the *National Institutes of Health* (NIH) issued a policy statement regarding the inclusion of women and minorities in clinical studies (U.S. Department of Health and Human Services, 1990). In 2000, the NIH Office of Extramural Research issued guidelines regarding the inclusion of women and minorities for extramural research. The NIH Office of Extramural Research oversees the grant process for research outside the National Institutes of Health. Extramural research accounts for about 84 percent of the NIH's annual $29 billion budget. In regard to gender composition, the NIH especially encouraged evaluations of gender differences, as evident in the following statement:

> Clinical research findings should be of benefit to all persons at risk of the disease, regardless of gender. ... Public concern requires that clinical studies include both genders in such a way that results are applicable to the general population; exceptions would be those diseases or conditions that occur only in one gender. ... Whenever there are scientific reasons to anticipate differences between men and women with regard to the hypothesis under investigation, applicants should consider the inclusion of an evaluation of gender differences in the proposed study. (U.S. Department of Health and Human Services, 1990, p. 1)

A *representative sample* includes individuals from each constituency in the target population, including women and ethnic minorities. If simple random sampling does not produce a representative sample, stratified sampling is an alternative to ensure representative samples.

CASE EXAMPLE

In a study of semantic representation and naming in children, McGregor, Newman, Reilly, and Capone (2002) recruited 32 participants in two groups: (a) 16 children with specific language impairment and (b) 16 typically developing children. They reported the ethnic make-up for both research groups as 70% Caucasian with 30% African American and Hispanic children. McGregor et al. (2002) noted that the United States population as a whole is about 75% Caucasian and 25% African American and Hispanic. Thus, they attempted to match their sample with the general U.S. population.

Sample Size and Power

Sample size refers to the total number of participants included in a study. Sample size is important because it contributes to the power of a research design. Power is the ability of a research study to detect significant treatment effects when they are present. Lipsey (1990) adopted the term "design sensitivity" to refer to this attribute of research studies.

If a study's sensitivity is too low, a treatment may be labeled as ineffective when it is effective. Shadish, Cook, and Campbell (2002) warned that low power is a major cause of false null conclusions in individual research studies. Indeed, a survey of research reports (outside communication disorders) found that statistical power was only 40–47%. This finding is well below the recommended 80% power for detecting moderate-sized effects (Jennions & Møller, 2003). A review of power in communication disorders research would probably yield similar results.

The sensitivity of a research design depends on its plan, implementation, and statistical analysis (Tatano Beck, 1994). Design sensitivity is affected by internal validity, measurement reliability, choice of statistical tests, and the sample size. When all else is equal, research designs with more participants will have more power to identify treatment effects. Exhibit 5.1 lists the factors that typically affect the sensitivity of research designs.

Computer-Generated Power Analysis

The computer software packages that perform power or sample-size calculations include NQUERY ADVISOR, PASS, STAT POWER, and G*Power (Thomas & Krebs, 1997). Some of these software packages are expensive, but G*Power is distributed as freeware. G*Power 3 performs power analysis tests for the most common statistical tests used in behavioral research (Institute für Experimentelle Psychologie, 2008). It is available for Windows XP/Vista and Mac OS 10.4 operating systems.

To calculate power with G*Power 3, users should know the following:

1. Type of statistical test planned, e.g., F, t, or X^2
2. Alpha value (typically 0.05)
3. Expected effect size, e.g., 0.50 (a half SD)
4. Proposed sample size (total number of participants)

EXHIBIT 5.1
Factors That Affect Research Design Sensitivity

***

THE INDEPENDENT VARIABLE
   1. Strength of the treatment
   2. Untreated or "low dosage" control condition for maximum contrast with the treatment condition
   3. Treatment group integrity—uniform application of the treatment condition to all participants
   4. Control group integrity—uniform application of the control condition to all participants

THE DEPENDENT VARIABLE
   1. Validity for measuring the expected change
   2. Precise units of measurement
   3. No floor or ceiling effects in the range of expected responses
   4. Consistency in measurement procedures
   5. Uniform response of participants to the treatment

STATISTICAL ANALYSIS
   1. Larger alpha for significance testing (0.05 is typical)
   2. One-tailed direction test of the hypothesis
   3. Statistical tests for interval or ratio levels of measurement
   4. Statistical controls for variance (e.g., blocking, pairing, or analysis of covariance) to reduce the influence of subject heterogeneity

SAMPLE SIZE
   1. Increasing the total sample size
   2. If all else has been done to maximize design sensitivity, using a *power analysis* to determine the minimum number of total participants needed for 80% power

***

Based on Lipsey, 1990; Thomas & Krebs, 1997.

Alternatively, users can enter the desired power level (e.g., 80%) and calculate the minimum number of participants needed to achieve that level. The values for power can be between 0.00 and 1.00, and values > 80% (0.80) are regarded as acceptable for most research plans.

The choice of effect size.   The choice of an effect size (ES) for power estimates depends on past experience with similar populations and like dependent variables. For example, a recent systematic review/meta-analysis of behavioral stuttering treatment (n = 12) yielded an average effect size of 0.91 (Herder, Howard, Nye, & Vanryckeghem,

2006). The dependent variables in Herder et al.'s (2006) systematic review were common outcome measures including speech fluency and assessments of psychological/emotional states. Based on their result, the 0.91 effect size might be adopted as a reasonable expectation for future studies with similar populations and like outcome measures. In other studies, average standardized effect sizes were reported for treatments of expressive phonology ($\overline{ES}$ = 0.67; Law, Garrett, & Nye, 2004) and aphasia ($\overline{ES}$ = 0.83; Robey, 1998). In the latter case, the average standardized effect sizes ranged from 0.66 to 1.15 depending on the timing of treatment (i.e., chronic, post-acute, or acute).

In other instances, there may be no systematic reviews or results from meta-analyses to provide effect-size guidelines for power analysis. However, there is evidence that half a standard deviation is a somewhat universal threshold for significant change in health-related quality of life (Norman, Sloan, & Wyrwich, 2003). Indeed, a standardized effect size of 0.50 (half a standard deviation) is equivalent to increasing success rate from 25% to 75%. An increase of this magnitude is likely to be an important outcome for a client (Meline & Harn, 2008a). If there is no clear evidence available for choosing an effect size for power estimates, 0.50 (i.e., half a standard deviation) is recommended as a general rule.

■ ■ ■ ■ ■

CASE EXAMPLE
Power Analysis

A case example with G*Power 3 computer-generated power analysis is shown in Exhibit 5.2. For this research plan, the researchers chose to calculate the minimum sample size needed to detect significance. The parameters entered were (a) effect size (0.50), (b) alpha level (0.05), (c) power (0.95), and (d) number of groups (2). Their calculation yielded a total sample size of 54 participants. In other words, a total of 54 participants (27 in each group) was the minimum number that they needed for statistical significance. Because the researchers anticipated the possibility of losing some design sensitivity (i.e., loss of 2 or 3 participants), they included a total of 60 participants in their study.

EVALUATING SELECTION PROCEDURES IN COMMUNICATION DISORDERS

An evaluation of an experiment is difficult if participants are not thoroughly described. A detailed description of participants is critical for evaluating an experiment's internal validity and enabling others to replicate the experiment for confirmation of results as well as for generalizing conclusions to real-life situations. Brookshire (1983) explained the effect of participant descriptions on outcomes as follows:

> When an investigator fails to describe adequately the subjects who participated in an experiment, the internal validity of the experiment suffers, because the reader cannot be certain that the observed effects resulted only from the action of the independent variable(s) and not from the action of uncontrolled and unreported subject variables. ...

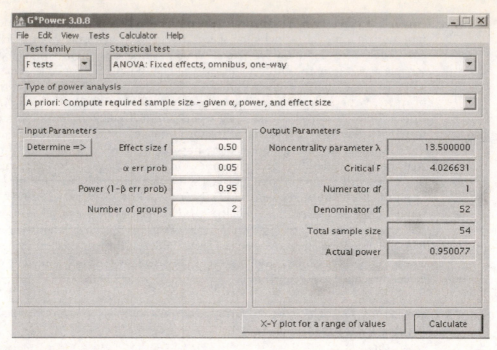

EXHIBIT 5.2
Case Example Utilizing G*Power 3 Computer-Generated Power Analysis

Reprinted with permission from Dr. Axel Buchner, Institut für Experimentelle Psychologie, Düsseldorf, Germany.

> Cursory description of subjects implies cursory consideration of subject characteristics that may have affected the results of the experiment. Careful description of subjects increases the reader's confidence in the believability of the results, and allows the reader to evaluate the outcome of the experiment. (p. 343)

In addition to descriptions of participants as a whole, individual descriptions are an important source of information. In this regard, Wertz, LaPointe, and Rosenbeck (1984) reflected on past studies of adults with aphasia:

> They [researchers] were careless with individuals within the group. Some patients were sacrificed—their performance submerged in the group mean—to protect, preserve, and promote what we were learning about the disorder. A few conservationists began to report on single cases that questioned the group data. We welcomed both, because without both the future was blank. (p. 51)

Schmitt and Meline (1990) examined 92 research reports with language-impaired children and found that only 30% of the studies included information about individual participants. Regarding the descriptions of adults with aphasia in research studies,

LaPointe (1985) noted that people with aphasia are not a homogeneous group, and studies that fail to describe participants in detail imply that homogeneity exists.

The scientific journals sometimes request detailed participant information in their editorial policies. For example, the journal *Aphasiology* advised contributors to include adequate participant description as outlined by Brookshire (1983). In addition, the journal *Aphasiology* requested specific participant information for each of 18 variables that included age, severity, time since onset, education, handedness, etiology, vision, intelligence, lateralization, mood, gender, and localization.

SINGLE-GROUP DESIGNS IN COMMUNICATION DISORDERS

Single-group research designs involve observing one group of participants in two or more conditions. Single-group designs are weak because they lack scientific comparability, which is a basic requirement for scientific inquiry. In addition, without a comparison group, an important control for extraneous variables is missing.

The most common single-group research design is the *pretest/posttest design*. The research design in Exhibit 5.3.1 includes an experimental treatment, a pretest observation, and a posttest observation. The importance of the outcome in pretest/posttest research designs is judged by comparing posttest results to pretest results. Typically, larger differences between posttest and pretest results are interpreted as more significant outcomes.

The research design in Exhibit 5.3.2 is the quasi-experimental counterpart of design 5.3.1. Research design 5.3.2 includes a naturally occurring event (i.e., preexisting condition), a pretest observation, and a posttest observation.

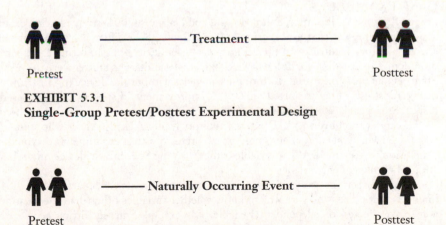

Pretest   Treatment   Posttest

EXHIBIT 5.3.1
Single-Group Pretest/Posttest Experimental Design

Pretest   Naturally Occurring Event   Posttest

EXHIBIT 5.3.2
Single-Group Pretest/Posttest Quasi-Experimental Design

To implement the quasi-experimental design depicted in Exhibit 5.3.2, researchers have to anticipate the occurrence of the naturally occurring event. Thus, they might pretest before the event occurs and posttest following the event. However, it is often difficult to anticipate events, so an alternative is to collect pretest data retrospectively. A retrospective study examines data that existed before the present study began. For example, Shriberg and Kwiatkowski (1987) studied 73 clinical records to discover variables related to the spontaneous generalization of speech. The purpose of studies of this type is usually exploratory. Exploratory studies often identify leads for future investigations. In Shriberg and Kwiatkowski's (1987) case, they identified additional variables and recommended investigating them in prospective studies.

Shortcomings in Single-Group Research Designs

The research designs in Exhibits 5.3.1 and 5.3.2 have one feature of comparability—participants are compared to themselves. In this way, individual differences are controlled. However, individual comparability alone is too weak to meet the scientific standard for comparability, because a large number of extraneous variables remain uncontrolled. The variables that remain uncontrolled are history, maturation, multiple-test effects, and statistical regression effects. History and maturation threats are related to the time interval between pretest and posttest observations. Longer intervals between pretest and posttest observations increase the likelihood that extraneous variables will influence the dependent variable. In addition, because these designs include more than one measurement, test-sensitization and test-practice effects are potential nuisance variables. Finally, if participants have unusually high or low pretest scores, a change in the dependent variable could be attributed to regression effects.

■ ■ ■ ■ ■

CASE EXAMPLE

Stuart, Kalinowski, Rastatter, Saltuklaroglu, and Dayalu's (2004) study is a case example of a single-group pretest/posttest experiment (see Exhibit 5.3.1). They investigated the effects of altered auditory feedback (via SpeechEasy ear-level device) on stuttering frequency during monologue and reading conditions. Male and female adults who stutter were the participants. Stuart et al. (2004) measured stuttering frequencies without the device (pretest) and with the device (posttest). They reported a 67–90% improvement in speech fluency. Based on the results, Stuart et al. (2004) concluded: "These findings support the notion that a self-contained in-the-ear device delivering AAF [altered auditory feedback] assists those who stutter" (p. 94).

Given what you know about single-group pretest/posttest experiments, do you think their conclusion was justified? What variables other than the SpeechEasy device might have influenced their dependent variable?

The most serious problem with single-group designs, such as Stuart et al.'s (2004) experiment, is that there is no sure way to know whether variables other than the treatment variable have affected the dependent variable. For example, merely fitting a device without turning it on could have caused a change in speech fluency (Rosenthal & Rosnow, 2008). Another possible explanation for the improvement in speech fluency is the "good subject effect." Rosenthal and Rosnow (2008) described the *good subject effect* as spontaneously displayed cooperative behavior—a trait that is especially common to volunteer participants. According to Rosenthal and Rosnow (2008), participants reason that "no matter how trivial and inane the experimental task seems to them, it must surely have some important scientific purpose or they would not have been asked to participate in the first place" (p. 221). Clearly, cause-effect conclusions that are based on single-group pretest/posttest experiments alone should be viewed with skepticism.

Based on what you know about Stuart et al.'s (2004) study, answer the following questions: Could the *good subject effect* have explained some or all of the improvement in fluency? Could the *fitting effect* have explained some or all of the improvement in fluency? What proportion of the 67-90% improvement in speech fluency would you guess is attributable to altered auditory feedback?

TWO-GROUP DESIGNS IN COMMUNICATION DISORDERS

Two-group research designs include observations of two groups of participants at different levels of the independent variable. In most cases, one level of the independent variable is a treatment condition, and the other level is a no-treatment (control) condition. The no-treatment condition is an important control for several potential nuisance variables. Because observations of the two groups are made at about the same time, time-related nuisance variables are usually adequately controlled. History and maturation effects may be present in the treatment group but should have a similar effect on the no-treatment group. Thus, these unwanted effects are balanced between treatment and no-treatment groups and are of no consequence when comparing outcomes. The potential threats of multiple-test effects and statistical regression are controlled in the same way. The purpose of two-group designs is usually to confirm the presence or absence of a treatment effect.

There are different types of two-group research designs that are employed in communication disorders research. Each type of design includes mechanisms for controlling the effects of nuisance variables, but each type also has advantages and disadvantages to consider.

Parallel Versus Crossover Research Designs

The groups in two-group research designs can be parallel to one another or they may cross over. The *parallel design* is the more common design in speech, language, and hearing research. In the case of parallel designs, participants are assigned to one of two groups. One group receives the treatment, while the second group serves as the control or comparison group.

In *crossover designs*, participants alternate between treatment and control conditions, with each participant acting as his or her own control (see Exhibit 5.4). Crossover designs are more economical because they require a smaller number of participants, though they are not recommended when researchers anticipate losing participants. However, the chief difficulty with crossover designs is the threat of carryover from

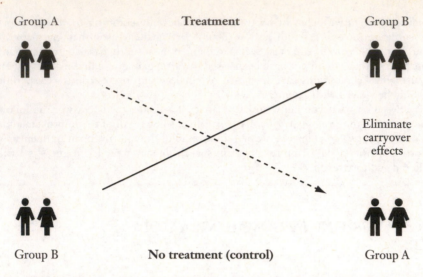

EXHIBIT 5.4
Randomized Two-Group Crossover Experimental Design

treatment to no-treatment conditions. This is especially true when the treatment has a known residual effect. For example, some pharmacological agents have residual effects that persist for weeks after the drug is withdrawn. In these cases, a wash-out period is necessary to ensure that there are no carryover effects.

CASE EXAMPLE

A case example of a crossover design in speech research is Stager, Calis, Grothe, Bloch, Berensen, Smith, et al.'s (2005) investigation of the effect of two medications on the speech fluency of 10 males and 1 female who stuttered. The two medications were *paroxetine*, a selective serotonin reuptake inhibitor, and *pimozide*, a selective dopamine antagonist. Their crossover design was 18 weeks in duration with a 6-week wash-out phase between the active phases. Stager et al. (2005) reported that two participants suffered severe side effects from the paroxetine and withdrew from the study. Even with the reduced sample size, significant improvement in speech fluency was reported for the pimozide trial; however, the pimozide was considered a risk for treating persons who stutter because of severe side effects (Stager et al., 2005). Based on what you know about crossover designs, answer the following questions: Why do you suppose Stager and co-investigators chose a crossover design as opposed to a parallel research design? Do you think that their wash-out phase was adequate to prevent carryover effects? Why should they have anticipated a loss of participants?

Independent Versus Related Research Designs

Two-group research designs can be categorized as either independent or related research designs. *Independent research designs* require the random assignment of participants to experimental and control groups. "Random assignment" means that each participant has an equal chance of being assigned to one group or the other. To assign participants to groups, a random sequence of events is generated by flipping a coin (heads or tails), rolling a die (1–6), drawing numbers from a hat, or with the help of specialized computer software. For example, the Number Generator in SPSS 16.0 (based on the Mersenne Twister algorithm) generates a set of random numbers. Once generated, the random numbers are used to allocate participants to groups without bias. Random assignment schedules like the one displayed in Exhibit 5.5 help to achieve random allocation of participants to treatment and control groups.

Why is randomization important?   In "simple randomization," participants are assigned to groups one at a time based on a single sequence of random assignments. Simple randomization and alternative procedures are intended to reduce the possibility of researcher bias and to ensure comparability between groups. *Blinding* is equally important because it ensures that all the participants (i.e., subjects, researchers, and others) will not unduly influence the outcome. According to Viera and Bangdiwala (2007), randomization and blinding are important because

1. *Randomization adds validity to statistical tests.*   One of several assumptions underlying the use of inferential statistics is that the differences between treatment and

EXHIBIT 5.5
Random Assignment Table Generated by Random Allocation Software (Saghaei, 2008)

0001: Control	0010: Treatment	0019: Control	0028: Control	0037: Control	0046: Control
0002: Control	0011: Treatment	0020: Treatment	0029: Treatment	0038: Control	0047: Treatment
0003: Treatment	0012: Treatment	0021: Control	0030: Control	0039: Control	0048: Treatment
0004: Treatment	0013: Control	0022: Control	0031: Treatment	0040: Control	0049: Treatment
0005: Control	0014: Control	0023: Control	0032: Treatment	0041: Treatment	0050: Treatment
0006: Control	0015: Treatment	0024: Control	0033: Control	0042: Treatment	
0007: Treatment	0016: Treatment	0025: Treatment	0034: Treatment	0043: Control	
0008: Control	0017: Control	0026: Treatment	0035: Control	0044: Treatment	
0009: Treatment	0018: Control	0027: Treatment	0036: Treatment	0045: Control	

control groups should behave like differences between two random samples from the population.

2. *Randomization minimizes confounding.* Randomization tends to produce groups that are similar in terms of known and unknown variables. *Confounding* is the bias that occurs when one group of participants has unique characteristics that affect the relationship between the treatment and outcome.

3. *Blinding reduces remaining biases.* The goal of blinding is to reduce or eliminate the potential biases of participants and investigators. If participants know their group assignment, they may alter their behavior. If investigators know the group assignments, they might consciously or unconsciously influence the outcome of one group more than the other.

4. *Ethical aspects.* Proper randomization and blinding should ensure that participants are treated equally on all accounts except the treatment under investigation. (pp. 133–134)

Schultz, Chalmers, Grimes, and Altman (1994) considered the following approaches to generating an allocation sequence as adequate: (a) computer-generated random assignment, (b) random number tables, (c) shuffled cards or tossed coins, and (d) minimization—an alternative to be discussed.

Simple Randomization and Alternative Balancing Procedures

The goals of randomization are to achieve two or more groups that are (a) balanced with regard to individual characteristics and (b) free of experimenter selection biases. Simple randomization achieves these goals when the sample size is sufficiently large. However, when sample size is fewer than 100, as it is in most experiments, simple randomization can cause a serious imbalance between groups. According to Lachin (1988), simple randomization guarantees a balance between groups only when the sample size is 200 or larger. For $n = 20$, the chance of a 60/40 imbalance or worse is about 50%. For $n = 100$, the chance of an imbalance is reduced to about 5%. If researchers choose simple randomization as their balancing method, they should decide on an acceptable level of risk for imbalance between groups before the study begins.

The alternatives to simple randomization are (a) block randomization, (b) stratified randomization, and (c) minimization. In experimental research designs with small samples, these alternative procedures can be used alone or in combination to achieve a fair allocation of participants to groups.

Block randomization. Instead of assigning participants to groups one at a time as is the case for simple randomization, *block randomization* assigns participants to treatment groups in blocks of predetermined size. Block randomization is a form of restricted randomization that enforces balance within each block. Though blocks can be of any size greater than one, the block size must be divisible by the number of groups. Suppose that an experiment includes 20 participants with experimental group A and control group B. If researchers choose a block size of four, there will be six different ways to arrange the blocks.

1. A-A-B-B
2. A-B-A-B
3. A-B-B-A
4. B-A-B-A
5. B-A-A-B
6. B-B-A-A

If the first roll of a die is 4, the corresponding block arrangement would be B-A-B-A. Thus, the first four participants would be assigned to treatment groups as follows:

Participant 1—Group B
Participant 2—Group A
Participant 3—Group B
Participant 4—Group A

Each of the six patterns has the same probability of being chosen. Additional rolls of the die will determine the assignments for the next four participants, and so on, until all the participants are assigned to groups A or B. This example would guarantee balance after every four participants.

A disadvantage for block randomization is that it may be possible to guess some participant allocations. This would lessen the effect of blinding as a means to control experimenter bias. The remedy is to blind investigators from group assignments.

An alternative procedure that helps preserve blinding is to randomize block size. Instead of a fixed block size, blocks are allowed to vary in size. Thus, participant allocations are difficult if not impossible to predict. To accomplish this feat, random-block-size algorithms are included in statistical software packages such as *Random Allocation Software* (see Exhibit 5.6).

Stratified randomization.   *Stratified randomization* is another alternative to the simple randomization procedure that is an appropriate choice for studies with small sample sizes. In small studies, some chance imbalance may occur that jeopardizes the interpretation of results—but, if researchers know which participant characteristics (strata) are important beforehand, they can create a separate block randomization list for each stratum. For example, "gender" and "ethnicity" may be important characteristics. In this case, the researchers can block randomize within each of the strata (gender and ethnicity). For example, the block randomization for the gender variable might look like the following:

| Female | A-B-B-A | B-A-B-A |
| Male | B-B-A-A | A-B-A-B |

Stratified randomization assures a balanced allocation of participants to groups for whatever strata are chosen. However, it is usually not practical to stratify for more

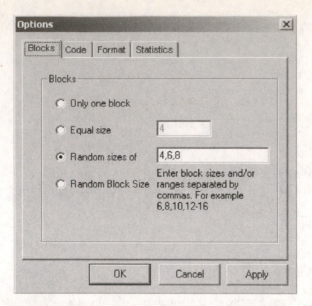

EXHIBIT 5.6
Random Allocation Software (Saghaei, 2008) Options Menu

Reprinted with permission from Mahmoud Saghaei, MD, Isfahan University of Medical Sciences, Isfahan, Iran.

than two or three variables (Altman & Bland, 1999). Scott, McPherson, Ramsay, and Campbell (2002) explained that "stratified randomization becomes unworkable as the number of prognostic factors increases, because the number of strata required can quickly exceed the number of patients in the trial" (p. 663). If there are more than two important characteristics to stratify, minimization may be a better choice for allocating participants to treatment groups.

Minimization procedures.   Minimization as a method for allocating participants to treatments in clinical trials was first proposed by Taves (1974). As with randomization methods, minimization's goal is to ensure balance between groups of participants. Treasure and MacRae (1998) argued that minimization is superior to randomization because "[the] similarity of the two groups is ensured, rather than hoped for" (p. 363).

Minimization is sometimes referred to as a nonrandom method because it eliminates almost all randomization from the process of balancing groups. Minimization procedures aim to minimize the total imbalance for all factors together instead of considering mutually exclusive subgroups as with stratified randomization (Scott et al., 2002). Scott et al. (2002) reported a systematic review on minimization that aimed to determine its use, advantages, and disadvantages compared with other allocation methods. They concluded that the minimization method, though rarely used in practice, is a highly effective allocation method. Advantages and disadvantages were as follows:

1. *Advantage*—It achieves balanced groups (with small samples as well as large samples).
2. *Advantage*—It encourages investigators to think about prognostic factors before the study begins.
3. *Advantage*—It can control confounding variables without splitting the sample into too many strata.
4. *Disadvantage*—It may violate the assumption of random allocation common to inferential statistics.
5. *Disadvantage*—Assignments of participants are easily predicted, so concealment is especially important.
6. *Disadvantage*—It may add organizational complexity and increased costs. (Scott et al., 2002, pp. 665–666)

To accomplish minimization, the first participant is randomly placed, but each subsequent participant is assigned to groups so that the imbalance between groups at that time is minimized. The primary advantage of minimization is that it can make small groups closely similar with respect to several participant characteristics. It is important that the minimization is done out of sight of any individual who could introduce bias. The necessary steps for minimization are as follows:

Step 1. Determine at the outset what characteristics you want to see equally represented in the two groups.

Step 2. Randomly assign the first participant to one of the groups.

Step 3. Assign each subsequent participant to one or the other group as they enter the study. Each participant is assigned to the group in which he or she will minimize any difference in the predetermined characteristics. For example, if group A has a higher average age and a disproportionate number of women, the next older woman is assigned to group B. If the next participant does not affect the imbalance, the assignment to one group or the other should be random.

Why is allocation concealment important?   Allocation concealment refers to hiding the assignment of participants to groups from investigators. If investigators know the assignment of participants, they might knowingly or unknowingly influence the experimental outcome. Without proper allocation concealment, treatment effects may be overstated. In fact, past randomized clinical trials with poor concealment have estimated the treatment effect to be as much as 40% higher than those with proper concealment (Viera & Bangdiwala, 2007). It is also possible for trials with poor allocation concealment to underestimate treatment effects. The bottom line is that randomized clinical trials with poor allocation concealment cannot be trusted to report accurate outcomes. Schultz et al. (1994) considered the following approaches to allocation concealment to be adequate: (a) central randomization such as by telephone to a trials office, (b) numbered or coded containers, and (c) sequentially numbered, opaque, sealed envelopes.

Experimental Versus Quasi-Experimental Designs

The design in Exhibit 5.7.1 illustrates the basic experimental design with randomization. The design in Exhibit 5.7.2 illustrates a basic quasi-experimental design without randomization. Random assignment of participants to groups is not possible in quasi-experimental designs, because the independent variable (a categorical variable) cannot be manipulated. The quasi-experimental alternative to random assignment is *matching*. *Matching procedures* attempt to establish group equivalence by matching the two or

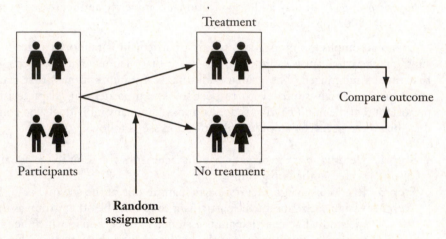

EXHIBIT 5.7.1
Randomized Two-Group Experimental Design

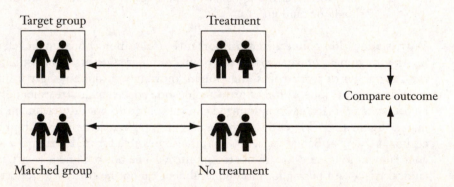

EXHIBIT 5.7.2
Nonrandomized Two-Group Quasi-Experimental Design

more groups on the basis of critical variables—variables other than the classification variable. The strength of a related two-group design depends on the success of selecting equivalent (i.e., matched) groups of participants.

The importance of the outcomes in two-group research designs is judged by comparing the experimental group's results with the control group's results. Typically, larger differences between experimental and control groups are interpreted as more significant outcomes. The statistical significance of experimental and quasi-experimental research outcomes usually relies on the *t*-test or *analysis of variance* (ANOVA) families of statistics. The choice of one or another statistic depends on the complexity of the research design, the number of independent and dependent variables, and the sample's characteristics.

Group Equivalence in Quasi-Experimental Designs

An important consideration in two-group designs is group equivalence. Two groups must be equivalent to satisfy the comparability requirement. If the two groups are not equivalent for relevant variables, such as age, gender, and intelligence, conclusions may be meaningless. In the case of independent designs, participants are usually randomly assigned to groups to achieve group equivalence. That procedure works for independent research designs, but related research designs must use matching procedures to achieve equivalence between groups.

To achieve equivalence in a related quasi-experimental design, two steps are necessary: (a) identify the relevant variables—those known to be related to the dependent variable—and (b) match the two or more groups of participants on the basis of these variables. For example, if the aim is to compare language-impaired children with a control group of typically developing children, the control group would be matched with the experimental group on the basis of relevant variables such as age, gender, and nonverbal intelligence.

Basic Two-Group Designs in Communication Disorders

The research design in Exhibit 5.8.1 is an independent two-group design with an experimental treatment. Its quasi-experimental counterpart (related two-group design) is depicted in Exhibit 5.8.2 and includes a preexisting independent variable such as a disease or prior clinical diagnosis. Research design 5.8.1 depends on the random assignment of participants to groups in order to achieve equivalency between the two groups. Alternatively, research design 5.8.2 utilizes matched subjects in experimental and control groups to achieve equivalency between the two groups.

The research designs depicted in Exhibits 5.8.1 and 5.8.2 are appropriate when pretest observations are not possible. Design 5.8.1 exercises control of extraneous variables through the random assignment of participants to experimental and control groups, so internal validity is relatively high.

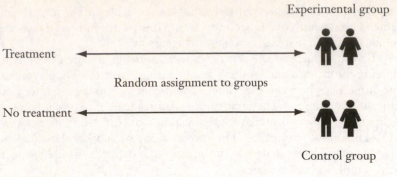

EXHIBIT 5.8.1
Independent Two-Group Experimental Design

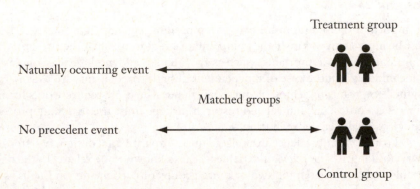

EXHIBIT 5.8.2
Related Two-Group Quasi-Experimental Design

Research design 5.8.2 is a weaker design because it relies on matching procedures to achieve group equivalency. The internal validity of design 5.8.2 depends on how well the researchers match groups based on relevant subject characteristics.

The research design in Exhibit 5.9.1 is a pretest/posttest design with two groups of participants. In addition, the groups are independent because participants are randomly assigned to the two groups. Research design 5.9.1 adds a pretest so that changes in behavior are observable. The pretest/posttest design with two groups of participants has several advantages over other two-group designs and is frequently used because it accounts for several extraneous variables. A potential problem with this design is the sensitizing effect of the pretest on participant performances. If the pretest sensitizes participants, external validity is weakened. When test procedures are unusual, difficult, or otherwise likely to affect performance on a subsequent test, pretest/posttest designs should be avoided unless satisfactory precautions can be implemented.

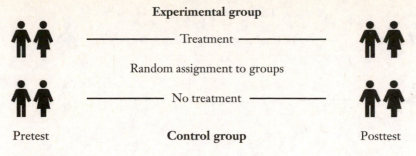

EXHIBIT 5.9.1
Pretest/Posttest Experimental Independent Design

CASE EXAMPLE

Justice, Chow, Capellini, Flanigan, and Colton (2003) adopted the pretest/posttest experimental design depicted in Exhibit 5.9.1, but the research team included two treatments and counterbalanced the order of treatments. This variation of the basic pretest/posttest experimental design is known as an alternating-treatment design.

Justice et al. (2003) randomly assigned participants to groups A and B. Both groups were given an emergent literacy pretest. Following the pretest, group A received a 6-week "experimental explicit" intervention program followed by a 6-week "comparison intervention program." Group B received the experimental and comparison intervention programs in reverse order. Thus, the order of treatments was counterbalanced across subject groups. Both subject groups were posttested at the end of the 12-week intervention period. In addition, interim tests were conducted between the two 6-week intervention periods. The researchers evaluated the overall effects of the two treatments after 12 weeks, and they evaluated the interim effects of the individual treatments after 6 weeks. Justice and co-investigators (2003) concluded that the experimental explicit program (name writing, alphabet recitation, phonological awareness) was superior to the comparison program (storybook reading).

Based on what you know about Justice et al.'s (2003) research methods, answer the following questions: Why did Justice et al. include two intervention programs in their pretest/posttest design? What is an advantage for the alternating-treatment design over a basic pretest/posttest experimental design? What are possible disadvantages in their use of the alternating-treatment design? They recruited 18 participants for their emergent literacy study. Was the sample adequate? What are some possible limitations associated with small samples?

The research design in Exhibit 5.9.2 is the quasi-experimental, related counterpart of the previous design. As in the design in Exhibit 5.8.2, the researcher must anticipate the occurrence of the treatment or must collect pretest data retrospectively. Research design 5.9.2 is significantly stronger because it includes a comparison group. However, weaknesses in the design persist when retrospective data are collected. Potential weaknesses may include problems with group equivalence as well as questionable pretest observations.

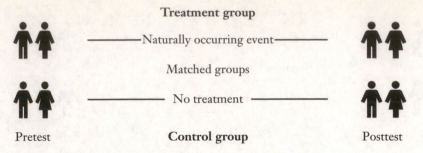

EXHIBIT 5.9.2
Pretest/Posttest Quasi-Experimental Related Design

MORE COMPLEX DESIGNS IN COMMUNICATION DISORDERS

The complexity of a research design is increased by (a) adding conditions to the independent variable, (b) adding independent variables, (c) increasing the number of groups, or (d) a combination of a, b, and c. Complex designs are elaborations of basic experimental and quasi-experimental designs.

Multivalent Research Designs

Multivalent research designs are complex designs that include more than two conditions or values of the independent variable. For example, if noise is the independent variable, the research hypothesis may require four or five levels of noise.

CASE EXAMPLE

Cox, Cooper, and McDade (1989) conducted a multivalent experiment. They used photographs of 10- to 14- year-old females pictured in one of three conditions: (a) wearing a body aid, (b) wearing a post-auricular aid, or (c) wearing no aid at all. College students who volunteered to be participants rated each photograph on a semantic differential scale. The independent variable (hearing-aid status) had three conditions: (a) body aid, (b) behind-the-ear aid, and (c) no aid. The dependent variable was "perceived achievement" as rated by the participants. The volunteers rated the two aided conditions about equally, but rated the unaided condition higher. Apparently, the presence of an aid was a factor that influenced the perception of achievement. In as much as this study was reported in 1989, do you think that the outcome would be different today?

Factorial Research Designs

Factorial designs include all possible combinations of the levels of two or more independent variables. In this way, the effects of two or more independent variables can be observed within a single study. Factorial designs attempt to model real-life events in which multiple variables coexist and may affect behaviors in combination. A combination of two or more variables sometimes produces a change in behavior that is not present when the effect of a single independent variable is observed.

CASE EXAMPLE

Mizuko and Reichle (1989) observed the interaction of two independent variables: (a) word categories and (b) graphic symbol systems. They observed that the effect of one independent variable changed as a function of the second independent variable. This is known as an *interaction effect*. Mizuko and Reichle's (1989) independent variables (i.e., *word category* and *symbol system*) appeared to interact. In other words, the relationship between nouns, verbs, and descriptors (independent variable one) changed as the type of symbol system changed (independent variable two). A look at the differences between means at each level of symbol system (Blissymbols, Picsyms, PCS) suggested an interaction effect. For example, the difference between nouns and verbs for Picsyms is significantly different from the difference between nouns and verbs for Blissymbols. Thus, an interaction effect can be described as a difference between differences. Exhibit 5.10 was constructed from summary statistics reported in Mizuko

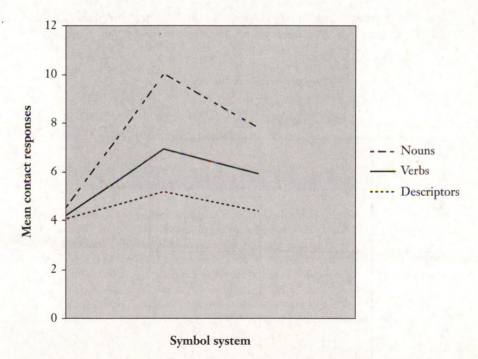

EXHIBIT 5.10
Graphic Depiction of an Interaction Between Two Independent Variables
Based on summary statistics in Mizuko and Reichle, 1989.

and Reichle's original article. Graphic displays such that as shown in Exhibit 5.10 are useful means for interpreting interaction effects.

Factorial research designs are generally classified in one of three ways: (a) related designs in which each participant experiences all treatment conditions, (b) independent designs in which matched groups of participants experience a single treatment condition, and (c) mixed designs that combine related and independent variables. Exhibit 5.11 models a two-by-two factorial design—a basic factorial design with two independent variables and two values for each independent variable. Factorial designs may have additional levels for each variable, such as 3×5, 2×4, and 4×5. A factorial design may also include additional independent variables, such as $2 \times 2 \times 2$ (three independent variables) and $2 \times 3 \times 4 \times 5$ (four independent variables). The number of possible interactions increases as the number of independent variables increases. Thus, results gathered from factorial research designs become increasingly difficult to interpret as the number of independent variables increases.

MULTIPLE-GROUP DESIGNS IN COMMUNICATION DISORDERS

Multiple-group research designs include two or more comparison groups along with an experimental or treatment group. Each comparison group typically serves as a con-

Independent variable A

	A_1	A_2
B_1	A_1B_1	A_2B_1
B_2	A_1B_2	A_2B_2

Independent variable B

EXHIBIT 5.11
Model of a Two-by-Two Factorial Design

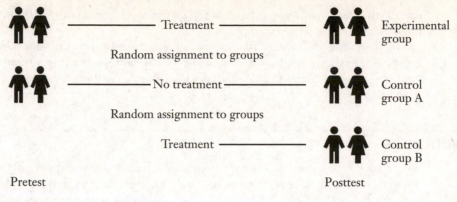

EXHIBIT 5.12
Three-Group Pretest/Posttest Experimental Design

trol for one or more nuisance variables. For example, the research design in Exhibit 5.12 includes one experimental group and two control groups.

In design 5.12, control group A controls time-related extraneous variables, such as maturation and history factors, whereas control group B controls pretest effects such as test sensitization and statistical regression. The addition of a second control group in design 5.12 manages the shortcomings inherent in pretest/posttest designs.

The Solomon four-group research design (not displayed) is an elaboration of the three-group design with two control groups depicted in Exhibit 5.12. The Solomon design adds a third control group (control group C), which is observed like control group B in Exhibit 5.12 but without the treatment. The additional control group in the Solomon four-group design is intended to control unknown nuisance variables that could possibly intrude during the time that passes between pretest and posttest observations. If the time interval between pretest and posttest phases is short (days or weeks), the additional control group is probably not needed—but if the time interval is months, it is probably a valuable control.

Variations of the Three-Group Design in Communication Disorders

A variation of the three-group research design is commonly found in research reports that include specific-language-impaired (SLI) children as participants. Leonard (1979) recommended two comparison groups when studying SLI children: a language-matched control group and an age-matched control group. The purpose of two control groups is to yield more meaningful results than permitted with only one comparison group. In a variation of the three-group research design (with two control groups), Eadie, Fey, Douglas, and Parsons (2002) recruited 29 children as participants in a study of grammatical morphology and sentence imitation. Their design included two experimental groups: 10 children with specific language impairment and 10 children with Down syndrome. Their control group was made up of 10 typically developing children.

Based on Eadie et al.'s (2002) study, answer the following questions: What criteria should they have adopted to ensure equivalence among the three groups? What is your evaluation of their sample? What are the factors that affect the power of a research design?

CONCLUSION

There are a wide variety of experiments and research designs, and virtually all types of designs are evident in speech, language, and hearing research. Kerlinger (1973) noted that the importance of studying and using research designs is to understand their strengths and weaknesses as well as their rationale and purpose. Kerlinger's advice is especially meaningful for students of research, prospective researchers, and clinicians who must evaluate the research literature for their evidence-based practices. The lessons to be learned are many. First, there are many different research designs, but they are not all suited to answering all questions. It is important that investigators choose research designs that fit their purpose. Second, not all research designs are appropriate for answering cause-effect questions. For example, questions about treatment efficacy require designs with comparison groups. Finally, it's apparent that planning is vitally important to good research. In order to achieve meaningful outcomes, researchers must devote extra effort to developing their research plans.

CASE STUDIES

Case 5.1: Weak or Strong Design?
Professor Toller and a research assistant plan a pretest/posttest design with one group of participants to test the hypothesis that oral-motor exercises are an effective treatment for speech articulation disorders. As a research consultant, what do you suggest to improve their research design?

Case 5.2: Do Thickened Liquids Work?
Two hospital-based researcher-clinicians are planning a study to determine the effectiveness of thickened liquids for treating oral pharyngeal dysphagia. Their goal is to generalize results to all individuals with dysphagia in the United States. What steps do you recommend for selecting participants?

Case 5.3: Problem of Matching Participants
Two audiologist-researchers are planning a two-group, pretest/posttest quasi-experiment with hearing-impaired children and normal-hearing children as participants. What are the relevant variables that should be considered for matching the two groups of children?

Case 5.4: How Many Participants?
The local research team asks you to join them to help prepare a grant proposal. Your first assignment is to determine the total number of participants needed for the proposed study. The plan, thus far, is to have two groups (i.e., experimental and control). The alpha level will

be set at 0.05, and the desired effect size is 0.75. The power to detect significant effects should be 80%. Give these criteria, how many participants are needed?

Case 5.5: Let's Be More Sensitive
In addition to asking you to recommend a sample size, the local research team (see Case 5.4) asks you to recommend ways to improve the research design's sensitivity. What type of design will you recommend? What tips will you give the team for improving the research design's sensitivity?

■ ■ ■ ■ ■ ━━━━━━━━━━━━━━━━━━━━━━━━━━━━━━━━━━━

STUDENT EXERCISES

1. Choose a research report with two or more groups of participants and describe its research design in detail. Why did the researchers include more than one group of participants?
2. Identify the participant selection criteria in one research article in a communication disorders journal. What are the selection criteria, and what is the purpose for including each criterion? What criteria would you have added or deleted from the selection criteria that the researchers specified?
3. Evaluate the selection criteria in a research report that includes a group of at least 20 participants. Given the characteristics of the research sample, what is the population to which the results can be generalized?
4. As you know, in experimental research designs, the random allocation of participants to groups is important. Suppose that the following methods are available for randomly assigning participants to experimental or control groups: (a) first letter of surnames, (b) patient room numbers, (c) student ID numbers, and (d) social security numbers. In what way might each of these methods result in a biased (nonrandom) allocation of participants to groups?
5. Choose a research report with 20 or more participants. How representative is the sample in relation to the United States population? What is the proportion of males and females? Did the study include ethnic groups such as African Americans, Asian Americans, and Hispanics? How did the researchers justify excluding particular subgroups in the population?
6. Locate an interesting research report from a recent journal. With your knowledge of statistical power, evaluate the method, participants, sample, and design for statistical power. What is the power associated with the study? Was the power adequate for detecting significant treatment effects? What could the researchers have done to increase the power of their research design?

CHAPTER 6

QUALITATIVE RESEARCH IN COMMUNICATION DISORDERS

> **triangulate** (trī-āng′gyə-lāt′) *v.* to make into three sides or
> points; to use a variety of data sources, different
> observers, multiple perspectives, multiple methods

Qualitative research refers to a family of more than 30 approaches and designs. It is rooted in anthropology, wherein anthropologists observed the day-to-day lives of people in their natural surroundings. Qualitative methods also have a long history in the social sciences, and their use is increasing in communication disorders. "Qualitative methods are first and foremost *research* methods. They are ways of finding out what people do, know, think, and feel by observing [them], interviewing [them], and analyzing documents" (Patton, 2002, p. 145).

The growing interest in qualitative methods is evidenced by topical papers, presentations, qualitative research reports in communication disorders journals, and special interest groups devoted to qualitative research. The *Qualitative Interest Group* at the University of Georgia (2004) characterized qualitative research as a general approach to scientific inquiry and more as follows:

The label "qualitative research" is used generically for approaches to inquiry that depend on elaborated accounts of what we see, hear, taste, touch, smell, and experience. It has roots in cultural anthropology, field sociology, and the professional fields. Qualitative research includes field research, case study research, ethnography, document and content analysis, interview and observational research, community study, and life history and biographical studies. Other names sometimes used as synonyms for qualitative research are interpretive, naturalistic, phenomenological, and descriptive. Qualitative research is associated with such theories as symbolic interactionism, constructivism, and ethnomethodology. Qualitative researchers have a lot of fun, which sustains them through the aggravation, frustration, uncertainty, and sheer slipperiness of most of the approaches to inquiry considered qualitative. (Qualitative Interest Group, 2004)

In contrast to the numbers and statistics in quantitative methods, qualitative methods depend largely on descriptions, categories, and words. Exhibit 6.1 compares the use of qualitative and quantitative methods for analyzing opinions, attitudes, experiences, and knowledge. As Exhibit 6.1 shows, qualitative and quantitative methods differ in many ways. The qualitative research method usually follows these seven steps:

1. Observe events or ask questions with open-ended answers.
2. Record what is observed, said, or done.
3. Interpret the data.
4. Return to further observe or ask more questions.

EXHIBIT 6.1
Qualitative Versus Quantitative Methods for Analyzing Opinions, Attitudes, Experiences, and Knowledge

QUALITATIVE METHODS	QUANTITATIVE METHODS
Explore a topic or idea; gain insight into lifestyle, culture, motivations, behaviors, and preferences	Quantify answers and generalize findings to a broader populace
Include focus groups, in-depth interviews, and reviews	Include surveys
Mostly inductive processes used to formulate theory	Mostly deductive processes used to test prespecified concepts and hypotheses that make up a theory
Mostly text and image based	Mostly number based
No statistical tests	Use statistical tests for analysis
Explore topics in-depth and in detail	Answer specific, prespecified questions.
More flexible as to locations and timing and often less expensive—typically involves fieldwork	Rigid in locations and timing and often more expensive—typically involves laboratory work
Validity and reliability depend on the skills and rigor of the researcher. The researcher is the primary instrument for data collection.	Validity and reliability depend on measurement. Data collection is mediated through standardized instruments and protocols.
Time costs are lighter on the planning end and heavier during analysis.	Time costs are heavier on the planning end and lighter during analysis.
Less generalizable to a broader populace	More generalizable to a broader populace.

Centers for Disease Control and Prevention, 2008.

5. Repeat steps 2–4 (iteration).
6. Develop formal theories to explain the data.
7. Formulate conclusions and generate hypotheses.

Quantitative data are numbers and statistics, whereas *qualitative data* are typically detailed, in-depth descriptions of the phenomena being studied. Qualitative data are derived from a variety of sources including field notes, clinical records, audio- and videotape transcriptions, photographs, and any other source that lends itself to understanding the phenomenon through firsthand experience. The purpose of qualitative research is to describe, explore, or generate ideas, thoughts, or feelings, and to form hypotheses that can be tested by quantitative research designs.

The qualitative research approach excels at understanding individual differences and similarities, whereas quantitative research excels at understanding group similarities and differences. Qualitative research is characterized by 10 interrelated themes or assumptions (Patton, 1990). The 10 themes are as follows:

1. *Naturalistic inquiry:*   Qualitative research focuses on persons, topics, locations, or events in their natural settings such as classrooms, homes, neighborhoods, or cultural milieus.
2. *Inductive analysis:*   Qualitative researchers begin with specific examples or facts, formulate questions, and end with general principles or theories.
3. *Holistic perspective:*   Qualitative researchers assume that the whole is greater than the sum of its parts. Whatever the focus of inquiry, each action, communication, or other aspect of the milieu is viewed as a part of the whole. The parts are dependent on one another and interrelated.
4. *Thick description:*   Qualitative researchers gather detailed information about the phenomenon of interest, and they typically *triangulate* data from multiple sources such as field notes, in-depth interviews, audiotapes, and other sources.
5. *Personal contact and insight:*   Because qualitative research requires direct experience with the phenomenon of interest, personal biases are unavoidable. Qualitative researchers are aware of personal biases, acknowledge them throughout the course of the study, and temper their influence.
6. *Dynamic systems:*   Qualitative research is a dynamic process wherein answers, questions, and theories are subject to change throughout the course of the study.
7. *Unique case orientation:*   Qualitative researchers assume that each case is unique and therefore deserves detailed and in-depth study.
8. *Context sensitivity:*   Qualitative researchers appreciate the contextual variables that influence the phenomenon of interest whether the topic of interest is a person, place, location, or other phenomenon.
9. *Empathic neutrality:*   Qualitative researchers are nonjudgmental and remain neutral observers throughout the course of the study.
10. *Design flexibility:*   Qualitative researchers redirect their focus, generate new questions, and explore other topics as they emerge during the course of a study.

Qualitative methods are superior to quantitative methods when individual perspectives are more important than group generalizations. The primary purpose is to explore or generate theories as opposed to testing hypotheses. According to Green and Britten (1998), the individual observations that characterize qualitative research are credible evidence for clinical practice. Green and Britten (1998) remarked:

> Clinical experience, based on personal observation, reflection, and judgment, is also needed to translate scientific results into treatment of individual patients. Personal experience is often characterized as being anecdotal, ungeneralisable, and a poor basis for making scientific decisions. However, it is often a more powerful persuader than scientific publication in changing practice. (p. 1230)

Clearly, qualitative methods are an appropriate choice for scientific inquiry in communication disorders. Furthermore, they have important implications for successfully translating research results into ideas for clinical practice.

FOUNDATIONS OF QUALITATIVE RESEARCH

The general approaches to qualitative research include (a) ethnography, (b) phenomenology, (c) field research, and (d) grounded theory. The major qualitative approaches are general ways of thinking about conducting qualitative research. Each approach typically specifies (a) the role of the researcher, (b) the stages of the research process, and (c) the methods of data analysis (Trochim, 2004). However, the various approaches may overlap, combine, and otherwise blend so that distinctions between the various approaches are blurred. The first of the several general approaches to qualitative research is known as *ethnography*.

Ethnography

The *ethnographic approach* has its roots in anthropology. Anthropology is the social science that studies the origins and social relationships of human beings. One of the most famous anthropologists was Margaret Mead, whose detailed descriptions of child development and adolescent behaviors in the Manus and Samoan cultures helped to define the ethnographic approach. Ethnographers typically focus on an entire culture of people. The definition of culture was once limited to geographic location and ethnicity, but it has broadened to refer to any group or organization, including clinical groups, schools, classrooms, and businesses. The most common ethnographic method is *participant observation*, wherein the researcher is immersed in the culture and becomes an active participant. Researchers assume *outsider* or *insider* perspectives depending on their qualifications. For example, an ethnographer who studies the culture of medical speech-language pathologists with no speech-language pathology training is an *outsider* and assumes an outsider's perspective. An ethnographer who conducts the same study with speech-language pathology credentials is an *insider* and assumes an insider's perspective.

Damico and Simmons-Mackie (2003) described ethnographic studies as flexible in the various approaches that they apply to data collection. Ethnographic researchers typically adopt many different methods for gathering data, such as in-depth interviews, focus groups, document analysis, audiotape analysis, videotape analysis, introspection, triangulation, and lamination. A case in point is Stillman, Snow, and Warren's (1999) study of SLP students and children with pervasive developmental disorder (PDD). They used individual interviews, focus groups, and video recordings to observe the interactions between the SLP students and children with PDD. This is an example of *triangulation*.

The term *triangulation* is used to describe efforts to corroborate the validity and reliability of observations and methods. Triangulation of the data involves comparing and contrasting data that are collected at different times, by different methods, and in different locations. Another technique for verifying data is referred to as *lamination*. Damico and Simmons-Mackie (2003) described lamination thus:

> When employing lamination, the researcher analyzes the collected data and forms tentative conclusions. Once this is done, the conclusions are verified through a different type of cross-comparison process; the researcher may ask the participants in the ethnography what they believe was happening when certain communicative or learning behaviors were observed. In this way, the researcher adds another layer of interpretation to the data so that the actual results or findings can be cross-referenced. In a sense, the term "lamination" is a metaphor for layering on different levels of interpretation. (p. 137)

The ethnographic approach has no preset limits as to what will be observed, and it has no prescribed ending point. The researchers determine when their study will conclude. Damico and Simmons-Mackie (2003) described ethnography as a promising approach in communication disorders because it is particularly well suited for investigating complex social and cultural phenomena such as diversity, development, classroom performance, rehabilitation, and service delivery.

Phenomenology

Another way of thinking about qualitative research is phenomenology. *Phenomenology* is a school of thought that focuses on individuals' experiences, perspectives, and unique interpretations of the world. The phenomenologist seeks to understand how the world appears to others. Phenomenology is more a philosophical understanding of the world than it is a methodological approach to qualitative research.

Phenomenologists typically reject speculation and the acceptance of unobservable phenomena, oppose the notion of *naturalism*—a metaphysical theory that holds that all phenomena can be explained mechanistically in terms of natural causes and laws—and believe that only objects in the natural world can be known. As an interpretative practice, phenomenology is a unique approach to qualitative research.

Cream, Onslow, Packman, and Llewellyn (2003) adopted the phenomenology approach to study experiences of people who stutter after therapy with prolonged speech techniques. *Prolonged speech* is the term applied to the speech patterns that result from therapies characterized as *smooth speech*, *easy speech*, and *precision fluency shaping*

(Cream et al., 2003). The Cream et al. (2003) research team described their methodology as follows:

> Phenomenology is characterized by the focus on phenomena as immediately experienced. The methodology as described by Van Manen (1990) was applied to this study, because none of the authors stutter, and could experience speech after PS (prolonged-speech] therapy directly. This approach incorporates other people's experiences and their reflections of their experiences were "borrowed" (Van Manen, 1990: 62) for the purpose of the investigation. The investigator aimed to assist participants to focus on the immediate experience on which they were reflecting, rather than on their accepted customary ways of interpretation. These verbal descriptions of experiences were transcribed into texts that provided data for the analysis. (p. 382)

Field Research

Another general approach to qualitative research is known as *field research*. Field research is a broad approach to qualitative research that is characterized by observations of phenomena in their natural state or context. Field researchers typically collect detailed notes that are subsequently categorized and analyzed in a variety of ways. Field research is integral to the ethnographic approach to qualitative research. As such, the field research approach is well represented in communication disorders research. One example is Bloom's (1970) classic study of children's early language development. Bloom collected tape-recorded conversations from several young children in naturalistic situations, e.g., eating, dressing, toileting, and during play with a peer.

Grounded Theory

Another general approach to qualitative research is *grounded theory*. The grounded theory approach aims to develop theories about the phenomenon of interest that are firmly grounded in observation. Overall, grounded theory prescribes a complex, iterative process of observation and verification. According to Damico and Simmons-Mackie (2003), grounded theory was proposed to accomplish three analytical strategies. They described the three strategies as follows:

> First, the researcher should periodically step back and ask, "What's going on here? and "Does what I think here fit the reality of the data?" Second, researchers should maintain an attitude of skepticism so that all information from any source is provisional in nature until it is checked out by "playing it against the data." [Third], in order to make best use of theoretical sensitivity, the researcher should follow specific procedures unique to qualitative research and its purposes. (Damico & Simmons-Mackie, 2003, p. 138)

Grounded theory does not prescribe a specific ending point for the study. Rather, the process of observation, verification, and iteration continues until the researcher is satisfied that the data are sufficient to develop a credible theory about the phenomenon of interest. There are few examples of the grounded theory approach in communication disorders. However, Damico and Simmons-Mackie (2003) characterized grounded theory as a promising approach for effectively analyzing phenomena in communication disorders. An example of research rooted in grounded theory is Reid, Hertzog, and Snyder's (1996) study. They described their rationale, method, and research question as follows:

> Finally, in looking at how a system functions, we need to consider process as well as outcomes. Therefore, a study was undertaken to explore and describe the perceptions of parents and ADHD children about their experiences with the school system. Grounded theory methods were used to develop a tentative model of the process and to suggest hypotheses concerning factors likely to influence the course of the process. Our investigation asked the question: "How do parents perceive the process they have gone through in obtaining services for their children with ADHD?" (Reid et al., 1996, p. 74)

QUALITATIVE RESEARCH DESIGNS AND METHODS

The six common qualitative research designs are (a) the case study, (b) discourse analysis, (c) kinesic analysis (d) direct observation, (e) participant observation, and (e) the unstructured in-depth interview. Each of the six qualitative research designs is distinguished by its methods for data collection and its methods for analysis. The analysis is often aided by the use of qualitative data analysis software (Exhibit 6.2). Qualitative

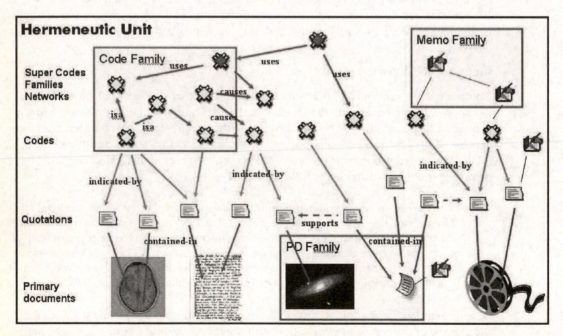

EXHIBIT 6.2
Qualitative Analysis Software for Data Structure for Research Projects (Atlas.ti, 2008)
Reprinted with permission of ATLAS.ti Scientific Software Development GmbH.

data analysis (QDA) software is designed to analyze "soft" data, i.e., material like the descriptions, text, and images found in qualitative research. ATLAS.ti is an example of QDA software. Exhibit 6.2 displays the hierarchy of objects inside ATLAS.ti's "Hermeneutic Unit," which provides the data structure for ATLAS.ti projects. Everything that is relevant to a particular study is included in the Hermeneutic Unit and resides in the electronic environment (ATLAS.ti, 2008).

The Case Study Method

A common design for collecting qualitative data is the *case study method*. A case study is an intensive observation of a person, topic, location, or event. Damico and Simmons-Mackie (2003) identified three types of case studies: (a) *Intrinsic case studies* seek to gather specific information about a person, place, or thing in a particular context; (b) *instrumental case studies* seek to better understand an issue, generate a theory, or develop or modify an existing theory; and (c) *collective case studies* seek to investigate a general phenomenon by way of combining several cases. The qualitative case study method has a long tradition in the social sciences, psychology, education, communication disorders, and other disciplines. Freud used the case study method to develop his theory of psychoanalysis, and Piaget used the case study method to develop a theory of cognitive development. Their observations were qualitative in nature, but many case studies are based on quantitative data or a combination of qualitative and quantitative data.

■ ■ ■ ■ ■ ▬▬▬▬▬▬▬▬▬▬▬▬▬▬▬▬▬▬▬▬▬▬▬▬▬▬▬▬▬▬▬

CASE EXAMPLES
The Case Study Method

Sapir, Spielman, Ramig, Hinds, Countryman, Fox, and Story (2003) studied the effects of an intensive voice treatment on one person, and their data were quantitative. In contrast, DePaul and Kent (2000) collected qualitative data in their case study that focused on speech intelligibility. DePaul and Kent (2000) described their case study as follows:

> This study describes the effects of listener proficiency and familiarization on judgments of speech intelligibility and speech severity associated with a progressive dysarthria. Speech performance was followed longitudinally for 39 months postdiagnosis for a man with ALS. The subject's spouse served as a highly familiar listener whose speech severity and intelligibility were compared to those of 24 unfamiliar listener-judges. (p. 230)

Several questions arise from DePaul and Kent's (2000) explanation. Based on what you know about their study, answer the following questions: Who were the participants in the DePaul and Kent (2000) case study? Was the primary focus of their study a person, a place, or a topic? DePaul and Kent (2000) concluded that their results suggest that speech-language pathologists should include listener training in their standards of practice for dysarthria treatment.

Strum and Nelson (1997) also used the case study method. They described their research design as follows:

> A multiple-case design was used to investigate the discourse of formal lessons in five classrooms at each of the grade levels—first, third, and fifth. The 15 participating class-

rooms were chosen to offer a "typical case" perspective on general education elementary classrooms (Bogdan & Biklen, 1992), without implying that they represent all elementary school classrooms. (p. 256)

Strum and Nelson (1997) selected 15 classrooms (locations) as the focus of their case study. Their study qualifies as a *collective case study* because it combines studies of several (15) different classrooms. Based on what you know about Strum and Nelson's (1997) study, why did they use the collective case study method?

Strum and Nelson's (1997) analysis goal was "[to] reduce the data across the multiple cases (classrooms) to patterns, categories, themes and to interpret the information that emerged into a larger consolidated picture" (p. 257). To that end, they identified 10 formal discourse rules, such as, "Teachers mostly talk and students mostly listen—except when teachers grant permission to talk." Based on their analyses, Strum and Nelson (1997) concluded that discourse and social interaction rules play a role in helping students know what to say, when to say it, and how to say it in whole-group discussions. Furthermore, they suggested that speech-language pathologists might collaborate with classroom teachers when a student has a problem with understanding discourse rules.

Overall, the case study method has a long history of generating theories and generating clinical practice ideas in communication disorders. The case study method is flexible in that it can focus on any one of several cases including clients, geographic locations, specific topics, or particular events. It is an especially effective method of scientific inquiry when combined with quantitative methods or other qualitative methods.

The Discourse Analysis Method

Discourse analysis is a general term that describes a number of approaches to analyzing written, spoken, and signed language use. As a method of scientific inquiry, it began in the 1960s. It is concerned with language use (spoken, signed, or written) beyond the boundaries of utterances or sentences in natural (not contrived) contexts.

TECHNOLOGY NOTE

The tape recorder is one of the first technologies used in qualitative research (Gibbs, Friese, & Mangabeira, 2002). Today, digital audio/video technologies record and analyze data with the help of powerful computer software. This software is collectively known as *computer-assisted qualitative data analysis* (CAQDAS). Software applications for text analysis include *Systematic Analysis of Language Transcripts* (SALT) (Language Analysis Lab, 2003) *and Computerized Profiling* (Long, 2003). Word processors have some text analysis capabilities, but more powerful text analysis is possible with *QDA Miner, WordStat, Open Text, Collate, TACT*, and *WordCruncher* (*ATLAS.ti*). A list of QDA resources is available at http://qualitativeresearch.uga.edu/QualPage/. Digital technology is a boon for most qualitative researchers, but some criticize its use (cf. Gibbs et al., 2002). What do you see as the advantages and disadvantages for CAQDAS?

The objects of discourse analysis are discourse, writing, talking, conversation, and other communicative events. Discourse analysis has cross-disciplinary roots and interests. It is practiced in a variety of social science disciplines, which include linguistics, anthropology, sociology, cognitive psychology, social psychology, communication studies, and speech-language pathology. Topics of interest in discourse analysis include the relationships among discourse and memory, turn taking, and other aspects of interactions, lexicon, style, rhetoric, persuasion, gestures, syntax, speech acts, pragmatics, and more.

CASE EXAMPLES
The Discourse Analysis Method

Culatta, Kovarsky, Theadore, Franklin, and Timler (2003) focused on early literacy instruction. Their purpose was to evaluate the effectiveness of language and literacy instruction with 31 children from Head Start classrooms. Culatta et al. (2003) combined aspects of the ethnographic approach with conversational analysis, a component of the discourse analysis method. Culatta et al. (2003) explained:

> This investigation drew upon two approaches to studying language as social interaction: the ethnography of communication and conversational analysis. Borrowing from the ethnography of communication, rhyming activities were analyzed as speech events; borrowing from conversation analysis, the instructional interactions were examined on a conversation turn by conversational turn basis. (p. 177)

Damico and Simmons-Mackie (2003) cited several examples of conversational analysis in the aphasia research literature. For one, Oelschlaeger and Damico (2000) applied the conversational analysis method to study a conversational partner's strategies when assisting with the word searches of an aphasic partner. They described their design as follows:

> The analytic objective of conversation analysis is examination of a focal conversational event to discover how it is systematically organized and accomplished by participants (Levinson, 1983). The basic analytic tool is a rich descriptive analysis of conversation sequences and the turns at talk within the sequences with findings inductively derived from these behavioral observations (Levinson, 1983). As in all varieties of qualitative research, extensive data collection, detailed description of the data collected, and various ways of comparing and contrasting these data serve to verify any findings. (Oelschlaeger & Damico, 2000, p. 208)

Discourse analysis methods have many applications in communication disorders research, including the exploration of conversational strategies with typically developing children and adults and those with disorders. Oelschlaeger and Damico (2000) summarized the importance of the investigation of partner strategies in the final paragraph of their report:

> The clinical contribution of this study (combined with Oelschlaeger's [1999] report) is the explication of how participatory word search strategies are accomplished in natural conversation. Clinicians should be able to use this information to determine whether conversational partners are using and capitalizing on strategies or may benefit from explicit training of strategies. (p. 219)

Given Oelschlaeger and Damico's (2000) concluding remarks, what are the options for continuing this line of research? Do you think there is a role for hypothesis testing in regard to training conversational strategies?

The Kinesic Analysis Method

Kinesiology is the study of communication through body movements, facial expressions, and gestures. *Kinesic analysis* examines what is communicated through these nonverbal movements, postures, and gestures. Kinesic analysis is usually combined with other qualitative methods such as discourse analysis in order to triangulate the data. The qualitative data collected in kinesic studies are usually systematically arranged into categories. For example, Ekman and Friesen (1969) classified nonverbal communications into five categories: emblems, illustrators, affective displays, regulators, and adaptors. These categories are as follows:

1. *Emblems* are nonverbal messages that have a verbal counterpart. The "OK" sign is an example of a hand gesture that has the verbal counterpart *okay*.
2. *Illustrators* are nonverbal body movements and gestures that do not have a clear verbal counterpart. They are usually used to illustrate what is being said.
3. *Affective displays* are body movements or facial expressions that communicate certain affective states or emotions. They are often used less consciously as illustrators.
4. *Regulators* are nonverbal signs that replace, modulate, and maintain the flow of speech during a conversation. Examples of regulators include nods of the head and eye movements.
5. *Adaptors* include postural changes and other body movements that are carried out at a low level of awareness. Examples of adaptors include sitting postures and general body orientation. Adaptors are easily misinterpreted. They are sometimes thought to be indicators of private thoughts. On the other hand, they are frequently used to resolve a specific physical situation such as to achieve a more relaxed seating position. (Ekman & Friesen, 1969)

Kinesics is an important part of communication, but body movements and facial expressions can be easily misinterpreted. Therefore, the analysis of kinesic data is often difficult—and credibility is sometimes questionable. Kinesics is also known to be culturally bound, so the potential for misunderstanding body movements and gestures increases across cultural boundaries.

The Direct Observation Method

Another method for qualitative analysis is known as *direct observation*. The direct observation method entails detailed and systematic observations of persons, locations, events, or topics of interest without the researcher's intrusion or participation in the scene. In this way, researcher biases are minimized. The direct observation method assumes that researchers will usually be detached from the scene. To this end, remote observations via one-way mirrors and video cameras help.

The direct observation method utilizes many techniques for collecting data, including note taking, video recordings, audio recordings, and photographs. Typically, data collection is triangulated from different sources to ensure the credibility of observations. Triangulation strengthens a study by combining methods. The logic of triangulation is based on the notion that no one method can adequately solve the problem of competing causal factors (Denzin, 1978). This can mean using several kinds of methods or data, including using both qualitative and quantitative approaches.

Denzin (1978) described four basic types of triangulation: (a) *data triangulation*, the use of a variety of data sources in a study, (b) *investigator triangulation*, the use of several different researchers or evaluators, (c) *theory triangulation*, the use of multiple perspectives to interpret a single set of data, and (d) *methodological triangulation*, the use of multiple methods to study a single problem or program.

Direct observation was the principle method employed by Piaget in his classic observations of infant behaviors and their cognitive development. Wadsworth (1989) offered the following description of Piaget's work in the context of the era in which Piaget lived.

In America, experimental research in psychology typically concerned itself with hypothesis testing, rigorous control of experimental variables, and treatment of data with sophisticated statistical procedures. Most of Piaget's research was not experimental in these ways. He did not typically employ elaborate statistics to test hypotheses or use control groups in his research. From his work in Paris in Binet's clinic, Piaget evolved a clinical-descriptive technique that became a trademark for his work. It essentially involved asking individual children carefully selected questions and noting their responses and their reasoning for those responses. In other cases, data were no more than the observation of infant behavior. It was difficult for American Psychologists to consider these techniques experimental because Piaget's methodology bore little resemblance to American experimental psychology. Piaget's work was basically observational, though it was invariably systematic and his analyses were exceedingly detailed; they were designed to detect developmental changes in cognitive functioning. (pp. 5–6)

CASE EXAMPLE
The Direct Observation Method

A contemporary example of the direct observation method and its application is described in Ukrainetz and Fresquez (2003). Their participants were 5 SLPs with 10 or more years of experience. The SLPs were chosen for two reasons: (a) They presented a contrastive picture to prior SLP participants, and (b) they had teachers who were willing to participate. Ukrainetz and Fresquez (2003) adopted purposeful sampling to choose participants for their study. "Purposeful sampling" selects information-rich cases that fit the purpose of the study, the available resources, and the questions being asked. There are at least 16 different types of purposeful sampling (see Exhibit 6.3). Based on what you know about their sampling approach, which of the techniques described in Exhibit 6.3 best matches Ukrainetz and Fresquez's (2003) purposeful sampling procedure?

EXHIBIT 6.3
Purposeful Sampling Techniques for Choosing Participants in Qualitative Studies

1. *Outlier Sampling.*   Choose extreme or deviant cases that are unusual examples of the phenomenon of interest, such as outstanding successes, notable failures, and rare events.

2. *Intensity Sampling.*   Choose information-rich cases that manifest the phenomenon intensely but not extremely, such as above-average or below-average persons, places, or events.

3. *Maximum Variation Sampling.*   Choose cases that represent a wide variety on the phenomenon of interest, such as persons who stutter from mildly to severely.

4. *Homogeneous Sampling.*   Choose cases that are alike with regard to the phenomenon of interest, such as having similar onset of a disease or like ethnic origin.

5. *Typical Case Sampling.*   Choose cases that are typical, normal, or average for the phenomenon of interest, such as children with specific language impairment who manifest typical language deficits.

6. *Stratified Purposeful Sampling.*   Choose cases that best represent the characteristics of various subgroups of a population such as subgroups of adult aphasia. This approach facilitates comparisons between groups.

7. *Critical Case Sampling.*   Choose cases that have a strategic importance in relation to the general problem. For example, to study infection rates, choose a workplace where safety regulations on cleanliness, air quality, and the like are met. This model workplace becomes a critical case. If the infection rate is high in this workplace, it is likely to be high in other workplaces that are less careful with safety regulations.

8. *Chain Sampling.*   Choose cases of interest from people who know what cases are information rich, good examples for study, or good interview participants.

9. *Criterion Sampling.*   Choose cases that meet set criteria, such as sixth-grade students, persons of 20 years of age, or SLPs with five years of experience.

10. *Theory-Based Sampling.*   Choose cases that fit the manifestations of a theoretical construct of interest such as a theory of stuttering.

11. *Confirmation Sampling.*   Choose cases that elaborate or deepen the initial analysis of some cases, seek further information, or confirm/disconfirm issues that are not clear.

12. *Opportunistic Sampling.*   Choose cases based on new leads that develop during fieldwork, such as the occurrence of an unexpected outcome.

13. *Random Purposeful Sampling.*   Randomly choose cases from a large, purposeful sample when the number of cases in the purposeful sample is too large to handle.

14. *Sampling for Political Importance.*   Choose cases that avoid persons or localities that are politically sensitive such as cases with a history of litigation.

15. *Convenience Sampling.*   Choose cases that are readily available such as the first 10 people you meet or your patients. This is the poorest way to gathering samples, yields the poorest information, and has the lowest credibility.

16. *Mixed Purposeful Sampling.*   Choose cases based on a combination of two or more sampling techniques. This technique aids triangulation.

Adapted from Patton, 2002, pp. 243–244.

Ukrainetz and Fresquez's (2003) method employed multiple data sources, which included open-ended interviews, historical data from written reports, and direct observations with field notes. They described the *direct observation phase* of their study as follows:

> One observation, with field notes, of 30–60 minutes, of each teacher and her class, and several observations of each SLP carrying out therapy. The SLP observations took place wherever therapy was occurring: speech room, resource room, or classroom. The first author transcribed the field notes, expanding and clarifying from the handwritten work within 2 days of taking the notes. (Ukrainetz & Fresquez, 2003, p. 287)

According to their description, Ukrainetz took field notes and then reviewed the notes within two days after the direct observation. Based on what you know about their method, what steps might have improved the credibility of their direct observations?

The Participant Observation Method

In contrast to the direct observation method, the participant observation method requires the researcher to become a participant in the culture or context being observed. The participant observation method is more demanding than direct observation because the researcher must acclimate to the situation and become an accepted member in the scene.

CASE EXAMPLE

A classic example of the participant observation method is Bloom's (1970) detailed account of her observations of young children acquiring language. Bloom's (1970) account was as follows:

> With a few brief exceptions, the investigator, who was well known to the children, was present in the observation sessions and interacted freely with the child. The mothers were present less than one-third of the time and the fathers only occasionally. The investigator's participation was necessary for noting features of behavior and environment in order to transcribe the tape recordings subsequently, and for maintaining the relative uniformity of the sessions for the three children. The samples were less than "naturalistic" to this extent. (p. 16)

Bloom (1970) suggested that the observations in the children's homes may have been less than natural because of her presence. Her observations began when the children were between 19 and 21 months of age. Based on what you know about Bloom's study, how did Bloom's presence affect the recorded observations? Did her presence have a substantial effect?

The *participant observation method* typically demands more time and resources than direct observation because of the need to immerse oneself into the context of the study. Thus, the high cost limits its use in communication disorders. Nonetheless, the participant observation method is a powerful method for observing cultural variables, language development, and other social behaviors from an insider's perspective.

The Unstructured In-Depth Interview Method

Another method for qualitative analysis is the *unstructured in-depth interview*. The unstructured interview is a widely used method in qualitative research circles for gathering data. The method is characterized by open-ended questions, no formal structure, and an iterative process of questions, answers, and generating more questions based on previous answers. Whereas structured interviews focus on answers to a narrowly defined set of questions, unstructured interviews focus on broad topics and concepts. The unstructured interviewing method is especially well suited for exploring sensitive, emotional, and personal issues. Unstructured interviews can be conducted with individuals or groups of participants.

Qualitative inquiry aims to minimize the imposition of predetermined responses when gathering data. To achieve this purpose, qualitative researchers ask questions that are open ended so that participants can respond in their own words. A truly open-ended question does not presuppose which dimension of feeling or thought will be salient for the interviewee. In contrast, *fixed-response questions* limit the response to a predetermined list of possibilities: for example;

How satisfied are you with your therapy?
  a. very satisfied
  b. somewhat satisfied
  c. not too satisfied
  d. not at all satisfied

In this case, the question format limits responses to a, b, c, or d. Thus, this is a fixed-response question. An alternative is to ask the same question without the list of alternative responses. However, the question is still not open ended, because it specifies the dimension of response (i.e., degree of satisfaction) and narrowly limits the respondent's response to the wording of the question.

As a contrast to fixed-response questions, *open-ended questions* follow the following format:

How do you feel about _____?
What is your opinion of _____?
What do you think of _____?

These truly open-ended questions permit those being interviewed to take whatever direction and use whatever words they want in order to express what they have to say (Patton, 2002).

Another type of interview procedure is the *focus group*. *Focus group interviews* involve small groups of people who focus on a specific topic. Groups are typically 6 to 10 people with similar backgrounds who participate in the interview for one to two hours. In a given study, a series of different focus groups may be used to get a variety of perspectives and increase confidence in whatever patterns emerge. Marketing researchers began using focus groups in the 1950s. Merton, Riske, and Kendall (1956) were the first to introduce the research-oriented focus group interview. Marketing researchers typically use focus groups of individuals with characteristics matching those of their consumers to evaluate products in various stages of development. In this way, the researchers seek to assess user needs, feelings, and preferences before a product is launched.

Focus group sessions are typically free-flowing and relatively unstructured, but the moderator must follow a preplanned script of specific issues and establish goals for the type of information to be gathered. Online forum discussions and newsgroups are sometimes used to approximate focus groups; however, at least two disadvantages are apparent: (a) Internet users may present an unwanted bias because of their unique attributes, and (b) confidentiality of online data is problematic. Stillman, Snow, and Warren (1999) used focus groups (in small-group discussions) in combination with individual interviews as means to gather data in their investigation of encounters between speech-language pathology students and children with pervasive developmental disorder (PDD).

CASE EXAMPLES
The Unstructured In-Depth Interview

Unstructured in-depth interviews are fairly common in communication disorders. In addition to their direct observations, Ukrainetz and Fresquez (2003) gathered data from other sources including open-ended interviews and student files. Their purpose was to examine how speech-language pathologists (SLPs) carried out their roles in schools. Ukrainetz and Fresquez (2003) described their interview protocol as follows:

> Audiotaped open-ended interviews with each SLP and teacher participant, transcribed by the second author and two research assistants, and a few clarifying questions by e-mail to the SLPs following the data collection periods. Topics included the following: education and work history; degree to which educational programs and practices were mandated; caseload, service structure, and assessment methods; teaching practices; explaining the terms *language* and *phonemic awareness;* role in reading and writing instructions; and roles and interconnections of the remedial educators. (p. 286)

Ukrainetz and Fresquez (2003) used email to follow up their face-to-face interviews of SLPs. Meline and Mata-Pistokache (2003) examined advantages and disadvantages related to the use of email in professional practices. Based on what you know about Ukrainetz and Fresquez's (2003) study, what do you think are advantages and disadvantages for the use of email in research studies?

Mastergeorge (1999) adopted an unstructured interview as the method of data collection in a study designed to "explore families' use of metaphoric language and its role as a mediator in revealing family members' perceptions of diagnosis and disorder" (p. 246). Mastergeorge (1999) described her interview procedure as follows:

> Family stories were collected about their experiences in coping with disabilities. Each family was interviewed twice, with each interview lasting approximately 3 to 4 hours. When possible, the families were interviewed in the privacy of their own homes by graduate students trained in ethnographic interviewing techniques. (pp. 247–248)

Mastergeorge reported that interviews were conducted in the families' homes when possible. Given what you know about Mastergeorge's (1999) study, answer the following questions: Why did she choose to interview families in their homes? If interviews had been conducted in schools or clinics, do you think the data would have been different? Mastergeorge (1999) concluded that metaphor is a powerful vehicle that families use to voice their experiences with disabilities.

CREDIBILITY AND TRANSFERABILITY IN QUALITATIVE RESEARCH

Lincoln and Guba (1985) proposed credibility and transferability as two criteria for evaluating qualitative research. *Credibility* is the criterion used for evaluating the believability of results. Qualitative research aims to understand phenomena from the participants' perspectives. A study's results and conclusions are credible to the degree that they accurately reflect the participants' feelings, opinions, intentions, and actions. Credibility is improved by employing multiple methods and triangulating data from different sources. Five techniques for evaluating credibility:

1. *Integrity of the observations.*   Factors to consider are the length and persistence of observations and the presence of triangulation of data by multiple sources.
2. *Peer debriefing.*   Factors to consider are the use of a devil's advocate perspective and the use of disinterested parties to assess conclusions.
3. *Negative case analysis.*   Factors to consider are revision of conclusions to account for known cases and recasting conclusions until they fit observed reality.
4. *Referential adequacy.*   Factors to consider are unanalyzed data set aside and analyzed after conclusions are drawn to see if they match.
5. *Member checks.*   Factors to consider are the sharing of conclusions with the participants and assessing the match between researchers' conclusions and the participants' reality.

The credibility of qualitative research is a basic requirement for its acceptance; however, transferability of the results and conclusions is also important, especially for clinical practice. *Transferability* refers to the extent to which results can be transferred from a study to other persons, locations, events, or other contexts. The transferability of qualitative research results is improved by detailed descriptions of research methods and thorough descriptions of the focus and context of studies. The ability to successfully transfer results to a person or location is determined by the consumer's evaluation. Thus, speech-language pathologists are responsible for evaluating the transferability of qualitative research results to their clinical practices—and audiologists are responsible for evaluating the transferability of results to their practices. The consumers (teachers, audiologists, and SLPs) evaluate the consistency of results and conclusions for the study at hand with other (independent) reports having the same focus. The decision to transfer results (or not) is based on (a) the consumer's local perspective and (b) the external consistency of the results and conclusions.

COMBINING QUALITATIVE AND QUANTITATIVE METHODS

Trochim (2004) professed that good research requires both qualitative and the quantitative methods. In fact, most qualitative research contains quantification in one form or another. An example is Bloom's (1970) qualitative study of early language development. Though the vast majority of the data was qualitative in nature, Bloom reported frequencies of occurrence (a quantitative measure) for the children's single-word utterances. Trochim (2004) observed that researchers are increasingly interested in blending the qualitative and quantitative traditions to get the advantages of each. The Office of Behavioral and Social Sciences Research of the National Institutes of Health (OBSSR, n.d.) recommended four models for combining qualitative and quantitative approaches within a single study.

The four models for combining qualitative and quantitative approaches are as follows:

1. *Sequential.*   Qualitative models serve for the first stage of knowledge building to discover key issues and elements for subsequent study using formal structured methods. For example, focus groups and preliminary pilot studies are conducted to refine a standardized instrument of clinical assessment for use in a new population or ethnic group.
2. *Parallel.*   Some models effectively conduct qualitative methods such as case studies, focused ethnographic observation, or multiple linked in-depth interviews (or a combination of these) in tandem with other methods.
3. *Coordinated substudies.*   Qualitative studies contribute under the umbrella of a larger program project or long-term study.
4. *Integrated.*   Methodologically diverse concepts and data are integrated at each stage within the study design to develop a robust evaluation of each emerging finding and set of data. (OBSSR, n.d.)

TECHNOLOGY NOTE

The Internet is the world's largest electronic archive of written material and probably the largest medium for interpersonal exchanges. *Chat rooms, listservs,* and *newsgroups* are rich sources of qualitative data, but Internet-based research raises some ethical concerns (Eysenbach & Till, 2001). For example, qualitative researchers can implement interviews, focus groups, and surveys online in order to collect their data. If an online site is a public place, *informed consent* may be unnecessary, but if a site is deemed to be private, informed consent is clearly required. The problem is that it's not easy to determine if a reasonable expectation of privacy exists on a particular website. The Internet also presents a challenge for the confidentiality of collected data. Based on what you know about the Internet and needs for confidentiality, what criteria would help to determine if an Internet site is private or public? Take a look at Eysenbach and Till's (2001) criteria.

CASE EXAMPLES
Combining Qualitative and Quantitative Methods

Culatta et al.'s (2003) study illustrates the *parallel model* for combining qualitative and quantitative approaches within a single study. They adopted the parallel model to study early literacy instruction. Culatta et al. (2003) explained as follows:

> Although quantitative procedures were used to evaluate the effectiveness of the literacy instruction in terms of performance measures, qualitative analyses provided information about children's engagement and participation in instructional activities and documented changes in performance over time. (p. 177)

Based on their quantitative results, Culatta et al. (2003) concluded that some treatment conditions were better than others. The qualitative results were summed up: "A qualitative examination of children's participation revealed their affective involvement and engagement in instructional activities" (p. 172). Thus, the combination of qualitative and quantitative methods yielded distinctly different but complementary information about literacy instruction.

Strum and Nelson (1997) reported another case of qualitative and quantitative approaches combined in a single study. They described the roles of qualitative and quantitative analyses as follows:

> The 15 classrooms were chosen to permit a rich description of both qualitative and quantitative aspects of formal classroom discourse. The qualitative analysis involved a series of multiple passes through the transcripts to develop a coding system, a series of themes, and eventually, a set of 10 rules to describe the interactions. The quantitative analysis involved compiling data such as numbers of words spoken and numbers of words per T-unit (or C-unit) by both students and teachers at each of the three grade levels. The frequencies of various communicative functions were also examined across grade levels. (Strum & Nelson, 1997, p. 256)

Given the four models for combining qualitative and quantitative approaches within a single study, which of the four models best fits the description provided by Strum and Nelson (1997)? Why do you think that combining qualitative and quantitative approaches might have yielded a richer analysis of Strum and Nelson's data?

CONCLUSION

Qualitative methods present a variety of powerful approaches and designs for exploring topics and ideas and gaining insight into lifestyles, cultures, motivations, behaviors, preferences, and more. Qualitative researchers typically collect data in the form of interviews, observations, and documents. To ensure credibility, qualitative researchers incorporate procedures such as triangulation and lamination. Researchers sometimes use several qualitative methods in combination, or they may combine qualitative and quantitative approaches. Before choosing one or another approach, prospective researchers should closely examine their research questions to be sure that they can be answered with qualitative methods. Patton (2002) offered 10 bits of advice for students

EXHIBIT 6.4
Advice for Students Considering a Qualitative Thesis

1. Be sure that the qualitative approach fits your research questions.
2. Study qualitative research methods in a couple books and original sources before proceeding.
3. Identify a thesis advisor who supports your proposal for a qualitative research design.
4. Understand that qualitative research follows a completely different logic from quantitative research. Really work on the design.
5. Practice interviewing and observation skills.
6. Plan your analysis before you gather the data.
7. Be sure that you are prepared to deal with the controversies of doing qualitative research.
8. Do it because you want to and are convinced that it is right for you.
9. Find a good mentor or support group.
10. Prepare to be changed. Looking deeply at other people's lives will force you to look deeply at yourself.

Adapted from Patton, 2002 pp. 33–35.

who are considering a qualitative thesis. This advice is summarized in Exhibit 6.4. For students and others, the issues addressed in Exhibit 6.4 are important to consider before beginning a qualitative study.

CASE STUDIES

Case 6.1: Why Speech-Language Pathology?
Justine, a graduate student in speech-language pathology, is developing a thesis proposal. Her timeline for completing the thesis is 12 months from today. Justine and her thesis advisor, Dr. Ferol, plan to answer the question, Why do students choose a career in speech-language pathology? What type of qualitative research design or combination of designs do you recommend for Justine's thesis?

Case 6.2: Let's Focus on AAC
Dr. Harvey is Jean's research mentor at the local university. Jean is a speech-language pathologist at the regional trauma center. Dr. Harvey has assigned Jean to plan and develop a focus group to evaluate a new product for augmentative/alternative communication use. You volunteered to help Jean with the project because you recently completed a research class. What steps will you and Jean follow to organize and conduct the focus group?

Case 6.3: To Email or Not to Email
A fellow student, Vincent, asked you to participate in an online interview. Vincent is completing a requirement for his senior research class, and he plans to conduct unstructured inter-

views with 10 students as participants. The research question is, What are students' attitudes and opinions about cheating on exams? Vincent plans to conduct the interviews solely by email exchanges. What questions should you ask?

Case 6.4: What's with Triangulation?
Two graduate students, Joan and Patrick, are planning a qualitative study with their professor and mentor, Dr. Strangelove. They are planning a series of direct observations of children on school playgrounds. The professor believes that Joan can collect the data in the form of detailed notes, but Joan and Patrick are concerned about credibility. They think that the professor, Joan, and Patrick each should make independent observations and then compare notes. What is the best argument for Joan and Patrick's case?

Case 6.5: Contemplating a Qualitative Thesis
Jack is contemplating a senior thesis, but he can't decide if a qualitative approach or a quantitative approach is best. At present, all the professors are inclined to use quantitative methods, but he may be able to convince Dr. Shirley to sponsor his qualitative thesis. What is your best advice for Jack? If he is otherwise well prepared to do a qualitative thesis, what are his options?

STUDENT EXERCISES

1. What steps would you take to triangulate data sources in a qualitative study that focuses on nonverbal communication?
2. How would you adopt the sequential model to plan a qualitative/quantitative study to develop a test of reading fluency for bilingual African American children?
3. Locate a report in the professional journals (online or print) that uses the case study method as the primary research design. Based on this report, answer these questions: Is the case study qualitative, quantitative, or a combination? What proportion of the study is qualitative and how much is quantitative?
4. How would you use lamination to verify your interpretation of data gathered by directly observing audiological evaluations?
5. Locate a qualitative research report in the speech, language, and hearing journals. Based on this report, answer these questions: What is the transferability of results? What steps did the researchers take to improve the transferability of results? What suggestions do you have for improving their study's transferability to clinical situations?
6. Write a brief proposal for a qualitative study. Your proposal should answer these questions: What is the study's purpose? Which qualitative approach will best answer your questions? Who do you anticipate as participants in your study? Which purposeful sampling technique will you use?

CHAPTER 7

SINGLE CASE DESIGNS IN COMMUNICATION DISORDERS RESEARCH

explore (ĭk splôr′) *v.* to investigate systematically; to make a careful examination or search

The family of single case designs includes both simple case studies and time-series designs. The *simple case study* is usually a thorough description of one or more children or adults. Most often, its results are rich descriptions rather than numbers and statistics. Simple case studies lack the controls that are included in experimental designs. Thus, they fall short of the rigorous standards that typify scientific inquiry. However, uncontrolled case studies are a legitimate choice when the sole purpose is to generate ideas. In that sense, uncontrolled case studies can be the seeds for future scientific inquiries.

In contrast to simple case studies, *time-series designs* typically include controls that meet the rigorous standards of scientific inquiry. Time-series designs observe a series of behaviors across some period of time, and they permit cause-effect conclusions; however, the conclusions are less robust than those from randomized-controlled group designs. For this reason, time-series designs are classified as quasi-experimental.

One use of time-series designs is to gather preliminary data before undertaking a randomized-controlled group experiment. In this sense, time-series designs are exploratory in nature. However, time-series designs provide strong evidence for clinical practice, especially when results from several independent studies are combined.

A special instance of time-series designs is known as the *single case design*. Single case designs are excellent alternatives to group designs for investigating phenomena in communication disorders. The unit of analysis in single case designs is usually a single individual, though it can be a dyad, small group of individuals, or a classroom. When the unit of analysis is a group, the data for analysis is often a group statistic such as a mean, median, or standard deviation. In these cases, researchers report individual results along with group results to show that the treatment affected most participants in the same way. In contrast, single case designs focus exclusively on individual participants.

The sequence of events in the single case design is depicted in series 1:

$$O_1 \quad O_2 \quad O_3 \quad I_1 \quad O_4 \quad O_5 \quad O_6 \qquad \text{(series 1)}$$

The symbol O represents the observation of a dependent variable, and the symbol I represents a one-time intervention. In this case, the series O_1–O_3 represents observations that take place in a baseline phase, and the series O_4–O_6 includes observations that follow the one-time intervention. More often, interventions are continuously applied throughout the intervention phase. In this case, the basic single case protocol is depicted in series 2:

$$O_1 \quad O_2 \quad O_3 \quad I_1 \quad O_4 \quad I_1 \quad O_5 \quad I_1 \quad O_6 \qquad \text{(series 2)}$$

In series 2, the O_4, O_5, and O_6 observations follow interventions (I_1) throughout the treatment phase. The use of a continuous treatment in single case designs is typical in communication disorders research. The family of time-series designs includes many variations of the basic designs depicted in series 1 and 2.

SINGLE CASE DESIGNS VERSUS GROUP DESIGNS

Single case research designs are unlike group research designs in many ways. First, they focus on individual performance, whereas group designs focus on group performance. Second, single case designs compare different conditions within one participant, and group designs compare a treatment group to one or more control groups. For internal validity, group designs rely on the external controls provided by comparison groups or no-treatment control groups. Single case designs rely on comparisons between different conditions or phases.

The comparisons in single case designs are made by presenting alternative conditions to a participant at different points in time. For example, a treatment might be evaluated by alternating periods of treatment and no treatment across time. Inferences are made about the treatment in single case designs based on the patterns of the data across the different conditions. A third way in which single case and group designs differ regards external validity and the ability to generalize results to the population of interest. Group designs depend on representative samples selected from the population for their external validity. In contrast, single case designs depend on replication with additional participants for their external validity. Single case designs are less rigorous in this regard because replication with two or more participants may suggest that an intervention is applicable to others, but it is not conclusive evidence. Fourth, single case designs require decision making regarding the course of the study as it progresses. Group designs are planned beforehand and carried out with little, if any, change in the original plan.

THE BASELINE PHASE IN SINGLE CASE DESIGNS

Single case designs begin with systematic observations of an individual's behavior for several sessions before the treatment is introduced. This period of time is known as the "baseline phase"—sometimes referred to as the pretreatment phase. The baseline phase has two purposes: (a) to describe the extent of the individual's problem or status of the target behavior as it naturally occurs and (b) to predict future behavior if intervention is not provided. To ensure the reliability of measurements and the validity of the baseline, a minimum of five observations is usually prescribed. However, the exact number of observations in the baseline phase depends on the stability or degree of variability of the dependent variable. Observations continue and data are collected until a predictable pattern of behavior is established. If the observed behavior is erratic and no stable pattern emerges, the experiment may conclude with no intervention. If the observed behavior is stable with a predictable trend, an intervention phase is initiated in the next session.

There are four basic types of single case designs: (a) the A-B-A(=B) design, (b) the multiple-baseline (changing baseline) design, (c) the changing-criterion design, and (d) the simultaneous-treatment design. However, there are many variations or elaborations for each of these basic designs.

THE A-B-A SINGLE CASE DESIGN

The *A-B-A single case design* is a prototype for single case quasi-experimental research. The A-B-A-B design is an extension of the A-B-A design that adds a B phase to the A-B-A sequence. The "A-B-A" notation represents a series of three phases that are implemented over time. The first *A* is an initial baseline phase wherein the dependent variable is observed in its natural state and data are collected until a stable baseline is clearly visible. The presence or absence of a stable baseline can also be confirmed by statistical analysis. The *A phase* is important because it is the basis for predicting the natural course of the behavior without intervention of the treatment. The *B* represents the intervention phase wherein the treatment is first introduced. The second *A* represents a second baseline condition wherein the treatment is withdrawn. In its extended form (A-B-A-B), the final *B phase* is a reintroduction of the intervention. The added B condition in the A-B-A-B design answers the ethical concern that the experiment might conclude without the benefit of intervention for the participant.

The A-B-A-B design has an additional advantage over the A-B-A design in that it replicates the A-B comparison (A-B + A-B). This internal replication of the A-B sequence provides additional support for a cause-effect relationship between independent (intervention) and dependent (behavioral) variables. Exhibit 7.1 displays the basic A-B-A-B single case design with fictitious data from the observations of some dependent variable.

The first phase is designated as A_1 in Exhibit 7.1. It illustrates the measurement of a participant's behavior across five sessions. The schedule for baseline probes depends on the nature of the target behavior and other factors, so the five sessions may

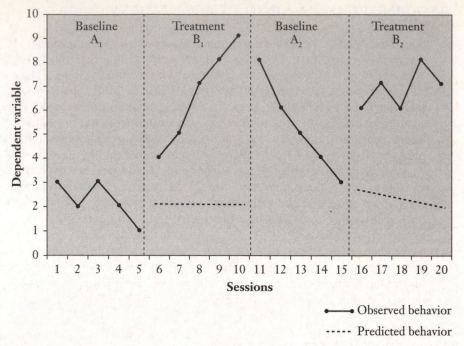

EXHIBIT 7.1
The Basic Single Case A-B-A-B Design

occur in one day or over the course of five consecutive days at prescribed intervals of time. In this illustration, the data recorded in the A phase are relatively stable with little variation observed from session to session. To conclude that a baseline is stable, the dependent variable should be relatively unchanging across at least three consecutive sessions. This is a critical assumption for time-series designs because it is the basis for predicting the future course of the dependent variable.

Once a stable baseline is established, the treatment phase begins with the first session in the B_1 phase and typically continues for five or more sessions until the experimenter is satisfied that the effect of the intervention (or noneffect) is evident. The broken line in Exhibit 7.1's phase B_1 depicts the prediction inferred by the pattern of observations in phase A_1.

The baseline data in phase A_1 predict that the observed behavior will continue on the same course for future sessions if a treatment is not introduced. This prediction is the basis of comparison as well as the internal control that provides scientific credibility for the experimental outcome. The solid line in the first treatment phase (B_1) represents the participant's performance across sessions 6 to 10. The treatment phase may continue for more than five sessions depending on the targeted behavior and the observed change (if any) in the participant's performance.

The effect of the treatment is inferred by comparing the solid line shown in the treatment phase B_1 to the broken line in the same phase—or alternatively, the solid line in A_1 to the solid line in B_1. In this case, a visual inspection of the results suggests that the change in behavior during the B_1 phase is not predicted by the baseline data in A_1. This is preliminary evidence for efficacy, but it lacks confirmation.

To test the assumption that the original baseline was an accurate predictor of future performance, a second baseline phase (A_2) is introduced by withdrawing the treatment but continuing to observe the behavior across sessions 11 to 15. The second A phase (A_2) is important because it tests the internal validity of the experiment by ruling out history and maturation effects (i.e., nuisance variables) as causes of the change in behavior observed in B_1. The second A phase is sometimes referred to as the *withdrawal phase* because the intervention is removed at this time.

When the intervention is withdrawn, the dependent variable's course is plotted. If the dependent variable moves toward the baseline, the experimenters might conclude that the treatment has a causal relationship with the dependent variable. However, if the dependent variable remains stable or trends upward, a cause-effect relationship is dubious. In the latter case, the investigators would probably halt the experiment. However, if a regression to baseline effect is observed in A_2, the intervention is reintroduced in B_2. Again, the course of behavior predicted by the previous phase is illustrated by the broken line in B_2, and the actual behavior observed is the solid line in B_2. The effect of reintroducing the treatment in phase B_2 is evaluated by comparing the actual performance (solid line) to the predicted performance (broken line). If reintroducing the treatment in B_2 results in a change in the dependent variable similar to the change observed in B_1, researchers are likely to conclude that the intervention caused the change in behavior. This does not necessarily mean that the intervention is the sole cause of the change, because extraneous variables cannot be totally ruled out. However, if extraneous variables are present, their contribution to the behavioral change is probably small.

The A-B-A and A-B-A-B designs include one independent variable (usually a treatment variable) to test the effect of an intervention. However, researchers in communication disorders may want to compare the effects of different treatments on a target behavior. For example, researchers may want to compare the effects of two instructional procedures for teaching reading to young children. A single case design for testing the effects of two treatment variables is the A-B-A-C single case design. In this design, the first treatment variable is designated as B, and the second treatment variable is designated as C. The A-B-A-C single case design is a useful design, but it requires care to avoid multiple treatment interference, which is a serious threat to internal validity.

Multiple treatment interference is a problem inherent in A-B-A-C single case designs because the effects of treatment B are likely to carry over to the C treatment. Thus, the C phase is contaminated with an unwanted nuisance variable. Multiple treatment interference is controlled in advance by recruiting additional participants and counterbalancing the order of treatments across participants. For example, if an A-B-A-C design includes four participants, treatments are counterbalanced across participants as follows:

1. A-B-A-C
2. A-C-A-B
3. A-B-A-C
4. A-C-A-B

In this case, the experiment's outcome is evaluated as the summative effect of treatments across the four participants.

Though experimenters may conclude that a treatment was cause for a change in behavior, conclusions based on one individual cannot be generalized to the target population. To provide evidence for the generalization of results to other cases (i.e., external validity), direct replication with additional participants is the usual choice. Thus, most single case experiments in communication disorders include three or more participants.

REPLICATION IN SINGLE CASE DESIGNS

In single case designs (and group designs), replication involves repeating the experiment with exactly the same conditions but with different participants. If the same intervention effect is demonstrated with two or more additional participants, experimenters might conclude that the intervention is effective with a variety of individuals. This is evidence for external validity. However, the evidence may fall short of proving that the intervention will benefit all children or adults who are like the participants in the study. At best, the successful replication of a single case experiment suggests that the results can be generalized, but it is less than conclusive. The best scientific evidence that a particular intervention is applicable to the population of children or adults is achieved by randomized-controlled experiments with (large) representative samples of participants randomly selected from the population. However, the synthesis of results from small *n* studies such as single case experiments is strong evidence as well.

■ ■ ■ ■ ■

CASE EXAMPLE
The A-B-A-B Single Case Design

To study the effects on children's speech rates when their mothers talked more slowly, Guitar and Marchinkoski (2001) chose an A-B-A-B single case design. Their units of analysis were six mother–child dyads that included three boys and three girls, 3 to 4 years of age. The researchers manipulated the speech rates of the mothers (independent variable) in the intervention phases (B_1, B_2) of the A-B-A-B single case design. The mothers' natural speech rates were observed in the baseline phases. In the first B phase (intervention), the mothers were trained to use a slow speech rate. The dependent variable was speech rate as measured in syllables per minute. Each phase in their A-B-A-B design was 10 minutes long with eight probes or measurements of the dependent variable. The researchers concluded that five of the six children reduced their speech rates when their mothers spoke more slowly. However, their conclusions were tentative because speech rates varied widely in some conditions. In other words, they failed to achieve a stable baseline with some of the cases. Guitar and Marchinkoski (2001) suggested that a replication of their study would benefit from extending the length of phases to achieve stable speech rates.

■ ■ ■ ■ ■

CASE EXAMPLES
The A-B-A-B Alternating Treatments Single Case Design

Mechling, Gast, and Cronin (2006) adopted the A-B-A-B design as their method of study; however, they alternated treatments between A and B phases. Their A phase was, in effect, the baseline for behavior because it represented a traditional approach, whereas the B phase was the experimental treatment. Participants were two children with autism spectrum disorder (ASD). The children were both boys, and their chronological ages were 13 years, 2 months; and 14 years, 4 months.

Mechling et al.'s (2006) rationale for their study was that children with ASD need to be motivated for the best task performance. They proposed an experimental treatment with two components: (a) The children chose the stimuli, and (b) the stimuli were presented in 1-minute video segments on computers. For the more traditional approach, teachers chose tangible stimuli, and photographs of the items were displayed one at a time prior to the task. Thus, the variables that differentiated the treatments were choice versus no choice and video presentation versus photographs. The dependent variable was the time needed to complete a task. Task duration was measured by one of the researchers by writing start and stop times on a data collection sheet. Though Mechling et al. (2006) did not state their hypothesis; they apparently expected the experimental treatment (video and choice) to result in shorter times to complete the tasks. Both of the participants completed three tasks across the conditions as shown in Exhibit 7.2. Visual inspection of the results shows that the boys completed the tasks in a shorter time when the reinforcement was video and choice. The researchers reported means and ranges for the task durations. For example, Jackson's mean for phase A_1 (tangible) was 53.8 minutes, and his mean for phase B_1 (video and choice) was 28.8 minutes—a difference of 25 minutes.

What limitations are apparent in the Mechling et al. (2006) single case study? First, the number of participants in their study was only two children with ASD. Although they did replicate their result with one additional participant, the evidence for extending the outcome to other students and different schools is weak. Second, there was a real possibility of experimenter bias. One or the other researcher conducted the protocol, measured the task duration, and collected the data. Thus, the researchers' bias could have affected the results. Finally, their experimental treatment included two elements (video and choice), so it was impossible to say how one or the other alone might have affected the outcome. Nonetheless, Mechling et al.'s (2006) study seemed to establish that type of reinforcement affects the performance of students with ASD. Their study also reinforced the need for further investigations of this kind. It will be left to future studies to better evaluate the specific causes and their effects.

Morrow and Fridriksson (2006) also used an alternating treatments approach to compare two techniques for "spaced retrieval," which is used to treat persons with anomia. According to Morrow and Fridriksson (2006), spaced retrieval requires stringent control of the intervals between stimuli to achieve positive outcomes. This technique doubles or halves the time between stimulus presentations depending on the patient's response accuracy. However, these researchers questioned whether such a strict control of the intervals was necessary. Thus, Morrow and Fridriksson (2006) set out to determine whether the timing of the stimulus presentation influenced treatment outcomes.

To answer their research question, Morrow and Fridriksson (2006) selected three persons with aphasia as participants. All had naming errors characterized as semantic paraphasia. They used an alternating treatments single case design to compare two presentation modes: (a) stringent control of time intervals and (b) random time intervals. The three participants

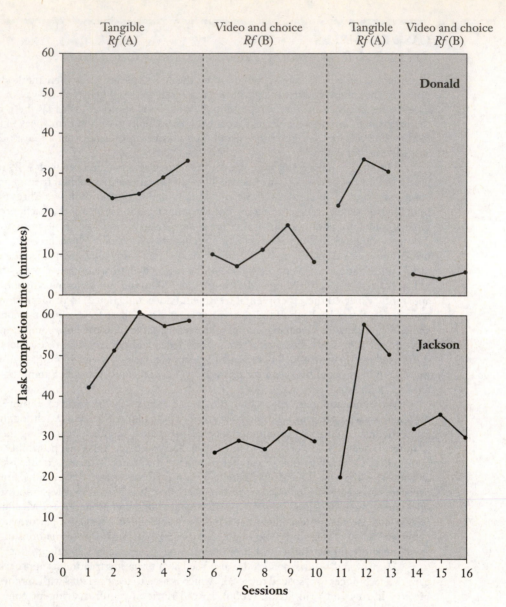

EXHIBIT 7.2
A Case Example: Alternating Treatments A-B-A-B Design (*n* = 2)

were instructed to name each of three target items. If they responded incorrectly, the clinician provided the correct name and instructed the participant to repeat it. In the first condition, the intervals between stimulus presentations were randomly varied from 1 to 8 minutes. In the second condition, the intervals were halved if the participant incorrectly responded and doubled when they correctly responded.

Morrow and Fridriksson's (2006) dependent measurement was the number of targets mastered (i.e., correctly named). The baselines were established for the three participants across the first three sessions. All the participants scored zero across the first three sessions, so their baselines were shown to be stable. The treatment conditions were alternated across 20 sessions with the addition of 3-week and 6-week probes at the end. The probes were included to demonstrate maintenance of the treatment effect. Morrow and Fridriksson's (2006) results indicated no real difference between the two approaches. Both approaches were successful in improving naming of the targets. Thus, the investigators concluded that either approach can be used. However, they noted that their participants had mild to moderate aphasia. Persons with severe aphasia may experience different outcomes. Furthermore, the small number of participants somewhat limited the applicability of results to real-life situations. Nonetheless, Morrow and Fridriksson (2006) made a noteworthy contribution to the clinical sciences. Future investigations will support or refute their conclusions.

VISUAL INSPECTION VERSUS STATISTICAL TESTS

To conclude that a treatment is effective in a single case design, researchers can choose *visual inspection*, statistical procedures, or a combination of both techniques. Visual inspection is the initial choice of most researchers because the phases in single case designs are easily graphed, and changes (or no changes) in the dependent variable are readily apparent. However, visual analyses are subjective, and interrater agreement regarding the presence or absence of a treatment effect in visual analyses typically averages 60% or less according to Robey, Schultz, Crawford, and Sinner (1999). Thus, the use of visual inspection alone to judge treatment effects in single case designs is not always reliable for analysis. The better practice is to use both visual inspection and statistics to analyze data in single case designs.

Because of the shortcomings inherent in visual analyses, researchers utilize statistical tests such as analysis of variance (ANOVA), *t*-tests, and the standardized effect size (ES). The problem with using ANOVA and *t*-test procedures with time-series data is that they assume the data for analysis are independent (i.e., unrelated to one another). However, because the data in time-series designs are collected from one participant, they are not independent. Statisticians refer to this form of dependence across observations as *temporal autocorrelation*. For this reason, ANOVA and *t*-test procedures can be subject to error when applied to time-series designs. Alternative procedures such as *Interrupted Time Series Analyses* (ITSA) and its variant, ITSACORR, yield a test of overall change, a test of change in slope, and a test of change in level (Robey et al., 1999). The ITSA and ITSACORR procedures account for the correlated nature of the data and yield a meaningful statistic (F) that tests the null hypothesis of overall change.

TECHNOLOGY NOTE

Statistical tools are useful for analyzing trends in time-series designs. Statistical software packages such as MINITAB and SPSS include trend analysis and autocorrelation functions for analyzing data in time-series designs. An online resource is Dr. Paul Jones's *Single-Case Research and Statistical Analysis* webpages. The Jones website includes statistical analysis tools with autocorrelation, chi square, nonparametric, time series, and *t*-test options. Program instructions on the website include features, general functions, and data-entry procedures. A "personal version" of the statistical analysis program is available for offline data processing. The *Single-Case Research and Statistical Analysis* website is located at www.unlv.edu/faculty/pjones/singlecase/scsaguid.htm.

The ES statistic is not a test of the null hypothesis, but it yields a measure of the overall magnitude of a change. An estimation of effect size for time-series data is relatively easy to calculate. The standardized ES is derived by the formula in equation 1 (Faith, Allison, & Gorman, 1997, p. 254).

$$ES = \frac{\bar{X}_B - \bar{X}_A}{S_A}$$

$$S_A = \frac{1}{n-1}\Sigma(x_i - \bar{x})^2$$

(eq. 1)

The subscripts "A" and "B" designate baseline and intervention phases respectively. The mean ($\bar{X}$) is the average for baseline (A) and intervention (B) data, and S is the standard deviation that is calculated from data in the baseline phase. If there is no variability observed in the baseline phase, the effect size cannot be estimated. The effect sizes derived from single case designs are not the same as the effect sizes computed in group research designs, so comparisons are not meaningful.

THE MULTIPLE-BASELINE SINGLE CASE DESIGN

The *multiple-baseline single case design* is sometimes referred to as a changing baseline. It is depicted as a series of A-B designs stacked on top of one another, with each baseline phase progressively longer. There can be three or more baselines, and each baseline represents a target variable. The multiple-baseline design includes a treatment variable and three or more target variables. Target variables are chosen carefully because they must be independent of one another. In other words, a change in the treated variable should not be accompanied by a change in an untreated variable.

The multiple-baseline design is a flexible design in that it can simultaneously analyze three or more target behaviors. It also avoids the ethical concern regarding withdrawal of treatment, because no withdrawal of treatment is needed. The multiple-baseline design is also an alternative when an A-B-A design is not possible because a dependent variable does not respond to withdrawal of the treatment due to carryover or long-lasting effects of the treatment on the dependent variable. This is known as the *generalized effects problem*.

Though multiple-baseline designs have some advantages, they also have disadvantages relative to the classic A-B-A designs. First, the multiple-baseline design is weaker than the A-B-A design because the controlling effects of the treatment variable on the dependent variable are not directly demonstrated as they are in the intervention and withdrawal phases of the A-B-A design. Second, multiple-baseline designs require a multitude of data collection over an extended period of time. Thus, the multiple-baseline design requires substantial resources for planning, implementing, and ensuring the cooperation of participants.

The multiple-baseline design includes three or more target variables with their respective baselines. The target variables may be any one of three types: (a) *different behaviors* for one participant observed in one setting or, alternatively, the sum of responses for more than one participant such as a dyad, small group of individuals, or classroom observed in one setting, (b) *different participants* who are observed in one setting exhibiting one behavior, or (c) *different settings* with one participant and one behavior. Following collection of the baseline data, the treatment variable is introduced to each of the target variables in turn (behaviors, participants, or settings). The introduction of the treatment variable to the second and third target variables is triggered by a predetermined level of performance. For example, if the dependent variable increases by a predetermined level of 50%, the treatment is applied to the second target variable while the first target variable continues to be treated and so on. Exhibit 7.3 illustrates the basic multiple-baseline design with two phases (A-B), multiple tiers, and fictitious data from observations of a dependent variable.

The symbol "A" represents the baseline phase wherein the dependent variable is observed in its natural state, and data are collected until a stable baseline is established. In this case, baseline data are collected concurrently on the three baselines. The symbol "B" represents the intervention phase wherein the treatment is introduced. Each of the tiers represents one target variable. The treatment is applied to each target variable but at different points in time. Thus, the treatment is applied to the first target variable, and when the response reaches a predetermined level, the treatment is applied to the second target variable, then the third target behavior, and so on until the treatment has been applied to all of the target behaviors. The multiple-baseline single case design demonstrates a treatment effect by showing that the response changes whenever the treatment is introduced at the different points in time.

■ ■ ■ ■ ■ ▬▬▬

CASE EXAMPLES
The Multiple-Baseline Single Case Design

To study the effect of typicality of exemplars on naming ability, two researchers (Kiran & Thompson, 2003) adopted a multiple-baseline-across-behaviors single case design. The behaviors in this case were different levels of typicality (e.g., typical, intermediate, and atypical) for specific semantic categories. For example, "parrot" was a typical referent in the bird category, but "penguin" was an atypical referent. The units of analysis were four adult

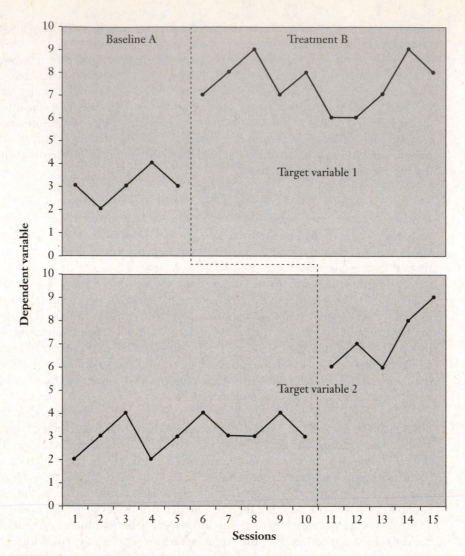

EXHIBIT 7.3
The Basic Multiple-Baseline Single Case Design

participants with fluent aphasia—three females and one male, 63–75 years of age. The researchers employed a semantic feature treatment as their intervention. The dependent variable was the number of items named correctly. The number of probes during the intervention phases ranged from 6 to 11. The researchers reported that three of the four participants demonstrated a stable baseline, which the researchers operationally defined as less than two points of fluctuation across sessions. The researchers observed positive changes in the dependent variable (naming ability) after treatment was introduced and also observed generalization from one typicality level to another.

Kiran and Thompson (2003) explored naming abilities for animate referents. Kiran (2008) reported a replication of the 2003 study with inanimate referents such as names for furniture and clothing. Again, Kiran (2008) utilized the multiple-baseline approach to investigate the effects of the typicality treatment. Kiran (2008) recruited patients with nonfluent aphasia from local hospitals as participants. The participants were four females and one male, 47–77 years of age. They met several selection criteria, including (a) a single left-hemisphere stroke, (b) onset at least seven months prior, (c) premorbid right-handedness, and (d) at least a high school diploma. According to Kiran (2008), the results extended Kiran and Thompson's (2003) conclusions to patients with nonfluent aphasia as well as to inanimate naming categories.

Given what you know about Kiran (2008) and Kiran and Thompson's (2003) studies, what aspects of the first study were replicated in the 2008 report, and which aspects were not replicated? Kiran (2008) noted that three participants showed strong generalization for improved naming, while two participants did not. How should this outcome be interpreted for clinical practice?

Another example of the multiple-baseline single case design is Lovelace and Stewart's (2007) investigation of print awareness in preschoolers with language impairment. Their participants were 4- to 5-year-old children—one boy and four girls. The target variable was the different participants. Lovelace and Stewart (2007) asked the question, "To what extent does the use of nonevocative, explicit print referencing cues during shared book reading in the context of language intervention facilitate print concept knowledge with language impairment? (p. 19)" To find an answer, they chose a multiple-baseline single case design. Lovelace and Stewart (2007) measured the children's knowledge of print concepts with an assessment tool of their design, *Concepts of Print Assessment*. The dependent variable was the percentage of correct responses on this assessment instrument.

Lovelace and Stewart (2007) established baseline measurements over three consecutive sessions and then introduced the experimental condition in sequence to one participant at a time until all the participants were receiving the treatment. The experimental condition (treatment) was a "scripted input," which consisted of the nonevocative strategies of commenting, tracking, and pointing to examples of 20 print-related concepts. All five participants demonstrated higher percentages of correct responses once the treatment was introduced. For example, Katrina's baseline was 25%, but she scored 45% in the first of five treatment sessions and 80% in the last session. Thus, Katrina's gain was immediate and progressively improved over the five sessions.

Lovelace and Stewart (2007) also included a generalization probe as a follow-up to treatment. The generalization probes followed the last treatment session and consisted of different tasks. The intent was to test the treatment effect's ability to generalize to different situations. Though the generalization probes showed some regression, the generalization scores were above the baseline scores. Lovelace and Stewart (2007) noted several limitations in their study. First, the participants' attendance was an issue. Three participants missed one session, but one participant missed eight sessions. The absences might have affected the fidelity of the experimental treatment. Second, their Concepts of Print Assessment tool was not proven to be reliable and valid. Third, the investigators used different storybooks during baseline and treatment sessions. Fourth, their participants were motivated toward book reading, but other children may be less motivated. Finally, the storybooks varied in their print. Some books included large, contextualized print while others did not. Though Lovelace and Stewart's (2007) study clearly had some important limitations, the results suggested that print awareness can be facilitated. Future investigations will benefit from the lessons learned in their study.

THE CHANGING-CRITERION SINGLE CASE DESIGN

The *changing-criterion single case design* is another time-series design that employs base-line and intervention phases to demonstrate a treatment effect while controlling extraneous influences. The changing-criterion design is especially well suited for solving clinical problems in which skills are practiced and achieved gradually, not abruptly. The sequence of events in the changing-criterion design is $A-B_1-B_2-B_3$ where A is the baseline phase, and the intervention phase B is divided into several subphases. A *maintenance phase* can follow the intervention as an optional phase. The addition of a maintenance phase is important for understanding whether the treatment's effect will persist in a different situation, time, or context. The basic changing-criterion design with fictitious data is shown in Exhibit 7.4.

As is typical with single case designs, the baseline phase of the changing-criterion design continues until the participant's responses are stabilized across three or more sessions. An intervention phase is divided into several subphases that include gradually changing criteria. The criterion for each subphase is the number of responses that need to be performed to achieve a particular consequence that is predetermined by the investigator. For example, the consequence may be a tangible reward of some sort that is awarded on a regular schedule within each session. In the changing-criterion design, the criterion is gradually changed at the end of each subphase of the intervention. The

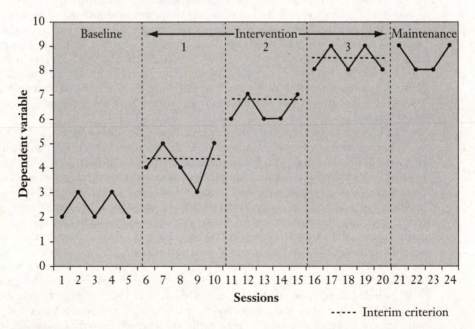

EXHIBIT 7.4
The Basic Changing-Criterion Single Case Design

criterion is typically increased so that the subject must demonstrate a slightly greater performance to earn the reward. The criterion is changed throughout the intervention phase until a terminal goal is achieved.

In the changing-criterion design, the treatment effect is demonstrated if the participant's performances match the criteria as they are changed. If performances closely match the criteria, the investigator may conclude that the intervention is responsible for changes in the dependent variable and extraneous variables are not.

A disadvantage of the changing-criterion single case design is the possibility of ambiguity if the subject's performance does not closely follow the positive changes in the criterion. A variation of the changing-criterion design includes *mini-reversal phases* wherein the investigator makes bidirectional changes in the interim criteria. In this case, the treatment effect is demonstrated if the responses match the criteria as they change direction. Overall, the changing-criterion design is appropriate for establishing a functional relationship between a treatment and behavior. However, it requires intensive planning and careful implementation for success.

THE SIMULTANEOUS-TREATMENTS SINGLE CASE DESIGN

The purpose of the *simultaneous-treatments single case design* is to compare the effects of alternate treatments on a dependent variable. It exposes one participant to two different treatments at the same time. To control for extraneous influences such as history and maturation effects, the order of treatments is counterbalanced. For example, the two treatments are alternated 1-2 on one day, 2-1 on the next day, and so on. In this case, the participant is exposed to both treatments in the same day but in different sessions. The basic simultaneous-treatments single case design with fictitious data is shown in Exhibit 7.5.

The baseline data are collected in both sessions prior to introducing the treatment. Once stable baselines are established, the intervention phase B begins with the first treatment introduced in session one and the second treatment introduced in session two. The presentation of treatments is subsequently counterbalanced from day to day for the remainder of intervention. If one treatment is shown to be superior to the other treatment, the superior treatment may be continued in both sessions during phase C. The intervention is concluded when the treatment effect is clearly demonstrated, and an optional phase D begins. Phase D is a maintenance phase wherein the investigators observe the treatment's carryover effect.

The simultaneous-treatments design is an alternative design for comparing the effects of two treatments applied concurrently, but it has some limitations. First, the design can include additional treatments, but it is difficult to balance more than two treatments at a time. Therefore, two simultaneous treatments are optimal. Second, multiple treatment interference is a threat to internal validity. The design depends on treatments that have little or no carryover effect from treatment to treatment, and multiple-treatment interference is sometimes difficult to detect.

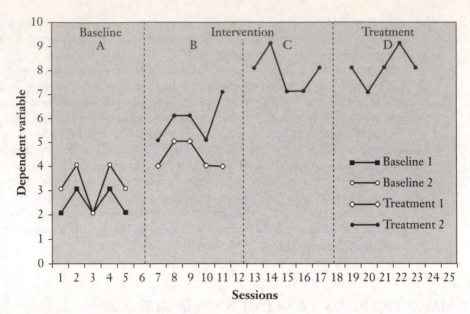

EXHIBIT 7.5
The Basic Simultaneous-Treatments Single Case Design

Overall, the simultaneous-treatments single case design is an alternative time-series design that is especially well suited for comparing two or more treatments. However, it requires diligent planning and careful implementation for valid results.

■ ■ ■ ■ ■

CASE EXAMPLE
The Simultaneous-Treatment Single Case Design

Meline, Gonzalez, Florez-Sabo, and Hinojosa (2004) employed a variation of the simultaneous-treatment single case design. Meline et al. (2004) examined the effects of two different treatments (modeling and paired reading) on third-grade children's reading performances, both reading accuracy and reading rate. Meline et al. (2004) counterbalanced reading passages as well as the two treatments of the independent variable.

Exhibit 7.6 displays Meline et al.'s (2004) results for one of the four participants. In this example, the dependent variable was reading rate. Baseline data are recorded in the A phase, and treatment data are recorded in the B phase. The baseline data (sessions 1–4) were horizontally stable, which indicated a stable baseline response. However, the overall slope across sessions 1 to 12 departed significantly from the horizontal plane, which suggested a positive treatment effect. The difference between the modeling and paired reading treatments did not prove to be significant.

Another indicator of treatment effects is known as the *percentage of non-overlapping data (PND)*. The PND is calculated as the percentage of data values in the treatment phase (phase B) that exceeds the largest data value in the baseline phase (phase A). In Meline et al.'s (2004)

TECHNOLOGY NOTE

Because single case research depends on visual displays of data for its interpretation, the production of suitable line graphs is important. There are numerous computer software packages with tools for creating graphs; however, most are not suitable for single case designs. An excellent resource for creating line graphs for single case designs is a technical article by Carr and Burkholder (1998). They described step-by-step instructions for creating *A-B-A-B* and *multiple-baseline* graphs with *Microsoft Excel*. The Carr and Burkholder (1998) examples were based on *Excel 97 for Windows/NT* and *Mac OS* operating systems, but their instructions are adaptable to newer versions of *Excel*. An advantage of preparing graphs in a spreadsheet program is that the data can be stored and analyzed in the same program.

case, 100% of the data in phase B exceeded the largest value in phase A. Thus, the treatment was evaluated as "very effective." Typically, a PND of greater than 90% is interpreted as "very effective"; a PND between 70% and 90% is "moderately effective"; and a PND of less than 70% suggests a weak effect or no effect at all. The PND is usually a reliable indicator of treatment effectiveness, but it is not a reliable indicator in every case (Scruggs & Mastropieri, 2001). For example, the PND metric is not sensitive to slope changes, and it is influenced by the number of observations.

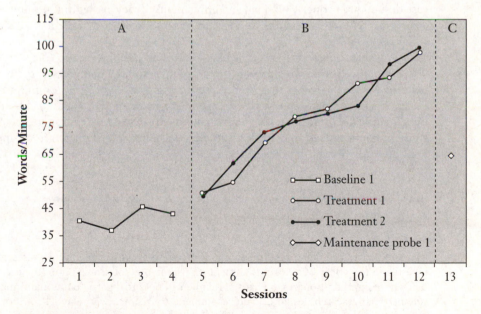

EXHIBIT 7.6
Case Example: The Simultaneous-Treatment Single Case Design with a Maintenance Probe
Meline et al. 2004.

In addition to the usual baseline and treatment phases, Meline et al. (2004) introduced a maintenance probe (phase C) (a) to test carryover effects with a novel reading passage and (b) to test the possible effect of "repeated readings." Though Meline et al. (2004) counterbalanced their presentation of reading passages in the treatment phase, repeated readings (a potential nuisance variable) may have contributed to the observed change in reading performance. Exhibit 7.6 shows that the participant's reading performance declined in phase C but remained significantly above the baseline performance.

Based on what you have learned, answer the following questions: What does the result in Exhibit 7.6's phase C suggest about carryover effects and the possible effects of repeated readings? How could Meline et al. (2004) have strengthened the maintenance phase in their study? How might you employ the simultaneous-baseline single case design to compare the effects of two different assistive hearing devices on speech discrimination?

CONCLUSION

The single case designs that we discussed are underutilized in communication disorders research. If you search the ASHA journals database, you may not find many contemporary examples of single case designs. It may be that veteran researchers and prospective researchers are less familiar with the elements of single case designs than traditional group designs. Another factor may be that some investigators view single case designs as inadequate for answering research questions. However, when single case designs are properly planned and implemented, they are legitimate alternatives for answering research questions in communication disorders—and they are superior in some respects.

A particular *strength* of single case controlled designs is their focus on individuals. A *limitation* is their weakness in generalizing results to members of the target population. A special strength of single case designs is the ability to examine treatment effects in a maintenance phase where carryover effects can be evaluated. Though carryover is clinically important, the maintenance of treatment effects is a neglected area of study in communication disorders. Single case controlled designs are an appropriate method for investigating these effects.

CASE STUDIES

Case 7.1: Problem of Limited Resources
Ms. McCarthy, a clinician-researcher, and Professor Schmitt are planning a research study to investigate the effect of a novel treatment on 6-year-old children's phonological behaviors. They have limited resources in terms of numbers of potential participants and time. As a consultant, what research design do you recommend to Ms. McCarthy and Professor Schmitt? What are the benefits and limitations of following your recommendations?

Case 7.2: Quest for Evidence of Maintenance
A team of four researchers are planning a collaboration to investigate the short-term and long-term carryover effects of a proven intervention for reading comprehension skills. What

are your recommendations for a plan to achieve their research goals? What benefits and limitations are related to your recommendations?

Case 7.3: Balancing Ethics with Scientific Inquiry
Mr. Scott, a clinician-researcher, and Dr. Salinas, a veteran research scientist, are collaborators in a study that aims to explore the effects of training on certain conversational behaviors. They planned to implement an A-B-A single case design, but objections were raised by the Institutional Review Board as well as from teachers of the prospective participants. What are the researchers' alternatives in this case?

Case 7.4: The Difficulty of Choosing a Design
Marilyn is highly motivated to do a thesis project, but she is debating the economics of different research designs. She wants to answer a question about the clinical value of two intervention approaches. Which approach is the most effective? Marilyn anticipates finding 5 to 10 patients who will volunteer for her study. What types of research designs would be most appropriate for Marilyn's thesis?

Case 7.5: Making Sense of Single Case Results
Joy has completed her senior thesis with the A-B-A-B single case design as her method of study. Though the visual inspection of results is favorable, she wants to use some quantitative measures to confirm her tentative conclusions. What do you recommend?

STUDENT EXERCISES

1. Search the communication disorders journals for a research report that includes a single case quasi-experimental design and evaluate the investigators' implementation of the design including baseline and intervention phases.

2. Locate an example of an A-B-A or A-B-A-B single case design in the communication disorders research literature. How did the researchers address the issue of external validity? How could they have evaluated carryover of the treatment effect?

3. Evaluate the investigators' conclusions in a research report that employs a single case design, such as an A-B-A-B or multiple-baseline design. How are the researchers' conclusions related to the results? Are the research conclusions accurately stated?

4. Search the communication disorders journals for a research report that includes a comparison of two groups of participants in a group design. Explain how the investigators might have used a single case design to answer their research questions—and discuss the advantages and disadvantages of each design choice (group vs. single case).

5. Locate a single case design in a research report and evaluate the researchers' interpretation of changes in the dependent variable from baseline to intervention (or intervention to baseline). Calculate an effect size for one of their baselines and interpret the result. HINT: You can estimate the values of the dependent variable from the visual displays of results. This task is easier if the figures are enlarged on a copier.

6. Deborah and Frank are asked to debate the relative merits of group versus single case designs for their research methods class. Deborah must argue the merits of group designs, and Frank will argue the merits of single case designs. What are the best debate points for Deborah? What are the best debate points for Frank?

CHAPTER 8

NONEXPERIMENTAL RESEARCH DESIGNS IN COMMUNICATION DISORDERS

observe (əb zûrv′) *v.* to contemplate, detect, discern, discover, distinguish, examine, inspect, perceive, recognize, study, survey, view

Though some researchers look for cause-and-effect relationships, many researchers aim to describe clinical anomalies, discover associations between variables, or document developmental patterns. In these cases, associations and descriptions are primary, and causation is secondary at the best. When cause and effect are not of primary importance, researchers may choose *nonexperimental methods* to answer their research questions.

DISTINCTIVE FEATURES OF NONEXPERIMENTAL APPROACHES

What makes a study nonexperimental? Research designs are nonexperimental when there is no control group or multiple measurements, and the purpose is something other than determining cause and effect. Nonexperimental methods provide rich descriptions of behaviors and associations between behaviors, but they rarely permit cause-effect inferences. Thus, if the purpose is to test the efficacy of a novel treatment or to compare different groups of people, the better choice is an experimental or quasi-experimental design. However, if the purpose is to describe phenomena, explore patterns, or verify associations, nonexperimental methods are the best choice.

To answer questions of a nonexperimental nature, there are many methods available. The most common nonexperimental methods in communication disorders are (a) case studies, (b) ethnographic designs, (c) historical designs, (d) correlational designs,

(e) developmental designs, and (f) surveys. *Case study* and *ethnographic research* types are distinguished by their thorough descriptions of one or more participants' behaviors and traits. The "case study approach" includes a single participant, whereas "ethnographic research" targets a group of individuals who share a common bond such as a specific disability or cultural trait. The following reports are typical of the case study and ethnographic approaches to research in communication disorders.

The Case Study and Ethnographic Approaches

Cox, Lee, Carey, and Minor (2003) adopted the case study approach for an in-depth description of the auditory and vestibular symptoms of one participant who was previously diagnosed with a rare syndrome. The prominent features of the participant's syndrome were vertigo and an opening in the bone above the semicircular canals.

In another study, O'Neil-Pirozzi (2003) applied the ethnographic approach to study education, health problems, and the speech-language abilities of 25 homeless mothers and their children. Both Cox et al. (2003) and O'Neil-Pirozzi (2003) studies were beneficial because they contributed immediate clinical applications as well as ideas for future studies. Case studies and ethnographic methods often lead researchers to investigate the same phenomena but with experimental methods.

The Historical Approach

Historical research is a nonexperimental method that collects data for analysis from existing records. The goals of historical research are to develop hypotheses and construct theories based on the historical evidence. For example, researchers might collect data from clinical records in order to evaluate clinical outcomes. Historical research along with case study and ethnographic approaches are retrospective designs that aim to explain unusual phenomena, construct theories, and serve as catalysts for prospective researchers.

Historical research is valuable in that it often sheds light on the long-term outcomes of clinical interventions. In communication disorders, we know a lot about short-term outcomes but much less about long-term outcomes. The historical approach is a means to examine long-term clinical outcomes. For example, what is the long-term effect of speech therapy on the lives of clients? A retrospective study that looks at historical evidence and includes a 20-year follow-up might answer this question.

The Correlational Method

The *correlational method* is another retrospective approach that is common in communication disorders. Correlational designs examine the degree of a relationship between two or more quantifiable variables. For example, researchers may be interested in the relationship between student grade-point averages (GPAs) and scores on the National Examinations in Speech-Language Pathology and Audiology (NESPA). The NESPA is designed to assess the mastery of professional concepts, so NESPA outcomes and GPAs should be related in some meaningful way. The correlational method evaluates the degree of a relationship between two or more variables without inferring the cause of an effect.

The Developmental Approach

Developmental research is a nonexperimental approach that measures behaviors over a specific period of time. The goal is to identify developmental trends by following a particular behavior over months or years. There are several ways to look at development over time. The differences between methods are mostly due to costs and available resources. If money, time, and other resources are unlimited, the longitudinal method is the best choice. However, most researchers are short of time, money, or other resources, so they rely on cross-sectional or semi-longitudinal approaches to developmental research. The goals are the same, but the latter approaches save considerable costs. Each approach to developmental research has its advantages and disadvantages.

The Survey Method

Survey research is another nonexperimental design with unique applications in communication disorders research. Its goal is to describe the attitudes, beliefs, or behaviors of a particular population of individuals. Surveys are used by pollsters and marketers to gather opinions and to evaluate consumer behaviors. A case example in communication disorders is the mail survey reported by Blood, Ridenour, Thomas, Qualls, and Hammer (2002). They used the survey method to evaluate the job satisfaction of speech-language pathologists (SLPs) in public schools. Based on a 60% return rate for the mailed survey, they concluded that a majority of SLPs are satisfied with their jobs. People's attitudes, opinions, and beliefs change with the influences of culture, economy, and society—so the same survey today could have different results.

Survey research is an effective means to learn about people and their opinions if appropriate methods are followed. However, surveys can be seriously flawed in ways that limit the conclusions or may provide useless information (see the Technology Note on "unfortunate consequences" related to poor survey research).

CORRELATIONAL RESEARCH IN COMMUNICATION DISORDERS

Researchers choose correlational methods to explore relationships because many variables can be examined at one time. The purpose of correlational research is "to discover significant variables in the field situation, to discover relations among variables, and to lay groundwork for later, more systematic and rigorous testing of hypotheses" (Kerlinger, 1973, p. 378). Correlational designs investigate both the direction and strength of a relationship between two variables. The variables are related if the measurement of one variable explains something about the measurement of the other variable.

A perfect relationship between two variables is depicted in Exhibit 8.1. By convention, the dimensions of the graph in Exhibit 8.1 are labeled "X" for the horizontal (abscissa) dimension and "Y" for the vertical (ordinate) dimension. In a visual display, the values of the two variables are plotted according to their coordinates $X_1 Y_1$, $X_2 Y_2$, $X_3 Y_3$, and so on. The solid line in Exhibit 8.1 that slopes upward and to the right depicts a perfect positive relationship between variables X and Y. A perfect positive

TECHNOLOGY NOTE

There are unfortunate consequences related to poor survey research. Because it is relatively easy to do, novices sometimes conduct surveys with good intentions but poor results. When survey methods are careless, the outcomes are of limited value to all. Several recent reports of surveys illustrate the point. Schwartz and Drager (2008) set out to answer the question; What do school-based SLPs know about autism? They emailed questions to more than 400 potential participants in all 50 states. The response rate was less than 20%. The size of response was inadequate to answer their question. Though low in cost, emailing surveys is hazardous. The hazards include incorrect addresses, participants ignoring emails as junk, and loss of emails in spam filters. A second example was a survey aimed at determining whether SLPs use nonspeech oral motor exercises to target children's speech sound problems (Lof & Watson, 2008). The authors reported that they randomly selected SLPs from a subset of the ASHA membership, but they did not explain the method of randomization nor did they identify the subset. Though they mailed surveys to 2,000 potential respondents, there were no follow-up reminders. The result was a response rate of 27.5%—too small for meaningful conclusions. Without careful planning and precise implementation, surveys may provide useless information.

relationship means that variable X increases as variable Y increases in exactly the same increments. The relationship is also linear because the XY coordinates are connected as a straight line, not a curve. If the XY coordinates described a curve, the relationship between the two variables would be curvilinear. The broken line sloping upward and to the left in Exhibit 8.1 depicts a perfect negative relationship between variables X and Y. A perfect negative (inverse) relationship means that variable X decreases as variable

—————— Positive Linear Relationship

- - - - - Negative Linear Relationship

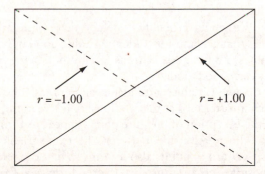

EXHIBIT 8.1
Perfect Positive and Negative Relationships

Y increases in exactly the same increments. The relationship is linear because the XY coordinates form a straight line.

The degree of relationship between two variables is measured along a continuum from –1.00 to +1.00. The sign "+" or "–" indicates the positive or negative *direction* of the relationship. The value of the correlation coefficient (0.00–1.00) indicates the *strength* of the relationship. The value 0.00 indicates no relationship, and the value 1.00 is a perfect relationship. The value 0.50 indicates a moderate relationship between two variables.

Researchers depend on statistical procedures to compute correlation coefficients. The *Pearson Correlation Coefficient* is the statistic of choice when the data are measured at interval or ratio levels. A correlation statistic that is appropriate for ranked data is the *Spearman Rank Correlation Coefficient*. The shorthand notation for Pearson's Correlation Coefficient is *r* (*rho*). The statistical significance of *rho* is evaluated with the *t*-test statistic. The *null* and *alternative* hypotheses for the statistical significance of *rho* are written as follows:

H_0: *rho* = 0
H_1: *rho* <> 0

A closely related statistic is the *index of determination* (rho^2). The index of determination is simply the arithmetic square of the correlation coefficient. It is interpreted as the proportion of variance in Y that is attributable to X. In other words, the index of determination expresses the degree of variance that is shared by two variables. The more two variables have in common, the better the prediction of one variable from the measurement of the other variable. A graph of two variables with shared variances is illustrated in Exhibit 8.2. The illustration depicts an increasing degree of shared variance from top (no overlap) to bottom (complete overlap).

Exhibit 8.3 displays hypothetical data from a class of 10 students. We might expect that grades and class attendance are related in some way. We can speculate that students who attend class regularly will perform better on exams. In this hypothetical case, the correlation between these two variables is calculated as $r = 0.68$. That translates into a 46% overlap (shared variance) between the two variables, which leaves 54% of the shared variance unexplained. In other words, class attendance explains a large proportion of grades but not all.

In this hypothetical case, we would probably conclude that, while attendance matters, there are other variables that account for students' grades, good or bad. Based on what you know about variables and their associations, what other factors are likely to determine whether students earn good grades?

Exhibit 8.4 is a graph of the two variables: attendance and grades. The points of intersection are scattered, which informs us that the relationship between the variables is not perfect. However, with the exception of one, the points appear to form a linear pattern. That informs us that the relationship between the two variables is best described as a straight line. The pattern of points also informs us that the relationship between the two variables is positive, because the pattern trends upward from left to right on the chart.

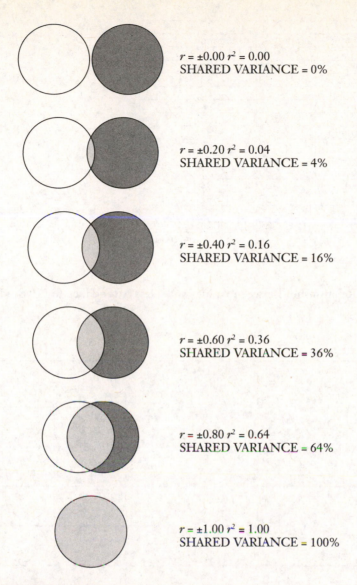

$r = \pm0.00 \; r^2 = 0.00$
SHARED VARIANCE = 0%

$r = \pm0.20 \; r^2 = 0.04$
SHARED VARIANCE = 4%

$r = \pm0.40 \; r^2 = 0.16$
SHARED VARIANCE = 16%

$r = \pm0.60 \; r^2 = 0.36$
SHARED VARIANCE = 36%

$r = \pm0.80 \; r^2 = 0.64$
SHARED VARIANCE = 64%

$r = \pm1.00 \; r^2 = 1.00$
SHARED VARIANCE = 100%

EXHIBIT 8.2
Associations Between Two Variables with 0% to 100% Shared Variances

Student	Grade	Attendance %	
Myra	88	94	
James	58	63	
Maggie	75	78	
John	66	97	
Hope	92	100	
Britney	98	97	
Rex	70	78	
Tanya	85	84	
Bria	80	87	
Jonah	87	84	
Sum =	799	862	
Mean =	79.9	86.2	
SD =	12.52065	11.39005	
			r = 0.68

EXHIBIT 8.3
Hypothetical Relationship Between Grades and Class Attendance for 10 Students

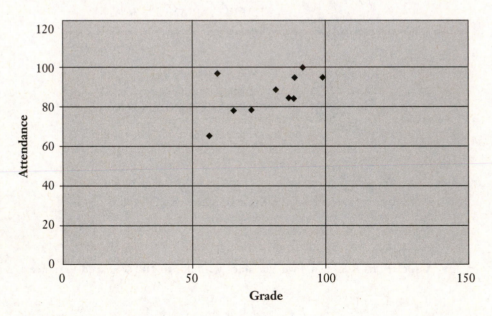

EXHIBIT 8.4
Scatterplot of the Hypothetical Relationship Between Grades and Class Attendance

HISTORICAL NOTE

A cousin to Charles Darwin, Francis Galton (1812–1911) established a laboratory to collect human statistics around 1885. Galton was the first to use correlation to measure associations between human features. He chose the symbol *r* as his index for correlation. While studying human features, Galton collected impressions of fingers in his lab. He determined that the patterns of loops, whorls, and arches could be used to identify individuals. His discovery was adopted by Scotland Yard in 1901. Fingerprint identification remains an important forensic procedure today. A further use of fingerprints that is becoming popular is using fingerprint readers to secure personal computers. A simple fingerprint scan can authenticate the user and unlock the computer system.

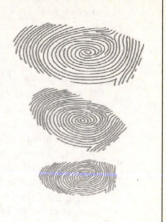

CASE EXAMPLE
Correlational Research

In a collaborative effort, Condouris, Meyer, and Tager-Flusberg (2003) investigated the relationship between scores on standardized tests such as the *Clinical Evaluation of Language Fundamentals* (CELF) and measures of spoken language such as "mean length of utterance" (MLU). They chose the correlation method to study relationships between 11 different variables. In their words, "The main goal of this study was to investigate the relationship between standardized and spontaneous speech measures of language in children with autism" (Condouris et al., 2003, p. 351). They examined associations among the 11 variables—not cause-effect relationships.

TECHNOLOGY NOTE

Correlational research designs require statistical analysis tools to compute the correlation coefficients and to test statistical significance. Statistical analysis tools for correlation are readily available in commercial software packages such as MINITAB, SPSS, and Microsoft Excel. Statistical analysis tools including Pearson's Correlation Coefficient are also available as freeware or shareware. Commercial software such as Microsoft Excel typically includes a worksheet with individual cells where the data are entered. Excel includes an "Analysis ToolPak" that is accessed by clicking "Data Analysis" on the Tools menu. If Data Analysis is not available on Excel's Tools menu, the Analysis Tool-Pak add-in program must be installed. Commercial software packages typically include help screens with examples for guidance.

Their research participants included 7 girls and 37 boys with autism. Condouris et al. (2003) reported 55 correlation coefficients, which ranged from a low of 0.21 (no statistical significance) to a high of 0.92 (statistically significant). The indexes of determination (rho^2) for these correlation coefficients are as follows:

$0.21 = (0.21)^2 = 0.04$

$0.92 = (0.92)^2 = 0.85$

In the latter case, 85% of the variance is shared by the two variables. In the former case, only 4% of the variance is common to both variables.

Condouris et al. (2003) reported a 0.49 correlation coefficient between the CELF and MLU. Though this result was statistically significant, the shared variance for these variables was only 24%—a relatively small degree of commonality. This result makes sense if the CELF and MLU variables measure different behaviors. Indeed, Condouris et al. (2003) speculated that in autism there may be dissociations between the structural and functional aspects of language. Apparently, the CELF and MLU measure somewhat different aspects of language, so clinicians should not rely on one to predict the other. Condouris et al. (2003) concluded their study with some clinical recommendations based on their results.

DEVELOPMENTAL RESEARCH IN COMMUNICATION DISORDERS

Developmental research includes designs that repeatedly measure behaviors over a period of time in order to record developmental trends. The independent variable in developmental studies is *maturation*, whereas the dependent variable is whatever behavior or trait the researchers choose to study. Maturation may be operationally defined as chronological age, but the underlying attributes are the physical and mental changes that take place over time. The basic developmental research types include: (a) longitudinal, (b) cross-sectional, and (c) semi-longitudinal designs. Each of these three developmental research types purport to accomplish the same task, but each one has features that distinguish it from the others.

Longitudinal Research Designs

Longitudinal research designs are actually a family of designs. They all observe the same subjects over some extended period of time. Longitudinal studies are typically one year or more in length. The exact length of a longitudinal study depends on (a) the nature of the behaviors or traits to be studied and (b) the goals established by the researchers. To conduct a longitudinal study, researchers develop a plan that specifies the length of the study and the intervals for measurements. For example, a longitudinal study might be two years in length with measurements of the dependent variable at two-week intervals. A research plan of this sort requires a total of 52 observations over the two-year period. Longitudinal research designs follow the same participants from the beginning of the study to its conclusion. This is a strength that is unique to longitudinal research, but it is also a limitation.

Limitations in longitudinal designs.   Two limitations are inherent in longitudinal research designs. First, the length of longitudinal studies increases the risk of losing participants; *subject mortality* is a known threat to internal validity. Longitudinal research designs are especially vulnerable in this regard. Because of the length of longitudinal studies, there is a significant risk that one or more participants will leave the geographic area or choose to withdraw from the study for personal reasons. Second, longitudinal studies require adequate human resources and finances to sustain the study for its duration.

CASE EXAMPLE
Longitudinal Research in Communication Disorders

Catts, Fey, Tomblin, and Zhang (2002) collaborated in what was a large undertaking: to examine reading outcomes for 570 children with language impairments. Their research method was longitudinal. Catts et al. (2002) began their study with a sample of 604 participants, but 34 of the 604 participants were lost to attrition. They collected data in kindergarten, second, and fourth grades. Thus, their study spanned a period of nearly five years.

Loss of participants is a special problem with longitudinal studies. The threat is proportionate with the length of the study. Longer studies have a greater likelihood of attrition. The loss of 34 of 604 participants (5½%) that Catts et al. (2002) reported is small for a five-year study. Researchers who undertake longitudinal studies must anticipate losses based on their participants' characteristics. If participants are likely to move away, expire, or otherwise drop out of the study, researchers recruit enough participants to make up for the expected loss.

Catts et al. (2002) successfully completed their longitudinal study and concluded that children identified as language impaired in kindergarten were at high risk for reading problems in the second and fourth grades. They could have used a different approach and saved costs but would have sacrificed in other ways.

Cross-Sectional Research Designs

An alternative that addresses the limitations in longitudinal studies but retains the features of developmental research is the *cross-sectional method*. The cross-sectional method lessens the threat of participant loss and reduces costs. Rather than observe the same participants over an extended period of time, cross-sectional designs include several different groups of participants. Each group of participants represents a different point in time along the developmental continuum. The time period for observation may be as short as one day or as long as several months.

Limitations in cross-sectional designs.   The cross-sectional method saves time and other resources but suffers from limitations of another kind. Whereas longitudinal designs risk a loss of participants, cross-sectional designs are relatively safe in that regard because of the shorter time period. However, cross-sectional designs include a threat to internal validity known as *nonequivalence*. Because cross-sectional designs include groups with different chronological ages, the participants must be carefully matched to ensure equivalence in all respects except age.

CASE EXAMPLE
Cross-Sectional Research in Communication Disorders

Preisser, Hodson, and Paden (1988) utilized the cross-sectional method in their study of phonological development. Preisser et al. (1988) collected evidence of children's normal phonological development from 18 months to 29 months of age. To accomplish this task, they recruited 60 children, with 20 children in each of three age groups: 18 months, 22 months, and 26 months. Participants were observed at preplanned intervals over a period of three months, so that phonological development was observed in group one from 18 to 21 months of age, group two from 22 to 25 months, and group three from 26 to 29 months. As a result, Preisser et al. (1988) recorded changes in phonological development over a span of 11 months; however, the task was completed in 3 months. To accomplish the same task, a longitudinal study would have taken 11 months to complete. The validity of their results depends on how effectively they matched participants.

Semi-Longitudinal Research Designs

The *semi-longitudinal method* combines features of the longitudinal and cross-sectional approaches. The semi-longitudinal approach requires more time to complete than cross-sectional designs but less than longitudinal designs. It includes two or more groups of participants who represent different points on the developmental continuum, similar to the way participants in cross-sectional designs are selected. The semi-longitudinal approach differs from the cross-sectional method in that it follows participants for an extended period of time such as 6 to 12 months.

Limitations in semi-longitudinal designs.   "Group equivalency" is a threat to the internal validity of semi-longitudinal studies, but the threat is lessened by the longitudinal component of the design. The semi-longitudinal approach is not as economical as the cross-sectional design, but it is less costly than the longitudinal approach. Overall, the semi-longitudinal method is a compromise approach that combines features of both cross-sectional and longitudinal approaches.

CASE EXAMPLE
Semi-Longitudinal Research in Communication Disorders

Williams and Elbert (2003) adopted the semi-longitudinal method to study phonological development in five late-talking children. They followed two participants at 22 months of age for a period of 10 months and three participants at 30–31 months of age for a period of 12 months. Williams and Elbert collected monthly language samples from each of the five participants. They reported that three of their five participants resolved their late onset of speech by 35 months of age, but two participants did not.

SURVEY RESEARCH IN COMMUNICATION DISORDERS

The primary goal of survey research is to investigate the characteristics of a population by collecting representative samples. If each and every member of a population is surveyed, the result is known as a *census*. To obtain a census, researchers must identify every member of a population and collect observations from each member. A census is rarely undertaken, because costs are prohibitive and not all members of the population can be contacted. For these reasons, researchers rely on samples to generalize results to populations, but the quality of a sample affects the quality of the inference. *Inference* is the act or process of reaching a conclusion about the population based solely on what is known about the sample.

Sampling Issues in Survey Designs

There are many types of sampling methods. The basic method is known as *simple random sampling*. To achieve an unbiased sample, researchers must ensure that every member of a population has an equal chance of being included in the sample. The simple random sampling method includes two steps: (a) Identify the members of the population such as all speech-language pathologists working in schools, and (b) randomly select a sample of members from the population.

Fairness is an important consideration in sampling research, and *bias* is a threat to the fairness of a sample. There are three common sources of bias in samples: (a) failure to identify all members of the population, (b) choosing a sample based on convenience such as students in a class or patients in a clinic, and (c) constituting a sample from volunteers. In the latter case, the sample may be biased if participants volunteer for personal reasons such as financial need or other reasons that make them fundamentally different from nonvolunteers.

No matter how much care is taken to achieve a representative sample from the population, there will be some *sampling error* as a result of simple random sampling. However, sampling error can be minimized by gathering a sample of adequate size. Thus, in a population with 1,000 members, a random sample of 100 participants is probably adequate to generalize results to the population. However, a random sample of 10 participants from the same population contains too much sampling error to allow inferences to the population.

Exhibit 8.5 displays *The Survey System*'s sample size calculator (Creative Research Systems, 2008). It is freely available online for determining how many people are needed to achieve results that represent the target population. The user must determine the precision of results that is needed by specifying the confidence interval. The

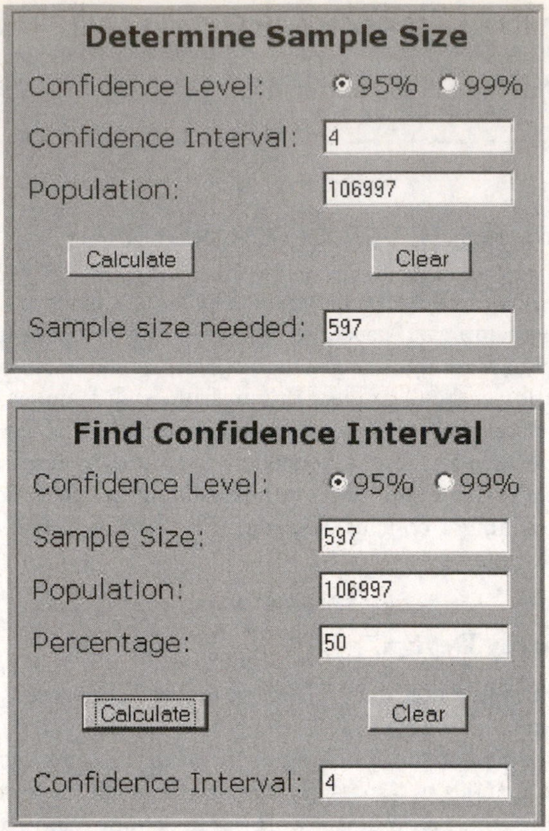

Determine Sample Size

Confidence Level: ⦿ 95%   ○ 99%

Confidence Interval: | 4 |

Population: | 106997 |

[Calculate]   [Clear]

Sample size needed: | 597 |

Find Confidence Interval

Confidence Level: ⦿ 95%   ○ 99%

Sample Size: | 597 |

Population: | 106997 |

Percentage: | 50 |

[Calculate]   [Clear]

Confidence Interval: | 4 |

EXHIBIT 8.5
Online Calculator for Determining Sample Size and Finding Confidence Intervals
Reprinted by permission from The Survey System (2008) by Creative Research Systems http://www.surveysystem.com

confidence level (95% or 99%) tells us how sure we can be of the results. The confidence interval sets the level of precision for our results. For example, if we choose 4 as the interval and 60% of the sample pick a particular answer, we can be confident that if the question had been asked of the entire population 56% (60 − 4) to 64% (60 + 4) of the population would have chosen that answer.

The example in Exhibit 8.5 illustrates the sample size needed if we were to sample the entire population of ASHA members ($N = 106,997$). In this case, the answer is 597. We would need a minimum of 597 responses from ASHA members to meet our needs. However, not every ASHA member that we contact is likely to respond, so we will have to estimate a reasonable response rate. If we estimate that our response rate will be 50% (a relatively high rate), at least 1,194 ASHA members will have to be contacted.

Minimizing Sampling Error

An approach to minimizing sampling error is the use of *stratified sampling*. Typically, stratified sampling is combined with simple random sampling to achieve a high-quality sample. The stratified sampling method divides the population into logical divisions to ensure that each of the divisions (strata) is fairly represented in the sample. For example, the United States is sometimes divided into geographic regions (strata) to ensure that each one is fairly represented in the sample. To ensure that the sample matches the proportion of males and females in the population, males and females are identified and sampled in proportions that match the population proportions (e.g., 105 males per 100 females under 14 years of age based on the 2000 U.S. census). The simple random sampling method is applied within each division to achieve a representative sample.

Other sampling methods are less common than the stratified sampling method. Each alternative method has its advantages and disadvantages. The alternatives to stratified sampling are *cluster sampling*, *purposive sampling*, *snowball sampling*, and *multi-stage sampling*. These methods are useful in special situations, but their limitations may increase sampling error.

Types of Survey Research Designs

The *instrument* that is used to collect data in survey research designs is known as a *survey*. A survey is any procedure that asks questions of respondents—usually taking the form of *questionnaires* or *interview instruments*. Survey instruments are designed to collect data about (a) sociological variables, such as age, gender, social economic status, education, and occupation, or (b) psychological variables, such as opinions, attitudes, and behaviors. Surveys are conducted through regular mail, email, telephone, face-to-face interviews, and webpages.

The questionnaires used in survey research are typically mailed to participants. Questionnaires are economical to administer, and they usually allow the respondent to complete the form at their convenience. However, questionnaires have two shortcomings: (a) The response rate is often poor, and (b) they are not reliable instruments for gathering detailed responses from participants. If the response rate is poor, the sample may not represent the population, and researchers will not be able to generalize results to the population. To maximize response rates, researchers should (a) minimize the

TECHNOLOGY NOTE

In 1986, Eric Thomas invented the automatic mailing list manager—now known as LISTSERV. Before LISTSERV, to join or leave a list, people had to write to the human administrator and ask to be added or removed. This was a time-consuming process especially as discussion lists became more popular. LISTSERV was freeware from 1986-1993, but is now a commercial product. However, a free version that is limited to 10 lists and 500 subscribers can be downloaded at the L-Soft website (http://www.lsoft.com). LISTSERV introduced the first spam filter in 1995.

costs for responding (in, e.g., time, effort, and money), (b) maximize the rewards for responding, and (c) establish trust that those rewards will be delivered. Edwards, Roberts, Clarke, DiGuiseppi, Wentz, Kwan, et al. (2003) recommended three steps to reduce the number of *nonresponders* to postal questionnaires:

1. Contact people before sending the questionnaire.
2. Send questionnaires by first-class mail or recorded delivery and provide a stamped return envelope.
3. Send one or more reminders with a copy of the questionnaire to nonresponders.

To ensure the validity of survey instruments, researchers must carefully choose the content, wording, format, and placement of questions. A successful survey requires substantial planning prior to its use. In contrast to the questionnaire format, interviews are more personal and allow the interviewer to probe for more information or ask follow-up questions. Furthermore, interviews are usually easier for the participants to complete. However, interviews are time consuming, and interviewers must be trained. To conduct a successful interview, interviewers must motivate respondents, mitigate concerns, judge the quality of responses, and avoid interviewer biases that may threaten the validity of the participants' responses. Overall, questionnaire and interview procedures are reliable means for collecting information about a population, but great care is needed to ensure their validity.

Types of Survey Response Formats

Before writing questions, survey researchers should decide what kind of response format best fits their purpose. Responses can be either "structured" or "unstructured." A survey could be all one format or a combination of the two formats.

Filter questions.   The first questions in a survey instrument are usually "filter," or background, questions. The purpose of filter questions is to determine if the respondent is qualified to answer subsequent questions. For example:

> Do you have any experience with children who are autistic? If YES, answer questions 10–15. If NO, skip to question 16.

These kinds of questions help to ensure the validity of responses by discouraging "false responses" from participants who may not be qualified to answer.

The structured response format.   The *structured response* is easiest for participants to answer and easiest for researchers to tabulate responses to. Thus, it is no surprise that most surveys use the structured response format. This format can be structured in many ways. The simplest responses are *fill-in-the-blank* and *true/false formats*. The fill-in-the-blank format requires the participant to indicate a response simply by checking a blank. For example:

> Please indicate the primary language spoken in your home.
>
> _____ English
> _____ Spanish
> _____ Other

An alternative response mode requires participants to state their preference.

Please indicate your preference for the following workplaces. "1" = first choice, "2" = second choice, and so on.

_____ School
_____ Hospital
_____ Private Practice
_____ Skilled Nursing Facility

Trochim (2008) recommended asking the following questions when using these formats:

1. Are all the alternatives covered?
2. Is the list of reasonable length?
3. Is the wording impartial?
4. Is the form of the response easy and uniform?

Another type of structured response involves *scaled choices*. In this format, participants are asked to indicate their response by circling a number. For example:

In-the-canal (ITC) hearing aids are best for most people with hearing loss.

1	2	3	4	5
Strongly Disagree	Disagree	Neutral	Agree	Strongly Agree

The unstructured response format.   There are few *unstructured response formats* from which to choose. The participant typically writes an answer in text. The format can vary from a small comment box (as shown below) to the detailed transcript of the response to an interviewer's question.

What is your opinion regarding mandatory continuing education for professional ethics?

Exhibit 8.6 includes a checklist of items that are useful to help ensure that issues related to (a) the target population, (b) the sample, (c) instrument design, (d) content, (e) possible biases, and (f) administration are addressed when preparing the survey instrument. The questions in Exhibit 8.6 were adapted from Trochim's (2008) survey

EXHIBIT 8.6
A Survey Feasibility Checklist

	YES	NO
POPULATION		
1. Can you obtain a complete list?	☐	☐
2. Is the target population able to read and write?	☐	☐
3. Will the target population cooperate?	☐	☐
4. Are there language or cultural barriers?	☐	☐
5. Are there geographic restrictions that could interfere with the feasibility of the survey?	☐	☐
SAMPLE		
6. Can you contact the sample participants?	☐	☐
7. Can all members of the population be sampled?	☐	☐
8. Are response rates likely to be a problem?	☐	☐
INSTRUMENT		
9. Do you expect to ask personal questions?	☐	☐
10. Will your questions require detailed responses?	☐	☐
11. Can you construct a reasonable sequence of questions?	☐	☐
12. Will you need screening questions (e.g., age, gender, experience)?	☐	☐
CONTENT		
13. Will respondents know about your survey's topic?	☐	☐
14. Will respondents be able to answer questions without help? (e.g., notes or records)	☐	☐
BIAS		
15. Will you be able to avoid the "social desirability" problem? (i.e., respondents may respond to make themselves look better)	☐	☐
16. Can you avoid false respondents?	☐	☐
17. Can you avoid interview/instrument bias?	☐	☐
ADMINISTRATIVE		
18. Can you justify the cost of the survey? (e.g., interview vs. mail)	☐	☐
19. Do you have enough time to gather responses?	☐	☐
20. Do you have sufficiently trained and motivated personnel?	☐	☐

Questions were adapted from Trochim, 2008.

research methods. Before planning a survey, students are advised to consult Trochim's (2008) webpages as well as textbooks that are devoted to the survey topic, such as Dillman's (2007) *Mail and Internet Surveys*.

■ ■ ■ ■ ■

CASE EXAMPLES
Survey Research in Communication Disorders

Case One: A Mail Survey

Kritikos (2003) constructed a 25-item questionnaire to survey speech-language pathologists' beliefs about the language assessment of bilingual/bicultural individuals. She was a doctoral student at the time of the survey. Specifically, Kritikos (2003) asked three questions:

1. Do SLPs differ in their personal efficacy? Personal efficacy involved their confidence in assessing the language of bilingual persons.
2. Do SLPs differ in their general efficacy? General efficacy involved their belief that most SLPs are skilled enough to assess the language of bilingual persons.
3. Do SLPs differ in their likelihood to recommend language intervention with bilingual input?

To answer these questions, Kritikos (2003) proposed a mail survey, but first she constructed a questionnaire with a combination of yes/no, multiple-choice, and scaled-response questions. To improve its validity, a pilot version of the questionnaire was tested and revised more than 30 times based on feedback from participants. Exhibit 8.7 lists examples from Kritikos's (2003) revised questionnaire.

The final version of the questionnaire was mailed to more than 2,000 bilingual SLPs. The population of bilingual SLPs was made up of names provided by state professional associations. From these lists of names, Kritikos (2003) randomly selected 150 SLPs from each of four states: New York, Texas, New Mexico, and California. According to Kritikos (2003), she surveyed only 101 bilingual SLPs in Florida because no more names than this were provided. In addition, 350 monolingual SLPs (236 in Florida) were randomly selected from the same five states.

Kritikos (2003) mailed the surveys with a cover letter, questionnaire, and stamped, self-addressed envelope for the return. There was no mention of incentive to return questionnaires other than the participant's goodwill and professionalism. It is not uncommon for consumer surveys to include a token incentive such as a dollar (sometimes more) to encourage responses. In Kritikos's (2003) case, this would have been expensive, because she mailed questionnaires to 2,337 SLPs. Apparently, it was also unnecessary, because the response rate was 44%—a fairly good response rate from one mailing. She probably could have increased the response rate by following up with a second mailing after four weeks or so. Because 213 of the returns were incomplete, they were discarded as unusable. Thus, the final tally was 811 usable surveys—35% of the total number mailed. Based on the survey results, Kritikos (2003) reported that many SLPs did not feel competent in assessing bilingual clients and recommended further research and education on the topic.

Case Two: A Telephone Survey

Mirrett, Roberts, and Price, (2003) used telephone interviews to collect data for their survey. Their purpose was to describe clinical behaviors, learning preferences, and communication

EXHIBIT 8.7
Selected Items from Kritikos's (2003) Survey Instrument

LEARNING ABOUT THE POPULATION THAT YOU SERVE

How often do you work in each setting?

	NEVER	NOT OFTEN	OFTEN	VERY OFTEN
a. School	1	2	3	4
b. Hospital	1	2	3	4
c. Clinic	1	2	3	4
d. University	1	2	3	4
e. Home Health	1	2	3	4
f. Other _____	1	2	3	4

LEARNING ABOUT YOUR ACADEMIC TRAINING ON BILINGUAL ISSUES

Based on your experience, circle the statement you agree with the most. Who should provide language assessment to bilingual individuals with language problems?

   a. Bilingual Education Specialists   1

   b. English as a Second Language (ESL) Specialists   2

   c. Speech-Language Pathologists   3

   d. Professionals should collaborate   4

   e. Other _____   5

Adapted from Kritikos, 2003, pp. 88–90.

problems of young males with fragile X syndrome (FXS). The target population was SLPs who were treating a child with fragile X syndrome. Specifically, Mirrett et al. (2003) had three goals:

   1. Survey the SLPs' impressions of communication skills.

   2. Survey SLP intervention goals and practices.

   3. Based on survey responses, identify commonly reported syndrome-specific strengths, needs, and behaviors.

     Their participants were 51 SLPs in North Carolina, Virginia, South Carolina, and Georgia who were referred by parents. Mirrett et al. (2003) constructed a 22-question interview form. Their questions were based on a review of the literature on phenotype and development in children with FXS. Examples of their questions are presented in Exhibit 8.8.

     Mirrett et al. (2003) concluded their report with a discussion of some limitations in their survey design as well as clinical implications based on their results. According to the authors, limitations included the small sample size and lack of a control group. However, they noted several themes that were reported by participants. For example, boys with fragile X syndrome

EXHIBIT 8.8
Selected Items from Mirrett, Roberts, and Price's (2003) Telephone Survey
Instrument

Do you or others have trouble understanding *CHILD's* speech?

Yes _____   No _____

a. Overall percent intelligibility (choose one):

   76%-100%   51%-75%   26%-50%   11%-25%   >10%

b. Single words (Choose most representative):

   Clear _____ Intelligible in context _____ Unintelligible _____

c. Generic phrases are:

   Clear _____ Intelligible in context _____ Unintelligible _____

d. Connected speech is:

   Clear _____ Intelligible in context _____ Unintelligible _____

e. Are speech errors developmental or related to a phonological disorder?

   Developmental _____ Dysarthria _____ Dyspraxia _____ Multiple process _____

f. Do you notice any voice quality problems? Yes _____   No _____

   If *yes:*

   Hoarseness _____ Harshness _____ High Pitch _____ Low Pitch _____ Other _____
   (explain) _____

g. Do you notice any rate problems? Yes _____ No _____ If *yes:* Too fast _____ Too
   slow _____

If another clinician called you and said that he/she had just been told he/she would be
working with a child with FXS, what would you tell this person is necessary in order to be
successful (e.g., special knowledge, assistance, strategies)?

Adapted from Mirrett et al., 2003, p. 331.

frequently had difficulty with transitions from task to task or location to location. Thus, they
appeared to benefit from predictable routines and structure. In addition, the boys with fragile X syndrome seemed to learn new concepts and communicate better with a combination of
visual and auditory inputs. Finally, Mirrett et al. (2003) recommended more research to confirm the preponderance of these characteristics in boys with FXS.

Case Three: A Web-Based Survey
Schwartz and Drager (2008) chose to explore the current status of training and knowledge in
autism among school-based speech-language pathologists. Schwartz was a graduate student
pursuing thesis research, and Drager was her advisor. Specifically, Schwartz and Drager (2008)
were interested in answering the following questions:

1. What do SLPs know about autism?
2. What training do SLPs have in autism?
3. How confident are SLPs about providing services for children with autism?

To find answers, they constructed a survey instrument with 52 items divided into four sections: (a) background information (personal information), (b) clinical and educational training (personal information), (c) characteristics of autism, and (d) competency in autism. The first two sections were mostly structured responses in the "check the answer" format. Examples of items from Schwartz and Drager's (2008) survey instrument are provided in Exhibit 8.9.

EXHIBIT 8.9
Selected Items from Schwartz and Drager's (2008) Survey Instrument

---

BACKGROUND INFORMATION

My typical session with a student with autism lasts:

( ) Less than 30 minutes   ( ) 30 minutes   ( ) More than 30 minutes

CLINICAL AND EDUCATIONAL TRAINING

Approximately how much time was spent discussing autism and intervention with students with autism in each of these classes (Check all that apply):

( ) 1 week   ( ) 2 weeks   ( ) 1 month   ( ) 1½ months   ( ) 2 months

CHARACTERISTICS OF AUTISM

The following questions follow a true/false format. Please circle the corresponding letter to your response.

Children must exhibit impaired communication skills to receive a diagnosis of autism.   T   F

COMPETENCY IN AUTISM

Please use the following scale to complete the following questions:

4 — Strongly agree

3 — Agree

2 — Disagree

1 — Strongly disagree

I feel competent that I have enough clinical and educational training to deliver effective intervention in children with autism. _____

Adapted from Schwartz and Drager, 2008, pp. 76–77.

The last two sections of Schwartz and Drager's (2008) survey instrument also included structured responses, but they were a combination of true/false items and scaled items as shown in Exhibit 8.9. The survey instrument was circulated to more than 400 school-based SLPs in 50 states, but the procedures were flawed.

Schwartz and Drager (2008) started with 1,000 potential participants, but they selected a sample of 400 to email. According to the authors, "the e-mail introduced the survey to potential participants and provided a Web link to the online survey" (Schwartz & Drager, 2008, p. 68). Unfortunately, the response rate (those who completed the survey) was only 10%. Schwartz and Drager (2008) addressed the following limitations in their survey of school-based SLPs:

1. The sample size was small.
2. Because the sample was small, only SLPs with an interest in autism may have responded.
3. Although 33 of 50 states were represented, only one state (New York) was represented by more than five participants.
4. The survey instrument did not ask about postgraduate training, such as workshops or other continuing education activities.
5. Some questions on the survey may have confused participants, such as the question that involved the length of time autism was addressed in course work (see Exhibit 8.9).

Based on what you know about Schwartz and Drager's (2008) survey of school-based SLPs, answer the following questions: How might they have increased their sample size? What steps could they have taken to improve their response rate? How would you redesign their question (about the length of time that autism was addressed in course work) to make it less confusing? Schwartz and Drager (2008) concluded SLPs could have benefited from additional training in autism. Is that a valid conclusion based on their results?

CONCLUSION

Not every research question is answered by experimental methods. Nonexperimental alternatives, such as case study and ethnographic approaches, correlation and developmental studies, and surveys are appropriate methods for answering important clinical and nonclinical questions. They are also means to examine phenomena that are not amenable to experimental methods or to explore new phenomena. It is important that investigators implement these methods with the same level of vigor, care, and planning that is common in experimental methods. Whatever the method of study, serious flaws will limit the study's conclusions—or the results may be of no value at all.

CASE STUDIES

Case 8.1: A Case of Too Little Too Late
Professor Little designed a survey instrument to investigate the opinions of students currently enrolled in communication disorders programs about research methods and their importance to clinical practice. A questionnaire was mailed to 1,000 students who were randomly selected

from college programs in a national database. Professor Little received 101 responses within the two months after mailing the questionnaires. What do you see as possible shortcomings in the research plan, and what are Professor Little's options?

Case 8.2: Case of the Chicken and Egg
SLPs Terrence and Mathis collected data for 10 variables related to reading performance, but they are not sure how to interpret the results. Terrence and Mathis believe that some of the variables are causally related to other variables. Their results included several statistically significant correlation coefficients with the values 0.72, 0.49, and 0.60. How should they interpret the results?

Case 8.3: The Long and the Short of It
Researchers Eggers and Gomez have done extensive planning for a longitudinal study of 80-year-old men with aphasia. They expect the study to last five years with measurements at one-month intervals. Eggers and Gomez have identified 22 participants and expect at least 20 to complete the study. As a consultant who specializes in research design, what problems do you foresee, and what alternatives do you recommend?

Case 8.4: The Problem with Spam Filters
Victor and Shirley are collaborating in a survey to determine attitudes toward people who stutter. They have designed a survey instrument and plan to email it to a representative sample of the target population. However, they know that email is sometimes ignored by recipients, or it can be intercepted by spam filters. What ideas can you give them to help ensure that their response rate will be at least 40%?

Case 8.5: How Many Participants Are Needed?
Beatrice expects to survey students who attend her school. There are a total of 14,670 students in the target population. Her survey instrument includes 25 true/false questions. Beatrice wants a 95% confidence in her sample and a precision interval of 5. Given these requirements, she is asking you to help her determine the minimum sample size. What is the minimum sample size needed in this case?

STUDENT EXERCISES

1. Assume that you are planning longitudinal research that will follow 20 adolescents to adulthood, a total of eight years. What can you do to counter the potential problem of subject mortality?
2. Random selection is necessary in survey research to ensure that the sample from the population is a fair sample (unbiased). How would you identify the population of kindergarten children with speech problems, and how will you select a random sample of the kindergarten children?
3. *Snowball sampling* was mentioned as an alternative for choosing samples from populations but was not discussed. What is snowball sampling, and how is it employed to sample a population?
4. Locate a correlational research design in a recent report in communication disorders. What is the independent variable? What are the dependent variables? How did the researchers explain the strength of the correlation coefficients?

5. Design a short questionnaire to survey opinions of classmates on a topic of your choice. Conduct a simple random sample of the population of students and analyze the results. Do the results represent the opinions of the population of students?

6. Locate a survey reported in one of the professional periodicals. Evaluate the population, the sample size, and response rate. Based on your findings, are their conclusions justified? Do the authors discuss the limitations of their study? What are they?

PART III

TESTING HYPOTHESES IN COMMUNICATION SCIENCES AND DISORDERS RESEARCH

CHAPTER 9

HYPOTHESIS TESTING IN COMMUNICATION DISORDERS RESEARCH

error (ĕr′ər) *n.* a mistake; the difference between a measured value and a true or theoretically correct value

Typically, researchers seek to discover relationships between two or more variables. To this end, they develop hypotheses about the variables of interest prior to beginning an experiment. What are hypotheses? *Hypotheses* are statements that describe the proposed relationship between two or more variables.

Hypothesis testing is a binary decision-making process. Hypotheses are either accepted or rejected based on statistical tests. The goal of hypothesis testing is to use the data that is collected from samples to accept or reject the hypothesis. The possibility of errors is important to researchers because scientific endeavors demand a high degree of reliability. For this reason, minimizing the risk of errors is critically important to the hypothesis-testing process.

THE HYPOTHESIS-TESTING PROCESS

Hypothesis testing begins with a statement of the hypothesis and ends with the decision to accept or reject the hypothesis. The hypothesis-testing process includes six steps: (a) state the hypothesis, (b) set a level of risk, (c) choose a sample size, (d) determine the critical value, (e) compute the test statistic, and (f) reject or accept the hypothesis. Each step requires careful planning to ensure that the standards of scientific inquiry are met.

Step One: State the Hypothesis

Hypotheses are an integral part of the class of mathematical measurement known as inferential statistics. The two major classes of statistics are called *descriptive* and *inferential*. *Descriptive statistics* serve to organize, summarize, and describe data without inferring anything about the population. In contrast, *inferential statistics* make conclusions about populations from sample data. To illustrate, researchers might hypothesize a difference between the group means of adults with aphasia and those without aphasia for memory skills. In doing so, researchers make suppositions about the whole population of adults with aphasia. To make reliable decisions about research hypotheses, researchers consider two opposing points of view. These opposing points of view are (a) the null hypothesis and (b) the alternative hypothesis.

The null hypothesis.   To test a statistical hypothesis, what to expect when the hypothesis is true must be known. Thus, researchers hypothesize the opposite of what they expect. For example, if researchers want to demonstrate that one treatment method is more effective than another, they could hypothesize that the two methods are equally effective. This is known as a *null hypothesis* (H_o) because the researchers hypothesized no difference between the two treatment methods. The null hypothesis is usually stated in terms of no relationship between variables or no difference between groups. Freund (1988) offered the following analogy to explain the null hypothesis.

> The idea of setting up a null hypothesis is common even in non-statistical thinking. It is precisely what we do in criminal proceedings, where an accused is presumed to be innocent until his guilt has been established beyond a reasonable doubt. The presumption of innocence is a null hypothesis (p. 289).

The alternative hypothesis.   The statement of the expected result of a research study is known as the alternative hypothesis (H_A). For example, Cannito and Kondraske (1990) hypothesized that participants with spasmodic dysphonia would perform significantly slower than participants without spasmodic dysphonia on complex motor sequencing tasks. The Cannito and Kondraske (1990) hypothesis was based on their extensive review of the existing research literature. In practice, researchers usually do one of the following: (a) state the null hypothesis, (b) state the alternative hypothesis, or (c) state no hypothesis at all. Most reports state the alternative hypothesis and leave it to readers to infer the null hypothesis. The best practice is to state the null hypothesis, alternative hypothesis, or both.

Step Two: Set an Acceptable Level of Risk

There are *four possible outcomes* when testing a research hypothesis: (a) the null hypothesis is accepted when it is true (correct decision), (b) the null hypothesis is rejected when it is false (correct decision), (c) the null hypothesis is rejected when in reality it is true (Type I error), or (d) the null hypothesis is accepted when in reality it is false (Type II error). Exhibit 9.1 shows the four possible outcomes when testing hypotheses.

Decision

	Accept H_0	Reject H_0
H_0 True	Correct Decision	Type I Error
H_0 False	Type II Error	Correct Decision

Reality

EXHIBIT 9.1
Four Possible Outcomes in Hypothesis Testing

The *decision box* in Exhibit 9.1 includes the two incorrect decisions and two correct decisions. The incorrect decisions are referred to as Type I and Type II errors. The probability of a Type I error is designated by the Greek letter α (alpha). The probability of a Type II error is designated by the Greek letter β (beta). Alpha is always specified by the researcher before data collection begins. However, the value of beta cannot be determined unless the population parameters are known. Beta is seldom specified, because research in communication disorders usually involves populations with unknown parameters. For example, disfluency is a common dependent variable, but its exact variation in the population is unknown. Even if beta cannot be specified, we know that the relationship between alpha and beta is an inverse one. If other factors are constant, an increase in alpha is accompanied by a decrease in beta, and a decrease in alpha is accompanied by an increase in beta.

A Type I error is considered the more serious of the two possible errors. In other words, the risk of rejecting a true null hypothesis (a Type I error) is potentially more damaging than making a Type II error. This is particularly true in medical research, where rejecting a true null hypothesis (i.e., committing a Type I error) can have serious consequences for human life. For this reason, alpha is conventionally set at the conservative level of .05 or less. Thus, researchers guard against the likelihood of concluding that a treatment works when it may not.

When α is equal to .05, this means that the researcher is willing to risk a Type I error 5 out of 100 times. Alternatively, when α is equal to .01, the researcher is willing to risk a Type I error only 1 out of 100 times. The best practice in communication disorders is to adopt the .05 level of confidence as the criterion for accepting or rejecting the null hypothesis.

Step Three: Choose the Sample Size

The sample size (n) determines: (a) the probability distribution to be used and (b) the power of the test. For example, the z *statistic* (i.e., standard normal distribution) requires relatively large samples ($n > 30$). However, the t *statistic* (and its distribution) is appropriate for small samples ($n < 30$) when certain assumptions are met. *Power* is defined as the probability of rejecting the null hypothesis when it is false—a correct decision. Sample size is one of several factors that influence the power of a statistical test. A larger sample usually results in a more powerful test of the null hypothesis. The conclusions drawn from studies with small samples such as $n < 10$ are a high risk for accepting the null hypothesis when it is false (Type II error).

Step Four: Determine the Critical Value

Statistical hypothesis testing requires a cutoff point that can be used to separate sample results that should lead to rejecting H_o from the sample results that should lead to accepting H_o. This cutoff point is known as the *critical value*. Critical values are found by using tables for the standard normal distribution or Student's t distribution. The critical value depends on (a) *alpha*—the level at which the researcher agrees to accept or reject H_o—and (b) the alternative hypothesis (H_A).

Alternative hypotheses.   There are two types of alternative hypotheses: (a) one-tailed (directional) and (b) two-tailed (nondirectional) hypotheses. A *one-tailed hypothesis* predicts the direction of results. For example, a researcher might hypothesize that treatment A is better than treatment B. This is a directional hypothesis. In contrast, a *two-tailed hypothesis* does not predict the direction of results. For example, a researcher might hypothesize that treatment A is different from treatment B but not predict which treatment is better. Exhibit 9.2 illustrates the sampling distribution for a one-tailed hypothesis test.

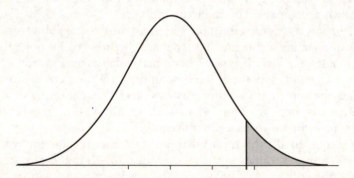

EXHIBIT 9.2
Sampling Distribution for a One-Tailed (Directional) Hypothesis Test

The rejection region.   The shaded area in Exhibit 9.2 extends from the cutoff point (i.e., the critical value) and divides the distribution into two regions. The area to the left of the shaded area is the rejection region while the shaded area is the acceptance region.

The rejection region can be located in either tail depending on the direction (+ or –) specified by the alternative hypothesis. If the expected result is a positive difference, the rejection region is located in the right tail. If the expected result is a negative difference, the rejection region is located in the left tail. When the test statistic (i.e., observed value) is less than the critical value, the null hypothesis is rejected. When the test statistic is greater than the critical value, the null hypothesis is accepted. Exhibit 9.3 depicts a two-tailed hypothesis test.

The two-tailed hypothesis test divides the rejection region equally between the two ends of the distribution. If other factors are constant, a one-tailed test is more powerful than a two-tailed test because the rejection region is larger—concentrated on one end of the sampling distribution. A two-tailed test divides the rejection region in halves—half in each tail. Thus, in the case of a two-tailed text, the probability of rejecting the null hypothesis is reduced.

In the case of the z statistic, the critical value is a standard score. For example, if $\alpha = .05$ and H_A is one-tailed, the critical value is -1.645 (1.645 standard deviation units below the population mean). If $\alpha = .05$ and H_A is two-tailed, the critical value is ± 1.96—almost two standard deviation units above or below the population mean. Because it is easier to reject the null hypothesis, a one-tailed test is more powerful. However, the use of one-tailed alternative hypotheses has been criticized for several reasons: (a) A one-tailed test ignores the possibility of an unexpected difference in the opposite direction; (b) a one-tailed test is more vulnerable to error if the distribution is not normal; and (c) a one-tailed test might be adopted when a two-tailed test is more appropriate.

Several guidelines are useful for planning research as well as for evaluating research reports. First, hypotheses should be two-tailed unless there is compelling evidence that the expected result will be directional. Second, the choice of directional or nondirectional hypotheses should be decided before a study begins. Third, researchers

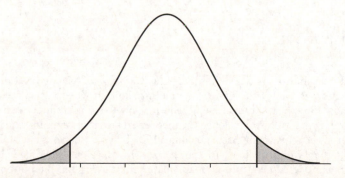

EXHIBIT 9.3
Sampling Distribution for a Two-Tailed (Nondirectional) Hypothesis Test

should provide a sound rationale when electing one-tailed hypotheses. An illustration is Yoder's (1989) study in which one-tailed hypothesis tests were elected. Yoder (1989) explained that one-tailed tests were justified because the purpose was to replicate the results of an earlier study, confirming a relationship between maternal speech and children's language learning.

Step Five: Compute the Test Statistic

The *test statistic* is a standard score such as z or a t statistic. These scores indicate the number of standard errors the sample statistic is from the hypothesized parameter. The general formula for a test statistic (i.e., observed value) is stated in equation 1.

$$\text{Test statistic} = \frac{\text{statistic} - \text{parameter}}{\text{standard error of the statistic}} \qquad (\text{eq.1})$$

The choice of a test statistic depends on several factors: (a) the hypothesis, (b) the distribution of the target population, (c) sample size, and (d) other sample characteristics. For example, if researchers hypothesize a difference between two sample means, the t statistic is an appropriate test statistic. However, if the population is not normally distributed, a nonparametric (distribution free) statistic may be more appropriate. *Nonparametric tests* are a special class of inferential statistics that do not depend on the population conforming to a prescribed shape, because the raw data are replaced by their ranks. A common nonparametric test is the Mann-Whitney U test (also known as the Wilcoxon rank sum test), but there are nonparametric tests to fit most experimental designs.

Step Six: Make a Decision About H_o

After the test statistic is calculated, it is compared to the *critical value*. If the test statistic's absolute value exceeds the critical value, the null hypothesis is rejected. If the test statistic does not exceed the critical value, the null hypothesis is accepted. If the null hypothesis is rejected, the alternative hypothesis is supported but not necessarily

TECHNOLOGY NOTE

The normal distribution is also known as the *Gaussian distribution* because Carl Friedrich Gauss was one of the first to use the distribution when he analyzed astronomical data in 1809, but Abraham De Moivre [du mwA'vru] is credited with the discovery circa 1733. De Moivre developed the theoretical distribution years before Gauss was born, but his paper was not discovered until 1924 by Karl Pearson. De Moivre also pioneered the theory of probability in *The Doctrine of Change* published in 1718. Born in Paris, Abraham De Moivre tutored mathematics for a living but died in poverty in 1754.

proven. Kerlinger (1979) described research outcomes as continually better approximations of the truth but never attaining complete truth. Furthermore, a result may be statistically significant but not of any practical value because statistical significance alone indicates the reliability of accepting a research hypothesis but not the importance of the result. In practice, clinicians are concerned with clinical relevance, and a statistically significant result may not be clinically relevant. Clinical significance is determined by several factors, and one of those factors is *effect size*, which is an indicator of practical significance. The notion of practical significance is an especially important one for evidence-based clinical practice (Meline & Paradiso, 2003).

THE NORMAL DISTRIBUTION

Many variables in communication disorders are continuously distributed as opposed to being placed into discrete categories. A *distribution* is simply a pattern of scores. The distribution of a variable provides information about individual cases as well as information about the group of scores. The distributions for categorical variables are displayed in bar graphs, whereas the distributions for continuous variables are usually displayed in line graphs or histograms.

The *normal distribution* is the most important one of many statistical distributions. The normal distribution is a theoretical distribution based on the general equation developed by the French mathematician De Moivre (1667–1754). It provides a model for evaluating the distributions of many real-life variables. In addition, normal distributions are useful for determining the probability of certain outcomes. De Moivre developed the general equation by observing games of chance. For example, a coin flip produces two possible outcomes: heads or tails. Each possibility has an equal chance of occurring. The probability of tails is 1:2, i.e., one possibility of tails divided by two possible outcomes. If enough coins are flipped, the distribution of outcomes should approximate De Moivre's normal distribution. In other words, half the outcomes will be tails and half will be heads. However, some of the coins in the sample will not be fair. For example, an individual coin may land heads 7 times out of 10 flips. Another coin may favor tails. Nonetheless, the pattern of outcomes for the totality of coins in the sample will approximate a normal distribution with a bell shape such as shown in Exhibit 9.4. The normal distribution has the following characteristics:

1. The normal distribution is *unimodal* (i.e., with one mode at the center). A bimodal distribution would have two modes.
2. The normal distribution is *symmetrical* (i.e., the right half mirrors the left half). It has its maximum height (ordinate) where Z is equal to zero and is symmetrical around that point. The mean and median are at the center, and 50% of the scores are below the center point, and 50% of the scores are above the center point.
3. The normal distribution of scores is *continuous* from one tail to the other.
4. The normal distribution is *asymptotic*—the curved line gets closer to the horizontal axis as it moves away from the center but does not meet the axis. Most of the scores are in the middle, with few scores at the edges.

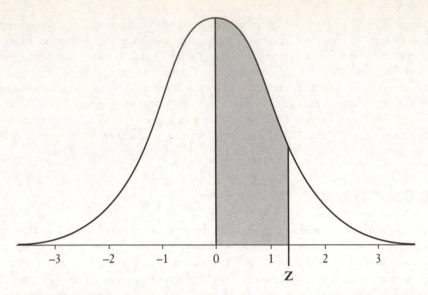

EXHIBIT 9.4
The Standard Normal Distribution

Because different variables have different means and standard deviations, an infinite number of distributions are possible. Although all of these distributions may approximate De Moivre's model, they are not comparable because of their different units of measurement. This problem is resolved by transforming all normal distributions to fit the standard normal distribution.

THE STANDARD NORMAL DISTRIBUTION

The standard normal distribution is a useful tool for describing a normally distributed variable. A normal distribution is a *standard normal distribution* when its scores are expressed in standardized scores (*z* scores). The notion behind the standard normal distribution is that all normal distributions can be converted to a common distribution with the same mean and standard deviation. This common distribution has a mean of zero and a standard deviation of one. The standard normal distribution is shown in Exhibit 9.4.

Because the standard normal distribution has a prescribed mean and standard deviation, the proportion of scores in a given area under the bell-shaped curve is always the same. Thus, the area between −1 and +1 standard deviations always includes 68% of the total distribution of scores. Likewise, the area between −2 and +2 standard deviations includes approximately 95% of the scores, and the area between −3 and +3 standard deviations includes about 99% of the scores. This information is important for determining the probability of an outcome. For example, the likelihood of a score falling ± 2 or more standard deviations from the mean is 5%, or 5 out of 100 times. The shaded area in Exhibit 9.4 includes about 40% of the scores in the total distribution of scores.

Standard Units

A single score in the distribution of scores can be represented by a standard unit of measure known as a *z score*. A z score (standard score) is derived from equation 2.

$$z = \frac{x - \bar{x}}{s} \hspace{4cm} \text{(eq.2)}$$

z = the standard value
x = any one score
$\bar{x}$ = mean of the sample distribution
S = the standard deviation of the sample distribution

The *z score* is a measure of individual location. In other words, it tells us where individual scores are located within a distribution of scores. The z score tells us how many standard deviations the corresponding value of *x* lies above or below the mean. By adopting a standard unit of measure such as the z score, we can easily compare variables that have different scores or units of measurement. For example, if a 5-year-old child obtains a raw score of 59 on the *Test for Auditory Comprehension of Language–3* (TACL-3; Carrow-Woolfolk, 1999) and a score of 60 on the *Peabody Picture Vocabulary Test–III* (PPVT-III; Dunn & Dunn, 1997), a comparison between scores is not meaningful because the test distributions are different. However, a clinician can compare the z scores from the two different assessments with the equivalent standard scores: –1.00 (TACL-3) and 0.00 (PPVT-III). In this example, the TACL-3 score is one standard deviation lower than the PPVT-III score, which could be interpreted as a significant clinical finding.

A table of values known as a *standard normal distribution table* is displayed in Exhibit 9.5. It contains z scores from 0.00 to 3.00 and proportions for the areas between means and *z scores*. For example, the proportion of the area between the mean and a z

TECHNOLOGY NOTE

Microsoft Excel's "NORMDIST" function returns the normal distribution for a selected mean and standard deviation. If the mean is 0 and standard deviation is 1, NORMDIST returns the standard normal distribution. The Excel function NORMDIST returns the standard normal distribution and the area under the normal curve for a given z score. NORMDIST can be used in place of a table of standard normal curve areas. For example, a z score of +0.67 returns an area of 75%, which is the proportion of scores that fall below the z score. A z score of –0.67 returns 25%—the proportion of scores below –0.67. The area between –0.67 and +0.67 is 50%.

Z	0.00	0.01	0.02	0.03	0.04	0.05	0.06	0.07	0.08	0.09
0.0	0.0000	0.0040	0.0080	0.0120	0.0160	0.0199	0.0239	0.0279	0.0319	0.0359
0.1	0.0398	0.0438	0.0478	0.0517	0.0557	0.0596	0.0636	0.0675	0.0714	0.0753
0.2	0.0793	0.0832	0.0871	0.0910	0.0948	0.0987	0.1026	0.1064	0.1103	0.1141
0.3	0.1179	0.1217	0.1255	0.1293	0.1331	0.1368	0.1406	0.1443	0.1480	0.1517
0.4	0.1554	0.1591	0.1628	0.1664	0.1700	0.1736	0.1772	0.1808	0.1844	0.1879
0.5	0.1915	0.1950	0.1985	0.2019	0.2054	0.2088	0.2123	0.2157	0.2190	0.2224
0.6	0.2257	0.2291	0.2324	0.2357	0.2389	0.2422	0.2454	0.2486	0.2517	0.2549
0.7	0.2580	0.2611	0.2642	0.2673	0.2704	0.2734	0.2764	0.2794	0.2823	0.2852
0.8	0.2881	0.2910	0.2939	0.2967	0.2995	0.3023	0.3051	0.3078	0.3106	0.3133
0.9	0.3159	0.3186	0.3212	0.3238	0.3264	0.3289	0.3315	0.3340	0.3365	0.3389
1.0	0.3413	0.3438	0.3461	0.3485	0.3508	0.3531	0.3554	0.3577	0.3599	0.3621
1.1	0.3643	0.3665	0.3686	0.3708	0.3729	0.3749	0.3770	0.3790	0.3810	0.3830
1.2	0.3849	0.3869	0.3888	0.3907	0.3925	0.3944	0.3962	0.3980	0.3997	0.4015
1.3	0.4032	0.4049	0.4066	0.4082	0.4099	0.4115	0.4131	0.4147	0.4162	0.4177
1.4	0.4192	0.4207	0.4222	0.4236	0.4251	0.4265	0.4279	0.4292	0.4306	0.4319
1.5	0.4332	0.4345	0.4357	0.4370	0.4382	0.4394	0.4406	0.4418	0.4429	0.4441
1.6	0.4452	0.4463	0.4474	0.4484	0.4495	0.4505	0.4515	0.4525	0.4535	0.4545
1.7	0.4554	0.4564	0.4573	0.4582	0.4591	0.4599	0.4608	0.4616	0.4625	0.4633
1.8	0.4641	0.4649	0.4656	0.4664	0.4671	0.4678	0.4686	0.4693	0.4699	0.4706
1.9	0.4713	0.4719	0.4726	0.4732	0.4738	0.4744	0.4750	0.4756	0.4761	0.4767
2.0	0.4772	0.4778	0.4783	0.4788	0.4793	0.4798	0.4803	0.4808	0.4812	0.4817
2.1	0.4821	0.4826	0.4830	0.4834	0.4838	0.4842	0.4846	0.4850	0.4854	0.4857
2.2	0.4861	0.4864	0.4868	0.4871	0.4875	0.4878	0.4881	0.4884	0.4887	0.4890
2.3	0.4893	0.4896	0.4898	0.4901	0.4904	0.4906	0.4909	0.4911	0.4913	0.4916
2.4	0.4918	0.4920	0.4922	0.4925	0.4927	0.4929	0.4931	0.4932	0.4934	0.4936
2.5	0.4938	0.4940	0.4941	0.4943	0.4945	0.4946	0.4948	0.4949	0.4951	0.4952

EXHIBIT 9.5
A Standard Normal Distribution Table

score equal to 1.50 is 0.4332 (43%). Because the distribution is symmetrical, the area between the mean and $z = +1.50$ is the same as the area between the mean and $z = -1.5$. Thus, the proportion of the area between −1.5 and +1.5 equals 86%.

Transformed Standard Scores

Because z scores include negative values and decimals, they are somewhat difficult to report and may be misleading to clients, parents, and others. For this reason, z scores are often transformed into a distribution of standard scores with a mean of 100 and a standard deviation equal to 15 units. The transformation is accomplished by multiplying each z score by 15 and adding 100 as shown in equation 3.

$$\text{Transformed score} = (15)\,(z) + 100 \qquad\qquad (\text{eq.3})$$

As a *clinical example*, the Peabody Picture Vocabulary Test-III (Dunn & Dunn, 1997) includes standard score equivalents (transformed standard scores) with a mean of 100 and a standard deviation of 15. The use of standard scores simplifies the interpretation of the scores. The mean is 100 and the standard deviation is 15, but the choice of values for the mean and standard deviation is arbitrary.

Shapes of Frequency Distributions

Data can be distributed in a variety of ways, taking on almost any shape or form. However, most frequency distributions can be described by a small number of standard shapes. The most important of these standard distributions is the bell-shaped normal distribution. However, even if a variable is normally distributed in the population, a sample of the population is not always normally distributed. Thus, other shapes are needed to describe distributions that are not normally distributed.

Skewed Distributions

One class of frequency distributions that are not bell shaped is known as *skewed distributions*. Skewed distributions are not symmetrical. Exhibit 9.6 illustrates the various shapes (i.e., skews) that distributions of data can form. For example, a negatively skewed distribution is pictured in Exhibit 9.6. Skewness is an indicator of symmetry or the lack of symmetry.

A graph is informative because it provides a picture of the degree of skewness. A positively skewed distribution has more scores with larger values toward the left tail, whereas a negatively skewed distribution has more scores with larger values toward the right tail. Note that the tails point in the direction of the skew. Typical positively and negatively skewed distributions are pictured in Exhibit 9.6.

Other Common Shapes for Frequency Distributions

Symmetrical distributions including the normal distribution are characterized by their kurtosis. *Kurtosis* is a measure of peakedness. It measures how fat or thin the tails of a

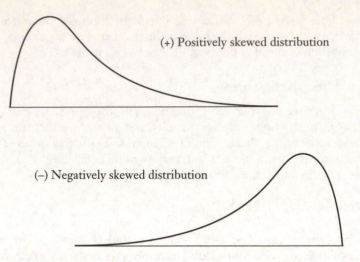

EXHIBIT 9.6
Positively Skewed and Negatively Skewed Distributions

distribution are relative to a normal distribution. A *mesokurtic distribution* such as the normal curve is characterized by a moderate degree of peakedness. If a large proportion of scores are located at the center of the distribution, the distribution is described as *leptokurtic*. *Platykurtic distributions* are characterized by a large proportion of scores in the tails. Exhibit 9.7 depicts the three common shapes for the distributions of scores.

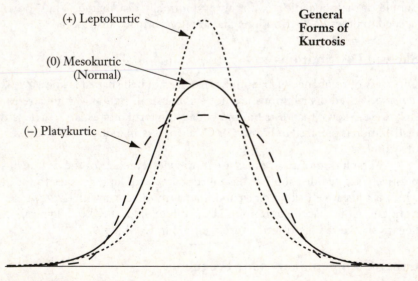

EXHIBIT 9.7
Common Shapes of Distributions

If research requires a precise measure of kurtosis, it is usually calculated as a coefficient of skewness. The tests for skewness and kurtosis are two-sided tests. The null hypothesis to be tested is that the skewness and kurtosis values are zero. One of several tests for skewness is the *Pearsonian coefficient of skewness* (SK). It is a simple statistic for comparing a distribution's mean and median to measure skewness. The formula for SK is shown in equation 4. If a distribution is perfectly symmetrical, the value of SK will equal zero. The distribution of scores becomes more skewed as SK approaches ± 3.00.

$$\text{Coefficient of Skewness (SK)} = \frac{3(\text{mean} - \text{median})}{\text{standard deviation}} \qquad \text{(eq. 4)}$$

THE DISTRIBUTION OF A SAMPLE STATISTIC

A distribution is defined as a pattern of scores. All variables have distributions. For example, height is a variable that is distributed in the population from low to high. Statistics such as means, medians, and standard deviations have distributions as well. *Distribution of a sample statistic* is a basic concept that underlies statistical inference.

Because the sample selected from a population is one of many possible samples, the statistic that is calculated from the sample is only one of many possible statistics. The distribution of a sample statistic tells us how often different values of that statistic should occur if samples of the same size are collected over and over from the same population. An example of the distribution of a sample statistic is known as the *distribution of sample means*.

The Distribution of Sample Means

As an example, consider a population with five cases ($N = 5$) and the scores [3, 5, 7, 9, 11]. The calculations of the population mean (μ) and standard deviation (σ) are shown in equation 5.

$$\mu = \frac{3 + 5 + 7 + 9 + 11}{5} = 7$$

$$\sigma = \sqrt{\frac{(3-7)^2 + (5-7)^2 + (7-7)^2 + (9-7)^2 + (11-7)^2}{5}} = 2.38 \qquad \text{(eq. 5)}$$

Given the population of $N = 5$, there are 10 possible random samples of size $n = 2$ that can be drawn from the population. Exhibit 9.8 lists the 10 samples and their means. The distribution of sample means from our example is displayed in Exhibit 9.9. Distributions such as the one in Exhibit 9.9 are known as probability distributions because they provide information about the chance occurrence of a particular outcome. The distribution of sample means is used to answer questions such as, How often should we expect to observe a mean IQ of 80 in a sample of 30 cases if the mean IQ in the population is 100?

EXHIBIT 9.8
Ten Possible Samples and Sample Means Drawn from a Population of Size N = 5

SAMPLE DATA	MEANS	SAMPLE DATA	MEANS
3, 5	4	5, 9	7
3, 7	5	5, 11	8
3, 9	6	7, 9	8
3, 11	7	7, 11	9
5, 7	6	9, 11	10

Based on the data in our example, what is the chance of observing a mean of 10 with a sample size $n = 2$ if the population mean is 7? Because the number 10 occurs only once in the distribution of 10 sample means, the answer is 0.10 (10%).

What is the chance of the sample mean differing from the population mean by more than 1? In this case, the answer is 40% because 4 of the 10 sample means differ from the population mean by more than 1. It is fairly easy to compute probabilities when the distribution of sample means is known. However, it is usually not practical to construct a distribution of sample means; because the target population is often large in number, the number of possible sample means is unwieldy.

The Standard Error of the Mean

It is not practical to collect all possible samples and then construct a distribution of sample means to determine the variation of a sample mean from the population mean.

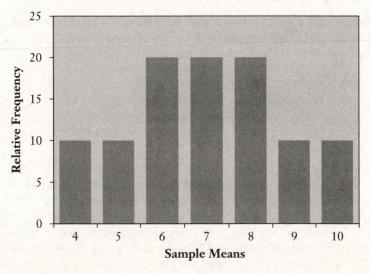

EXHIBIT 9.9
Distribution of Sample Means for a Population of N = 5

However, the information that we need is derived from two theorems that express essential facts about the distributions of sample means. The first of the two theorems says that (a) the mean of the distribution of sample means equals the population's mean, and (b) the distribution of sample means is less variable than the population. In the example, the population's mean equaled 7. The *mean of the sample means* is calculated in equation 6.

$$\mu_z = \frac{4 + 5 + 6 + 6 + 7 + 7 + 8 + 8 + 9 + 10}{10} = 7 \qquad \text{(eq. 6)}$$

Thus, the supposition that the mean of the sample means (μ_x) equals the population mean is supported ($\mu_x = \mu$). The second part of the theorem says that the standard deviation of the sample means is smaller than the standard deviation of the population. The standard deviation of the sample means is known as the *standard error of the mean*, which is abbreviated as *S.E.M.*

To calculate the exact standard deviation of the sample means, the standard deviation of the population (σ) is needed along with the number of cases in the sample (n). The left-most equation in equation 7 expresses the necessary calculation for populations of infinite size. The right-most equation adds a correction factor for finite populations of size N.

$$\text{Exact } S.E.M. = \frac{\sigma}{\sqrt{n}} \text{ or } \frac{\sigma}{\sqrt{n}} \times \sqrt{\frac{N - n}{N - 1}} \qquad \text{(eq. 7)}$$

Because the example involves a finite population ($N = 5$), the second of the two formulas is the correct choice. The standard error of the mean is calculated as 1.73, and the standard deviation of the population is 2.83. Thus the proposition that the distribution of sample means is less variable than the population is supported ($\sigma_x < \sigma$). However, speech-language pathologists and audiologists usually do not know the population parameters for the variables of interest. Fortunately, the second of the two theorems provides a solution. It is known as the *central limit theorem*.

THE CENTRAL LIMIT THEOREM

The central limit theorem (CLT) proposes that the distribution of sample means will be approximately normal if the sample is large enough. Even if a variable is not normally distributed in the population, the sampling distribution will be approximately normal with a large sample. A sample of size $n > 30$ is generally regarded as sufficiently large. Computer simulations involving large sets of data and many sample means are used for demonstrating the validity of the central limit theorem. In fact, with the help of computer simulation, Norušis (1988) has shown that even a uniform distribution has a distribution of sample means that approximates a normal distribution. Thus, the central limit theorem justifies the use of normal-curve methods for solving many statistical problems. It does not matter if the variable of interest is normally distributed in the population, because the means calculated from samples will be normally distributed anyway. On the other hand, if the variable is normally distributed in the population, the distribution of sample means will be normal for samples of any size.

Estimating Population Parameters

If the characteristics of a target population are unknown, the population parameters can be estimated from sample characteristics. This is possible because the central limit theorem says that a sampling distribution of sufficient size is approximately normal. Thus, the standard error of the mean is estimated from the standard deviation of the sample in equation 8.

$$\text{Estimated } S.E.M. = \frac{SD}{\sqrt{n}} \qquad\qquad\qquad \text{(eq. 8)}$$

Point Estimates Versus Interval Estimates

A single number derived from a sample and used to estimate a population value is called a "point estimate." In equation 8, the point estimator was the standard deviation of the sample. However, point estimates present a problem because sample statistics reflect the population parameter but also contain *sampling error*. The sampling error is the difference between the population value and the sample value. Thus, calculations based on point estimates are not exactly correct. Sampling error cannot be eliminated, but it can be managed by using another kind of estimation known as *interval estimation*. Interval estimation builds on point estimates to establish a range of values that we can say with some confidence contains the population parameter. This range of values is known as a *confidence interval* (CI). The general equation for constructing confidence intervals is shown in equation 9.

$$\text{CI} = \text{statistic} \pm (\text{critical value}) \, (\text{S.E. statistic}) \qquad\qquad \text{(eq. 9)}$$

To construct a confidence interval for the population mean, a critical value is chosen. Because the distribution of sample means is assumed to be normally distributed, 95% of the sample means are expected to fall within ± 2 standard errors of the population mean. Thus, the critical value equals 2 for a 95% confidence interval. The critical value will depend on the level of confidence chosen by the researcher. For example, a 90% confidence interval requires a critical value of 1.65. The lower limit of the CI is calculated by subtracting two standard errors from the estimated mean. The upper limit of the CI is determined by adding two standard errors to the estimated mean. For example, if the sample mean is 8 and the S.E.M. equals 1.5, the 95% confidence interval is calculated as shown in equation 10. In this case, the interval is expected to contain the true population mean 95 out of 100 times. The best practice is for researchers to report confidence intervals along with their point estimates.

$$\text{CI}_{95} = 8 \pm (2) \, (1.5) = 6.5 \text{ to } 9.5 \qquad\qquad\qquad \text{(eq. 10)}$$

STUDENT'S *t* DISTRIBUTIONS

For samples of size $n = 30$ and larger, the distribution of a sample statistic can be assumed to be normal. However, samples smaller than 30 present a problem. Fortunately, an alternative distribution is available for small samples. William Gossett, a young chemist who worked on quality control at a brewery in Dublin, made an important discovery circa 1900 (Pearson et al., 1990). Gossett found that, in the case of small samples, the sampling distributions were substantially different from the normal distribution. Gossett also noted that the sampling distributions increasingly approximated the normal distribution as the sample size increased. From these observations, Gossett derived a family of distributions that change as sample size changes. To ensure his anonymity, Gossett published his results in 1908 under the pseudonym "Student." Thus, this family of distributions came to be known as *Student's* t *distributions*. Like the normal distribution, Student's *t* distributions are symmetrical, bell shaped, and centered on the mean—but they change as their sample sizes change. Because research in communication disorders often involves small samples ($n < 30$), researchers usually depend on Student's *t* distributions to test hypotheses.

CONCLUSION

Hypothesis testing is the core of scientific discovery. To achieve closer and closer approximations of the truth, scientists depend on hypothesis testing conventions to test their ideas. It should be apparent that best practice requires careful and deliberate planning prior to an experiment's beginning. There are many decisions to be made such as choosing a sample size, determining a critical value for rejecting the null hypothesis, and determining if a one-tailed or two-tailed test is appropriate. We have also seen that the results of statistical tests are typically expressed as point estimates, but best practice dictates that researchers should also report interval estimates. Because sound clinical evidence is seldom based on one or two studies, it is important that each building block (experiment) is solidly constructed and based on the best scientific principles. Good hypothesis testing will lead to replication, and experimental replication will lead to the best clinical evidence for practitioners.

■ ■ ■ ■ ■

CASE STUDIES

Case 9.1: Adam's Dilemma
Adam is planning a student research project, but he is in a quandary about choosing the direction for the research hypothesis. Adam plans to investigate a hypothesized relationship between vocal tremor (the dependent variable) and chronological age (the independent variable). As a colleague and fellow student, what is your advice for Adam?

Case 9.2: A Clinical Case for Priscilla
Priscilla's clinical supervisor, Dolores Goodbody, assigned a preschool child to Priscilla for a comprehensive evaluation. After completing the evaluation, Priscilla was asked to chart a com-

parison of outcomes for three standardized test instruments, all designed to measure development of speech and language skills. The problem is that each of the three tests reports results in different units of measurement. How can Priscilla compare the outcomes for the three different test instruments?

Case 9.3: Question of Parameters

Steven is planning a senior thesis. His method is a comparative study of two groups of four children as participants. He is anticipating an analysis of the data with the help of inferential statistical procedures. Steve's first choice for a statistical analysis is the *t*-test procedure. As a consultant, what is your best advice for Steven?

Case 9.4: The Importance of Interval Estimates

Carol is an AuD candidate completing a thesis project. Because her study includes a sample of 30 subjects, she believes that point estimates for her statistical conclusions will be enough. What is wrong with her reasoning? Should she include interval estimates along with the point estimates?

Case 9.5: Carl's Sampling Distribution

Carl sampled the behaviors of 22 children with autism—all 7 years of age. He thinks that the distribution of scores is normally distributed but is not sure. How can you help Carl to test his sample's distribution?

STUDENT EXERCISES

1. Search the current volume of the *Journal of Speech-Language-Hearing Research* for a quantitative research report. What is the hypothesis? Is it stated as the null or alternative hypothesis? Is the hypothesis directional or nondirectional?

2. Identify a contemporary research report and evaluate the authors' steps for testing the hypothesis. Evaluate how the researchers accomplished each of the six steps in the hypothesis testing process.

3. Computer applications are an important asset for research data analysis. Acquaint yourself with Microsoft Excel's NORMDIST function and generate the standard normal distribution using NORMDIST.

4. Find a contemporary research report that utilizes distribution-free inferential statistics in its analysis-of-data section. Why did the researchers choose a nonparametric statistic? Do you think that their choice of a nonparametric statistic was justified?

5. Search the current reports of research for a table of data from the measurement of a variable. Calculate the means, the median, the standard deviation, and the Pearsonian coefficient of skewness (SK). Evaluate the distribution of scores for skewness.

6. Locate a sample of 10 research reports from your favorite journal(s). How many of the reports include interval estimates along with the point estimates? For the reports that report only point estimates, why are the point estimates possibly deceiving? Why might point estimates alone without interval estimates lead us to the wrong clinical conclusions?

CHAPTER 10

QUANTITATIVE ANALYSIS IN COMMUNICATION DISORDERS RESEARCH

analyze (ăn′ə-līz′) *v.* to examine, investigate, interpret; resolve problems by reducing the conditions in them to equations; to study the exact relations existing between quantities or magnitudes.

Most investigations rely on quantitative measurements of some kind to document one or more behaviors of interest. In some cases, descriptive statistics such as means, medians, and standard deviations are sufficient to explain results—but in most cases more sophisticated analyses are necessary. This is particularly true with group designs, where the answers to research questions are found by comparing two or more groups of participants.

With descriptive statistics, researchers aim to describe the features and characteristics of their participants alone. However, group research designs, especially clinical-outcomes research, aim to generalize or conclude something about the whole population. The participants in a study may be few in number, but the population could include thousands of children or adults. For example, Reynolds et al. (2003) devised the following research hypothesis: "Children between the ages of 37 and 54 months who participate in lessons designed to teach them to identify and produce rhyming words [will] make greater gains in their awareness of rhyme than will a similar group of children who do not receive this training" (p. 42). Though Reynolds et al. (2003) focused on a small subset of the population (10 males, 6 females); their aim was to generalize the outcome to other children with similar needs and similar characteristics. In this way, their results might benefit a wide range of clinical practices.

The problem with generalizing study results to the whole population is that the sample (a subset of the population) may not accurately represent the population as a whole. The goal is to have a sample that is representative of the target or theoretical population. Ideally, the sample is a small replica of the population—it possesses all the key variables in the same proportion as they are found in the target population. For example, if the population of interest includes twice as many boys as girls, the sample should replicate this feature of the population. However, researchers sometimes find it necessary to narrow their focus because the "accessible population" (those they can locate) is different from the population as a whole. For example, if the accessible population includes only girls, the researchers will have to limit their study and its conclusions to girls.

Though it is desirable to replicate as many key variables in the population as possible, in reality the accessible population may not permit a perfect replication. In instances where the sample is an imperfect replica of the population as a whole, researchers should explain this as a limitation in their study. An imperfect sample does not negate the value of a study, but it does limit the study's conclusions.

The purpose of an experiment is to test one or sometimes several hypotheses about some characteristic (i.e., parameter) of a target population. As a case in point, Reynolds et al. (2003) hypothesized that teaching rhyming words would increase the awareness of rhyme in a sample of 16 children. In this case, the characteristic of the population was the effect of teaching rhyme on awareness. Their small sample ($n = 16$) most likely limited their ability to generalize or infer the results to the population as a whole. Nonetheless, small studies are often a point of departure for larger studies to come. Important research questions are rarely if ever answered within the context of one study, but a single study may lead to a series of studies that confirm a clinical or other outcome.

Based on what you have learned about Reynolds et al.'s (2003) study, answer the following questions: What was the population that they targeted? Do you think that their sample population was representative of the population as a whole? Why do you

TECHNOLOGY NOTE

Many statistical software packages are available for analyzing quantitative data on desktop computers. The most commonly used statistical software packages are *SPSS*, *SYSTAT*, and *Minitab*. Each is available for both Windows and Macintosh operating systems, and each is menu driven, making them user-friendly and relatively easy to learn. SYSTAT and SPSS are general-purpose statistical packages that offer a variety of data manipulations, statistical analyses, and graphing tools. Minitab is a basic statistics and graphics package that is often used for student instruction in introductory statistics courses. The current version of Minitab is Release 15, and it includes basic statistics, multivariate analysis, nonparametric tests, graphics, and more (www.minitab.com). The current SPSS package is version 16.0 (www.spss.com). The current SYSTAT package is version 12 (www.systat.com). *SPSS* and SYSTAT include descriptive statistics, correlation, resampling, regression, inferential statistics, factor analysis, graphing, and more.

think they included an uneven number of boys and girls? What would you recommend to make their sample more representative of the population?

TESTING HYPOTHESES WITH INFERENTIAL STATISTICS

Descriptive statistics describe the characteristics of participants in a study based on the data at hand. *Inferential statistics* go beyond the data at hand by inferring characteristics about the whole population. Inferences are based on the subset of the population that we refer to as a *sample*.

What Are Inferential Statistics?

With inferential statistics, we estimate some characteristic of the population based on what we know about the sample. The validity of the inference depends on the quality of the sample. If the sample is a good representation of the population, the inference is likely to be good as well.

A case in point is Reynolds et al.'s (2003) study, which included a sample of 16 children. If they had inferred that all children who are taught to identify and produce rhymes will make substantial gains in their awareness of rhyme, they would probably have been wrong. A sample of only 16 children is not likely to represent the whole population of children, so such a broad conclusion would not be justified. Most samples are less than perfect, so it is not unusual for some aspects of the sample to limit a study's conclusions in one way or another.

How Do I Choose a Statistical Test?

To test hypotheses about populations, quantitative researchers should choose analytical procedures that match their study's design. For example, a pretest-posttest design usually involves two observations of the same subjects—one before treatment and one after treatment. In this case, a statistical procedure that matches the pretest-posttest design is a test for differences between two conditions—also known as a *related-samples test* because the same subjects are observed both before and after treatment.

The selection of analytical procedures for testing research hypotheses depends on the *level of measurement* for the dependent variable (nominal, ordinal, interval, or ratio) as well as the experimental design. Most quantitative analyses in communication disorders research are performed with one of two statistical procedures: either the *t-test* or *analysis of variance* (ANOVA). Both of these procedures are known as *parametric statistics* because they infer something about the population on the basis of the sample. Typically, *t*-test and ANOVA procedures require continuous data—usually interval- or ratio-level measurement or suitably transformed data. The *t*-test and ANOVA are the preferred statistical analyses when circumstances permit their use. They are convenient and powerful methods for testing the null hypothesis, i.e., the likelihood that the population means represented by the two or more samples are equal.

The most popular statistical procedure for testing differences between two groups of subjects in communication disorders is Student's t-test. Student's t-test was devised by Gossett in the early 1900s, and he published the work under the pseudonym "Student." Gossett's work was a solution to the problem of small samples ($n < 30$). Gossett devised distributions of scores based on degrees of freedom, and as the degrees of freedom increased in number, the distributions approximated a normal distribution of scores. For small samples, the t distribution is typically bell shaped but narrower than the normal distribution (i.e., leptokurtic). For samples of 30 or more observations, the t distribution is about the same as the normal distribution of scores.

The t-test is designed for testing hypotheses based on small samples ($n < 30$). If samples are large enough ($n > 30$), z can test the hypothesis of "no difference" between means. The z-*test* is based on the normal distribution of scores, otherwise known as the *normal curve*. The proportions of area under the normal curve are found in Exhibit 10.1. This distribution and 21 others are available on SISA's (2008) Simple Interactive Statistical Analysis webpage.

There are many simple and complex research designs and a variety of t-test and ANOVA procedures to match. Because t-test and ANOVA procedures are inferential statistics that purport to infer something about the population as a whole, their use presumes that the samples are randomly selected from the population. *Random sampling* implies that each member of the population has an equal chance of being selected. If samples are not randomly selected, the experimental results are limited to some degree. In the case of Reynolds et al. (2003), the investigators selected 16 children enrolled in a local daycare center as participants. Their sample was not randomly selected because children from other daycare centers were not eligible to be selected. When researchers choose participants on some basis other than random selection, their conclusions are limited in scope—sometimes in a small way and sometimes in a big way.

There are times when one or another variable of interest is categorical in nature. In these cases, the *chi-square* (χ^2) test is usually the best choice for statistical analysis. The chi-square test is a widely used nonparametric statistic. It is sometimes known as the *test of independence*. The chi-square test is typically used to analyze data that are too weak to analyze with t-test or ANOVA procedures. For this reason, the results are somewhat less reliable. However, it is simple to calculate and fairly easy to interpret.

Investigators report their t-test, ANOVA, and chi-square statistics in the results section of articles. However, authors do not always describe their results in detail, and sometimes the results are inaccurate. Consumers should evaluate results for their accuracy rather than simply accepting them as valid.

TESTS OF DIFFERENCES BETWEEN TWO GROUPS/CONDITIONS

Many research questions in communication disorders, especially those that pertain to clinical efficacy, are investigated by testing the difference between two groups or conditions. For example, a question about the efficacy of a specific therapy technique might be tested by randomly assigning subjects to experimental and control groups. In

EXHIBIT 10.1
Values of z and Associated One-Tailed Probabilities (p)

Z	.00	.01	.02	.03	.04	.05	.06	.07	.08	.09
					SECOND DIGIT OF Z					
0.0	.5000	.4960	.4920	.4880	.4840	.4801	.4761	.4721	.4681	.4641
0.1	.4602	.4562	.4522	.4483	.4443	.4404	.4364	.4325	.4286	.4247
0.2	.4207	.4168	.4129	.4090	.4052	.4013	.3974	.3936	.3897	.3859
0.3	.3821	.3783	.3745	.3707	.3669	.3632	.3594	.3557	.3520	.3483
0.4	.3446	.3409	.3372	.3336	.3300	.3264	.3228	.3192	.3156	.3121
0.5	.3085	.3050	.3015	.2981	.2946	.2912	.2877	.2843	.2810	.2776
0.6	.2743	.2709	.2676	.2643	.2611	.2578	.2546	.2514	.2483	.2451
0.7	.2420	.2389	.2358	.2327	.2296	.2266	.2236	.2206	.2177	.2148
0.8	.2119	.2090	.2061	.2033	.2005	.1977	.1949	.1922	.1894	.1867
0.9	.1841	.1814	.1788	.1762	.1736	.1711	.1685	.1660	.1635	.1611
1.0	.1587	.1562	.1539	.1515	.1492	.1469	.1446	.1423	.1401	.1379
1.1	.1357	.1335	.1314	.1292	.1271	.1251	.1230	.1210	.1190	.1170
1.2	.1151	.1131	.1112	.1093	.1075	.1056	.1038	.1020	.1003	.0985
1.3	.0968	.0951	.0934	.0918	.0901	.0885	.0869	.0853	.0838	.0823
1.4	.0808	.0793	.0778	.0764	.0749	.0735	.0721	.0708	.0694	.0681
1.5	.0668	.0655	.0643	.0630	.0618	.0606	.0594	.0582	.0571	.0559
1.6	.0548	.0537	.0526	.0516	.0505	.0495	.0485	.0475	.0465	.0455
1.7	.0446	.0436	.0427	.0418	.0409	.0401	.0392	.0384	.0375	.0367
1.8	.0359	.0351	.0344	.0336	.0329	.0322	.0314	.0307	.0301	.0294
1.9	.0287	.0281	.0274	.0268	.0262	.0256	.0250	.0244	.0239	.0233
2.0	.0228	.0222	.0217	.0212	.0207	.0202	.0197	.0192	.0188	.0183
2.1	.0179	.0174	.0170	.0166	.0162	.0158	.0154	.0150	.0146	.0143
2.2	.0139	.0136	.0132	.0129	.0125	.0122	.0119	.0116	.0113	.0110
2.3	.0107	.0104	.0102	.0099	.0096	.0094	.0091	.0089	.0087	.0084
2.4	.0082	.0080	.0078	.0075	.0073	.0071	.0069	.0068	.0066	.0064
2.5	.0062	.0060	.0059	.0057	.0055	.0054	.0052	.0051	.0049	.0048
2.6	.0047	.0045	.0044	.0043	.0041	.0040	.0039	.0038	.0037	.0036
2.7	.0035	.0034	.0033	.0032	.0031	.0030	.0029	.0028	.0027	.0026
2.8	.0026	.0025	.0024	.0023	.0023	.0022	.0021	.0021	.0020	.0019
2.9	.0019	.0018	.0018	.0017	.0016	.0016	.0015	.0015	.0014	.0014
3.0	.0013	.0013	.0013	.0012	.0012	.0011	.0011	.0011	.0010	.0010
3.1	.0010	.0009	.0009	.0009	.0008	.0008	.0008	.0008	.0007	.0007
3.2	.0007									
3.3	.0005									
3.4	.0003									
3.5	.00023									
3.6	.00016									
3.7	.00011									
3.8	.00007									
3.9	.00005									
4.0	.00003									

this case, the experimental group would receive the therapy, and the control group would receive a salutary treatment or no treatment at all. The *observed outcome* would be the difference between the two groups (experimental vs. control)—the difference is usually between means. However, the statistical analysis also accounts for the amount of individual variability within each group. Though the difference between means may be large, a large amount of variability within the groups could minimize the effect. The variability is sometimes large enough for the scores of the two groups to overlap. Researchers are less likely to find significant differences when two groups overlap.

If the difference between two groups is too small for statistical significance, researchers usually conclude that the proposed therapy is not likely to be effective in clinical practice. However, if the difference between the two groups is large enough to be statistically significant and the experimental group benefits from the treatment, they would likely conclude that the therapy will be effective in clinical practice.

An alternative to between-subjects designs is the *pretest-posttest design*, which is popular in communication disorders—in part because of it mirrors the clinical model. In pretest-posttest designs, a baseline measurement is established during the pretest stage, an experimental treatment is introduced in the second stage, and a posttest measurement is performed in the final (outcome) stage. If the posttest measurement of the dependent variable exceeds the pretest measurement, researchers might conclude that the intervening treatment was responsible for the change. Research designs that employ pretest-posttest observations with an intervening treatment are known as *related-measures* designs because the two samples (pretest and posttest) are composed of the same subjects. The related-measures design is also known as a *within-subjects design* because the comparison is between two or more conditions within the same group of participants.

Independent-Samples Designs

Research designs that include two groups of subjects as participants are known as *independent-samples designs* because the two samples (i.e., experimental subjects and controls) are composed of different participants. It is also known as a *between-subjects design* because the comparison is between two groups of subjects.

TECHNOLOGY NOTE

William Sealy Gossett introduced the *t*-test as a way to cheaply monitor the quality of beer brews. He was employed as a statistician for the Guinness brewery in Dublin, Ireland. In 1908, Gossett published the *t*-test in the journal *Biometrika*, but he used the pseudonym "Student" because Guinness regarded the use of statistics in brewing to be a trade secret. In all likelihood, Gossett would have lost his job if Guinness had known that he published the *t*-test in *Biometrika*. As a result of the deception, Gossett kept his job—and it was many years before his identity was know to fellow statisticians. Gossett died in 1937. The Guinness Brewery continues to be a major brewer in Ireland.

The *t-test for independent samples* is appropriate for answering the question, Is an observed difference between two groups of subjects attributable to chance? If the answer is "no," the alternative hypothesis is accepted. Another use for the *t*-test is to test the equivalency (or nonequivalency) of two groups of subjects. For example, Reynolds et al. (2003) randomly assigned 16 children to experimental and control groups. However, the children in the control group were slightly older (mean = 46 months; *SD* = 6.5) than children in the experimental group (mean = 42.4 months; *SD* = 5.1)—3.6 months difference. Because group equivalency was an important consideration, Reynolds et al. (2003) asked, Is the difference between mean ages for the experimental and control groups a significant one?

To test the hypothesis that the difference was not significant, Reynolds et al. (2003) used a *t*-test for independent samples. Their result was not significant, $p > .05$. The .05 (5%) level of confidence is the conventional cutoff point for accepting or rejecting the null hypothesis. If $p = .05$, the probability is that 5 times out of 100 you would find a statistically significant difference between means by chance even if there were none. The .05 level is considered a tolerable level of risk, but anything greater than .05 is questionable.

An evaluation of the difference between means should include a confidence interval. Confidence intervals are statistical procedures for establishing the precision of a result as well as deciding whether to accept or reject the null hypothesis. If the confidence interval contains zero, the null hypothesis is accepted. The width of the confidence interval indicates the precision of measurement, which depends on sample size. The 95% confidence interval for the Reynolds et al. (2003) difference between means is $CI (95\%) = -9.33 <$ difference $< +2.13$. The confidence interval tells us that the true difference between means could be anywhere between -9.33 and $+2.13$. However, because the confidence interval includes zero, the null hypothesis is true. Thus, Reynolds et al. (2003) correctly concluded that their groups were similar in age.

TECHNOLOGY NOTE

The choice of parametric statistics carries the burden of meeting certain assumptions to ensure a valid test: (a) normality of sample distributions and (b) homogeneity of sample variances. The simplest method to evaluate normality is to visualize the frequency distribution histogram. A second method is to examine the values of skewness and kurtosis for sample distributions. Microsoft Excel includes the histogram function in Tools/Data Analysis menus and includes "KURT" and "SKEW" functions in the statistical functions menu. Statistical applications such as Minitab and SPSS include similar functions. A third method for testing normality is the *Kolmogorov-Smirnov Test* included in Minitab and SPSS applications (alternatives are *Anderson-Darling* and *Ryan-Joiner* tests). Tests for homogeneity of variance include the *F*-test for two samples and *Bartlett's* and *Levene's* tests for multiple samples. These tests are included in many statistical software applications.

Based on what you have learned about the Reynolds et al. (2003) study, answer the following questions: Why did their two groups differ by 3½ months of age even though they used random assignment to constitute their experimental and control groups? If the study was replicated, how could a smaller difference in chronological age between experimental and control groups be achieved?

The z formula in equation 1 is appropriate when testing the hypothesis of "no difference," and samples are $n_1 > 30$ and $n_2 > 30$. A z of 1.65 equals the one-tailed probability (p) value of 0.05 (see the values in Exhibit 10.1).

$$z = \frac{\left(\overline{X}_1 - \overline{X}_2\right)}{\sqrt{\dfrac{s_1^2}{n_1} + \dfrac{s_2^2}{n_2}}} \qquad \text{(eq. 1)}$$

The problem in communication disorders is that many studies include samples with fewer than 30 observations, so the samples are too small to approximate the normal distribution. For small samples, Student's t-test is the correct statistical procedure. The outcome of Student's t-test is known as the t-*ratio*. The t-ratio is the ratio of the difference between the means of the two groups of subjects divided by the standard error of the difference (S.E.D.) as shown in equation 2.

$$\text{Student's } t = \frac{mean_1 - mean_2}{S.E.D.} \qquad \text{(eq. 2)}$$

The standard error of the difference is a measure of the variability or dispersion of the scores attributable to error. In the case of independent samples, the standard error of the difference is estimated from the square root of the pooled variances for the two groups as indicated in equation 3.

$$S.E.D. \text{ independent samples} = \sqrt{S_1^2/N_1 + S_2^2/N_2} \qquad \text{(eq. 3)}$$

Equation 4 is the working formula for Student's t-test when samples are independent of one another, as in the case of two different groups.

$$t = \frac{\overline{X}_1 - \overline{X}_2}{\sqrt{\dfrac{(n_1 - 1)s_1^2 + (n_2 - 1)s_2^2}{n_1 + n_2 - 2} \bullet \left(\dfrac{1}{n_1} + \dfrac{1}{n_2}\right)}} \qquad \text{(eq. 4)}$$

In this case, we test the hypothesis of "no difference," and the degrees of freedom (df) are $n_1 + n_2 - 2$. Thus, if both samples (n_1, n_2) include 15 observations, $df = 10 + 10 - 2 = 18$. Exhibit 10.2 displays the critical values of the t distribution for various probability levels. To test the null hypothesis, we compare the observed value for t to the critical value from Exhibit 10.2. Assuming that ours is a two-tailed test of the hypothesis, the critical value would be 2.10 for $p = 0.05$ (see Exhibit 10.2). If the observed value of t is equal to or greater than 2.10, then we can say that the hypothe-

EXHIBIT 10.2
Critical Values of *t* for Significance at Various Probability (*p*) Levels

	PROBABILITY LEVEL (*p*)				
	.10	.05	.025	.005	ONE-TAILED
df	.20	.10	.05	.01	TWO-TAILED
1	3.08	6.31	12.71	63.66	
2	1.89	2.92	4.30	9.92	
3	1.64	2.35	3.18	5.84	
4	1.53	2.13	2.78	4.60	
5	1.48	2.02	2.57	4.03	
6	1.44	1.94	2.45	3.71	
7	1.41	1.89	2.36	3.50	
8	1.40	1.86	2.31	3.36	
9	1.38	1.83	2.26	3.25	
10	1.37	1.81	2.23	3.17	
11	1.36	1.80	2.20	3.11	
12	1.36	1.78	2.18	3.05	
13	1.35	1.77	2.16	3.01	
14	1.35	1.76	2.14	2.98	
15	1.34	1.75	2.13	2.95	
16	1.34	1.75	2.12	2.92	
17	1.33	1.74	2.11	2.90	
18	1.33	1.73	2.10	2.88	
19	1.33	1.73	2.09	2.86	
20	1.33	1.72	2.09	2.85	
21	1.32	1.72	2.08	2.83	
22	1.32	1.72	2.07	2.82	
23	1.32	1.71	2.07	2.81	
24	1.32	1.71	2.06	2.80	
25	1.32	1.71	2.06	2.79	
50	1.30	1.68	2.01	2.68	
100	1.29	1.66	1.98	2.63	
1000	1.28	1.65	1.96	2.58	

sis of "no difference" is rejected. By rejecting the null hypothesis, we accept the alternative hypothesis.

To correctly use the t-test with independent samples, several assumptions are necessary. First, subjects should be randomly and independently sampled. Second, the two groups should be independent and unrelated. Third, the distribution of differences between the means must be normally distributed. This is not a problem when sample size is > 30 but may be a problem with smaller samples. Typically, researchers inspect the pattern of the data for its distributional characteristics. If a distribution of scores is not symmetrical, researchers may choose to transform the data to achieve a more normal distribution. *Transformations* are the mathematical operations, such as square, square root, reciprocal, and log, that replace each of the original data values with transformed values but retain the important characteristics of the data. A drawback to transforming data is that it changes the unit of measure in which the data are analyzed. As a consequence, the results may be difficult to interpret and less easily understood.

A fourth assumption requires the groups to have equal or near-equal variances. This is known as *homogeneity of variance*. The F *statistic* (equation 5) provides a simple test for homogeneity of variances.

$$F \text{ statistic } = \frac{SD_1}{SD_2}$$

and

$$df_{NUMERATOR} = n_1 - 1, \quad df_{DENOMINATOR} = n_2 - 1 \qquad \text{(eq. 5)}$$

Its application is straightforward. The calculation of F includes the standard deviations (SDs) for the two samples. For example, Reynolds et al. (2003) randomly assigned 16 subjects to two groups, but variance for chronological age was greater in the control group ($SD = 6.5$) versus the experimental group ($SD = 5.1$). To test for homogeneity of variances, the larger value is entered into the numerator and the smaller value into the denominator as shown in equation 6.

$$F = \frac{6.5}{5.1} = 1.27$$

$$\qquad \text{(eq. 6)}$$

$$df = 7, 7$$

To evaluate this result, the observed value (1.27) is compared to the critical value from a *table of critical values* for the F distribution. Exhibit 10.3 displays the critical values of F for significance at various probability levels. The precise probability values associated with F can be calculated on the VassarStats website (Lowry, n.d.). The table of critical values is entered with the degrees of freedom associated with the F ratio's numerator and those associated with its denominator. In the Reynolds et al. (2003) case, the critical value for F is 6.99. If the observed value equals or exceeds the critical value, the null hypothesis is rejected. In this case, the observed value of 1.27 is less than the criti-

EXHIBIT 10.3
Critical Values of *F* for Significance at Various Probability (*p*) Levels

df DENOMINATOR	*df* NUMERATOR									
	1	2	3	4	5	6	7	8	9	10
2	18.51	19.00	19.16	19.25	19.30	19.33	19.35	19.37	19.38	19.40
	98.50	**99.00**	**99.16**	**99.25**	**99.30**	**99.33**	**99.36**	**99.38**	**99.39**	**99.40**
3	10.13	9.55	9.28	9.12	9.01	8.94	8.89	8.85	8.81	8.79
	34.12	**30.82**	**29.46**	**28.71**	**28.24**	**27.91**	**27.67**	**27.49**	**27.34**	**27.23**
4	7.71	6.94	6.59	6.39	6.26	6.16	6.09	6.04	6.00	5.96
	21.20	**18.00**	**16.69**	**15.98**	**15.52**	**15.21**	**14.98**	**14.80**	**14.66**	**14.55**
5	6.61	5.79	5.41	5.19	5.05	4.95	4.88	4.82	4.77	4.74
	16.26	**13.27**	**12.06**	**11.39**	**10.97**	**10.67**	**10.46**	**10.29**	**10.16**	**10.05**
6	5.99	5.14	4.76	4.53	4.39	4.28	4.21	4.15	4.10	4.06
	13.75	**10.92**	**9.78**	**9.15**	**8.75**	**8.47**	**8.26**	**8.10**	**7.98**	**7.87**
7	5.59	4.74	4.35	4.12	3.97	3.87	3.79	3.73	3.68	3.64
	12.25	**9.55**	**8.45**	**7.85**	**7.46**	**7.19**	**6.99**	**6.84**	**6.72**	**6.62**
8	5.32	4.46	4.07	3.84	3.69	3.58	3.50	3.44	3.39	3.35
	11.26	**8.65**	**7.59**	**7.01**	**6.63**	**6.37**	**6.18**	**6.03**	**5.91**	**5.81**
9	5.12	4.26	3.86	3.63	3.48	3.37	3.29	3.23	3.18	3.14
	10.56	**8.02**	**6.99**	**6.42**	**6.06**	**5.80**	**5.61**	**5.47**	**5.35**	**5.26**
10	4.96	4.10	3.71	3.48	3.33	3.22	3.14	3.07	3.02	2.98
	10.04	**7.56**	**6.55**	**5.99**	**5.64**	**5.39**	**5.20**	**5.06**	**4.94**	**4.85**

The first entry is the critical value of *F* for the .05 level of significance; the second entry (**boldface**) is the critical value for the .01 level of significance.

cal value of 6.99, so the null hypothesis is accepted. Thus, the variances for experimental and control groups in Reynolds et al. (2003) can be assumed to be homogeneous.

If assumptions of normality or equal variances cannot be met, there are alternatives for testing the difference between means. The alternatives are *nonparametric procedures*, also known as distribution-free tests. The Mann-Whitney *U* test is an appropriate nonparametric statistic for independent samples with two means. Nonparametric tests are often used with ranked data and are not dependent on the usual assumptions of normality and equal variances. The main advantage for nonparametric tests is that they provide more power than parametric tests when the samples are from highly skewed distributions. However, they provide less power than parametric tests when the distributions are near normal. The power of a test is the probability of correctly rejecting the null hypothesis when it is in fact false. The Mann-Whitney *U* test is an available option in SPSS, Minitab, and other statistical packages.

TECHNOLOGY NOTE

Microsoft Excel provides statistical analysis tools in its Analysis ToolPack—including analysis of variance, the F-test for homogeneity of variances and t-test and z-test procedures. However, Excel's application for statistical analysis is limited (cf. www.practi-calstats.com/xlsstats/excelstats.html). An alternative is statistical software packages such as *Analyse-it* (www.analyse-it.com)—a statistical add-in for Excel. *Analyse-it* replaces Excel algorithms and provides additional statistical resources. Statistical software applications that stand alone include SPSS version 16.0 and Minitab Release 15. Both SPSS and Minitab packages include spreadsheets and a comprehensive array of statistical options.

Related-Samples Designs

The t-*test for related samples* is used to answer the question, Is an observed difference between two conditions within the same subjects attributable to chance? If not, the alternative hypothesis is accepted. In the case of related samples, data are naturally paired. The data are naturally paired when the same subjects are measured twice, as is true for (a) pretest-posttest designs and (b) same-subjects designs with two conditions.

To correctly use the t-test for related samples, several assumptions are important. First, participants should be randomly sampled from the population. Second, the two sets of scores must be correlated (related). Third, the sampling distributions should be normally distributed. The t-test for related samples is computed as the mean of the differences in scores between pairs of subjects divided by the S.E.D.

A case example is Hubbard's (1998) study of the effect of syllabic stress on stuttering behaviors. Hubbard recruited 10 adults who stuttered as participants and asked them to read aloud 40 sentences that varied in locations of syllabic stress. Hubbard (1998) compared the frequency of stuttering with the same subjects in two conditions—stressed and unstressed syllables. The statistical analysis was accomplished by using a t-test for related samples. Hubbard (1998) reported no significant difference between the two conditions ($t = -0.44$, $p = .67$). Hubbard's (1998) t-test included both tails of the t distribution (two-tailed test), but Smith-Olinde, Besing, and Koehnke (2004) chose a one-tailed t-test because they hypothesized "poor performance by the group with hearing loss [vs. the normal hearing group]" (p. 86). The Smith-Olinde et al. (2004) directional hypothesis increased the power of their statistical analysis because the probability of rejecting the null hypothesis increased. In Hubbard's (1998) case, only half of the t distribution is considered, so the probability value is also halved ($p = .335$).

The formula in equation 7 is used when the samples are related, i.e., when there is one sample that has been tested twice (i.e., repeated measures) or when two samples have been matched. We perform the calculations on the difference score (D) for each pair of lined-up scores. M_D is the mean of the $D = X_1 - X_2$ scores, and N is the number of D scores (lined-up pairs). S_D^2 is the unbiased estimate of the population value. The result is the observed value for the related-samples *t*-test, which is compared to the critical value in Exhibit 10.2. The degrees of freedom (*df*) are equal to $N - 1$, where N is the number of paired scores. If the observed value of *t* equals or exceeds the critical (tabled) value at a predetermined probability level, the null hypothesis is rejected. By rejecting the hypothesis of "no differences," we automatically accept the alternative hypothesis.

$$t \frac{M_D}{\sqrt{\left(\dfrac{1}{N}\right) S_D^2}}$$

and

(eq. 7)

$$S_D^2 = \frac{\sum (D - M_D)^2}{N - 1}$$

The nonparametric alternative to the *t*-test for related samples is the *Wilcoxon signed-rank test* for paired data. The Wilcoxon test is an appropriate choice when sample distributions are highly skewed. The Wilcoxon test is included as an option in SPSS, Minitab, and other statistics packages.

TESTS FOR DIFFERENCES AMONG MULTIPLE GROUPS/CONDITIONS

Most research in communication disorders has progressed beyond the stage where only two groups (i.e., experimental and control) or two conditions are compared to

TECHNOLOGY NOTE

As an alternative to local computer-based applications, there are many web-based applications (*webapps*). Webapps are accessed via a Web browser over the Internet. Webapps are popular because they are available anywhere Internet access is available. They are also easily updated without distributing and installing software on local computers. There are many webapps for *t*-tests, simple analysis of variance, and other statistical operations. For example, the *Simple Interactive Statistical Analysis* (SISA) webpage includes an interface for calculating *t*-tests with the input of means, sample sizes, and standard deviations. It also calculates confidence intervals. The SISA's webpage is www.quantitativeskills.com/sisa/statistics/t-test.htm. Another online *t*-test calculator is www.graphpad.com/quickcalcs/index.cfm. It allows various data entry choices and the choice of related, unrelated, and Welch-Satterthwaite versions of the *t*-test. An interactive calculator for simple analysis of variance is available at www.physics.csbsju.edu/stats/anova.html.

each other. Typically, contemporary experiments in communication disorders are more complex because researchers attempt to account for the complexities of natural events. By far, the majority of statistical procedures reported in communication disorders are some variant of the analysis of variance (ANOVA) approach to statistical analysis (Meline & Wang, 2004). The outcome of analysis of variance is the F *statistic* (or *F* ratio). The *F* statistic is named in recognition of R. A. Fisher's contributions to statistics. The analysis of variance is so named because it compares variances in order to test for differences between means.

ANOVO procedures are accompanied by assumptions similar to those for *t*-tests. The results of the ANOVA are less reliable when assumptions are violated. The *general assumptions* for analysis of variance procedures are as follows:

1. Data are continuously measured—usually at interval or ratio level of measurement.
2. Participants are randomly sampled from the population.
3. Data are sampled from populations with normal distributions as estimated by sampling characteristics. However, the ANOVA is generally robust to violations of normality when the sample size is large (e.g., $n > 30$).
4. Data are sampled from populations with equal variances as estimated by sample variances. The ANOVA is especially vulnerable to violations of equal variances when sample sizes are unequal. Tests for equal variances such as Levene's test for multiple samples are available in most statistics packages.

Whereas the *t*-test procedure is limited to analyzing two groups or comparisons at one time, ANOVA analyzes many groups or makes many comparisons at one time. In the special case of two sample means, the analysis of variance procedure is equivalent to the *t*-test ($F = t^2$). As with the *t*-test, there are many different ANOVAs to match the many experimental designs in communication disorders. Analysis of variance procedures are classified as *one-way* (i.e., with one grouping factor), *two-way* (i.e., with two grouping factors), *three-way* (i.e., with three grouping factors), and so on. Analysis of variance with multiple factors is generally known as multifactor analyses of variance. Thus, the ANOVA is broadly classified as either (a) simple analysis of variance procedures or (b) complex analysis of variance procedures.

Simple Analysis of Variance

The purpose of *simple analysis of variance* is to determine the probability that the means of some groups of scores deviate from one another by sampling error alone. To accomplish this purpose, the simple ANOVA separates variance into two distinct parts: (a) within-group variability and (b) between-groups variability. Variances are partitioned so that researchers can ascertain how much of the total variance is attributable to sampling error and how much is due to the treatment effect. The within-group variability is the portion of total variance that cannot be explained by the research design. In the simple ANOVA, this variability is known as the *mean square for error* (MS_{ERROR}) and is the denominator in the *F* ratio. The between-groups variability is the portion of total variance that is attributable to group membership. In the simple ANOVA, between-groups variability is known as the *mean square for effect* (MS_{EFFECT}) and is the numerator in the F ratio. Thus, the F statistic is computed as the ratio between MS_{EFFECT} and MS_{ERROR} as shown in equation 8.

$$F \text{ statistic} = \frac{MS_{effect}}{MS_{error}}$$

$$\text{(eq. 8)}$$

The two variances (MS_{EFFECT} and MS_{ERROR}) are compared in order to test whether the ratio of the variances is significantly greater than 1.

CASE EXAMPLES

Erler and Garstecki (2002) investigated women's perceptions of hearing loss and hearing-aid use. Their purpose was to "examine the degree of stigma associated with hearing loss and hearing aid use among women in three age groups (35–45 years, 55–65 years, and 75–85 years)" (Erler & Garstecki, 2002, p. 83). As a preliminary to examining perceptions of stigma associated with hearing loss and hearing-aid use, Erler and Garstecki (2002) gathered demographic data from 191 participants. The demographic data for years of education, general health, and health handicap were measured on a continuous scale, so the researchers employed several one-way ANOVAs to test for differences between the three age groups. Erler and Garstecki (2002) reported significant differences for years of education ($F = 6.2$, $p < .01$) and health handicap ($F = 3.2$, $p = .05$) but no significant difference between age groups for reports of health status ($F = 0.053$, $p > .05$). Based on the ANOVA results, the investigators concluded that women in the 75- to 85-year-old group reported fewer years of education and were more likely to report a health handicap. Based on what you learned about Erler and Garstecki's (2002) study, answer the following questions: Did the researchers meet the assumption of normality? What information is needed to evaluate the remaining assumptions for ANOVA?

A second example is Stuart's (2004) investigation of word list equivalency for auditory testing in different noise conditions (i.e., signal-to-noise ratios). Stuart (2004) selected one-way analysis of variance to evaluate the differences between noise conditions. However, the dependent variable was measured as "percentage of words correctly recognized." Their data were expressed as proportions, and proportions usually require some transformation before the statistical analysis is done in order to satisfy the assumptions of analysis of variance. This is especially true when a large number of proportions are small (< 0.20) or large (> 0.80). Stuart (2004) chose the arcsine transformation, which is the conventional transformation for proportions. *Arcsine* is the trigonometric function known as the *inverse sine*. Following the transformation, Stuart (2004) successfully analyzed the data.

The *nonparametric alternative* to the one-way analysis of variance is the *Kruskal-Wallis test*. It is used to compare three or more independent groups of sampled data. The test statistic for the Kruskal-Wallis test is H. The Kruskal-Wallis test is typically used when samples are very small ($n < 10$) or when sample sizes are seriously unbalanced. The Kruskal-Wallis test is included in SPSS, Minitab, S-Plus, and other statistics packages.

Complex Analysis of Variance

One-way, or simple, analysis of variance includes one independent variable with several levels, but *complex analysis of variance* procedures include two or more independent variables (factors). By including two or more factors, researchers are able to evaluate the interactions among factors (i.e., interaction effects) as well as the separate effects of each factor (i.e., main effects). The presence of a significant interaction effect means that the main effects cannot be relied on to tell the whole story. A general way to express interactions is to say an effect is modified by another effect. Fisher first used the term "interaction" circa 1926.

■ ■ ■ ■ ■

CASE EXAMPLE

Research questions in communication disorders often include more than one factor, as in an experiment reported by Turkstra, Ciccia, and Seaton (2003). They recruited 50 participants (13–20 years of age) including 24 females, 26 males, 21 African Americans, and 29 Caucasians. Turkstra et al. (2003) asked if race and gender were related to frequency of conversational turns. To answer this question, the investigators chose a multifactor ANOVA. Turkstra et al. (2003) reported a significant main effect for gender on frequency of turns ($F = 5.66$, $p < .05$). Males took significantly more turns than females. No other main effect was significant, and the investigators found no significant interaction effect.

Turkstra et al. (2003) relied on the main effect alone for their interpretation of results because there was no interaction effect, but factors sometimes interact to produce an effect. As an illustration, Exhibit 10.4 depicts an interaction effect in a fictitious study of aphasia treatments and time post-onset for the initiation of treatment. In this case, subjects were given either treatment A or treatment B, and treatments were initiated at two different times; one month post-onset and four months post-onset. As a result, the treatment effect was modified by the time post-onset for initiation of therapy. When treatments were initiated at four months, there was little difference between treatments A and B (82% vs. 80%). However, when treatments were initiated at one month post-onset, there was a significant difference between treatments A and B (80% vs. 92%).

To further evaluate research results for interaction effects, *simple line graphs* are useful for depicting the course of the dependent variable across two factors. The presence of interaction is indicated by nonparallel lines. If the lines cross, or if the lines would cross if extended, there is probably an interaction effect. The data reported in Exhibit 10.4 are displayed as a

EXHIBIT 10.4
Interaction Effect in a Fictitious Study of Aphasia Treatments and Time Post-Onset

TIME POST-ONSET	TREATMENT A MEAN	TREATMENT B MEAN	ROW MEAN
One Month	80%	92%	86%
Four Months	82%	80%	81%
Column Mean	81%	86%	

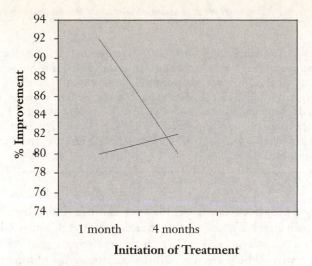

EXHIBIT 10.5
Interaction Effect Depicted in a Graph

graph in Exhibit 10.5. The lines in Exhibit 10.5 are clearly not parallel. This result is a strong indication that there is an interaction effect. Based on the data provided in Exhibit 10.4, answer the following questions: Which treatment is most efficacious—treatment A or B? Based on the same data, would you conclude that it is better to initiate treatment at one month or at four months post-onset?

The *nonparametric alternative* to the two-way ANOVA is *Friedman's test*. Friedman's test is based on an analysis of variance using the ranks of the data. It does not evaluate interaction effects. As is the case for other nonparametric tests, Friedman's test is an alternative when assumptions about normality and homogeneity of variance are seriously violated. Friedman's test and the multifactor ANOVA are included in SPSS, Minitab, S-Plus, and most statistics packages.

Post Hoc Comparisons

When multifactor ANOVAs identify significant effects, the location of the effect is not always evident, because many means are being compared. A significant main effect indicates the presence of at least one significant difference between means, but it does not identify specific pairs of means. There could be a significant difference between one pair of means or several pairs of means. To remedy this problem, researchers utilize post hoc comparison tests that analyze pairs of means for significance. As a result, the post hoc tests identify the specific pairs of means that are significantly different.

There are a variety of post hoc comparison tests for analysis of variance. The most popular are the *Bonferroni*, *Tukey HSD*, *Newman-Keuls*, and *Scheffé tests*.

■ ■ ■ ■ ■

CASE EXAMPLE

A good example of post hoc comparisons is Stuart's (2004) experiment. In one aspect of the study, Stuart (2004) examined the effect of broadband noise with a signal-to-noise ratio of –5 dB on different lists of words used in auditory testing. The one-way ANOVA procedure was the choice for statistical analysis. The independent variable included four different word lists, so there were a total of six comparisons between means. Stuart (2004) chose the Tukey HSD (honestly significant difference) test for the post hoc analysis. As a result, Stuart (2004) identified three mean comparisons that were statistically significant. The other three mean comparisons were not significantly different.

The choice of one post hoc comparison test over another is not straightforward and is sometimes controversial. There is little difference between Tukey's HSD and Newman-Keuls post hoc comparisons, but Bonferroni and Scheffé tests are criticized as being overly conservative. There are several Internet sites with information about post hoc comparisons and resources for their calculation. One is the GraphPad.com website. GraphPad.com includes an online post-test calculator (QuickCalcs) where investigators can enter the mean square, degrees of freedom, and means for each paired comparison. Following the data entry, QuickCalcs provides online results.

TESTS FOR ANALYZING CATEGORICAL DATA

In some cases, investigators collect categorical data in the course of their studies. Categorical data are also known as *count data*. The measurement for count data is nominal level.

■ ■ ■ ■ ■

CASE EXAMPLE

Erler and Garstecki (2002) collected categorical data from participants in their study of women's perceptions of hearing loss and the use of hearing aids. The investigators asked participants to answer questions such as, (a) Are you currently married? (b) Are you currently providing care to others? (c) Are you currently employed? The yes/no responses classified participants by categories, such as *married*, *not married*, *employed*, or *not employed*. Thus, the data that were subsequently analyzed were clearly nominal-level measures.

The analysis of categorical data is accomplished with statistical procedures known as *chi-square tests*. There are a variety of chi-square tests that are appropriate for different experimental designs, including between-subjects or within-subjects designs and unrelated-samples or related-samples designs. The purpose of chi-square tests is to determine whether the observed frequencies (counts) differ significantly from the frequencies expected by chance. Chi-square tests are accompanied by several assumptions and limitations:

1. Individual observations must be independent of one another, i.e., the response of one subject should have no influence on the response of another subject.
2. The observations for analysis must be count data, not percentages or other forms of data.
3. The sum of the expected frequencies must equal the sum of the observed frequencies.
4. The categories must be exclusive of one another.
5. The expected values for any one cell in the contingency table must not be too small (such as < 5), but this restriction varies with the type of chi-square test and its degrees of freedom.

Contingency tables are the rows-by-columns tables that are used to organize the data for chi-square analysis. Exhibit 10.6 is an example of a rows-by-columns contingency table with data from Erler and Garstecki's (2002) study of women's perception of hearing loss and their use of hearing aids.

The general formula for the chi-square test is provided in equation 9.

$$\chi^2 = \sum \frac{(O - E)^2}{E}$$

(eq. 9)

O = observed frequency
E = expected frequency
df = (columns-1)(rows-1)

The formula for calculating expected frequencies is stated thus: "the expected frequency for a cell equals [column total by row total] divided by the grand total." Erler and Garstecki (2002) recruited 191 women with age-normal hearing who were subsequently divided into three age groups: (a) younger women, (b) middle-aged women,

EXHIBIT 10.6
Example of a Rows-by-Columns Contingency Table

	YOUNG WOMEN	MIDDLE-AGED WOMEN	OLDER WOMEN	TOTALS
Married	40 (33)*	42 (36)*	21 (33)*	103
Not Married	22 (29)*	25 (31)*	41 (29)*	88
Totals	62	67	62	191

Adapted from Erler and Garstecki's (2002) results.
*Observed (expected) values.

and (c) older women. As a part of their investigation, the researchers analyzed demographic data that were gathered by a questionnaire. Only the data for one category (*married/not married*) are included in Exhibit 10.6. The calculation of chi-square requires several steps.

The *first step* for calculating the chi-square statistic (equation 9) is as follows: The column total (62) is multiplied by the row total (103) and divided by the grand total (191) to equal the expected value for cell one (33). The expected values for the remaining cells are calculated in the same fashion. The *second step* involves calculating the difference between the observed and expected value in each cell, squaring the difference, and dividing by the expected value. Thus, in the case of the first cell (Young Women, Married) in Exhibit 10.6, the computation is $(40 - 33)^2 / 33 = 1.48$. The computations are performed for the remaining cells in like fashion. The *third step* involves summing the results from each cell of the contingency table. The outcome is known as the *observed value* of the chi-square statistic. The observed value is compared to the critical value for chi-square based on the appropriate degrees of freedom, $df = 2$ in this example. The critical values of χ^2 are listed in Exhibit 10.7.

Erler and Garstecki (2002) reported the result of their chi-square analysis as $\chi^2 = 14.9, p < .01$ ($df = 2$). Exhibit 10.7 shows that the critical value for 2 degrees of freedom and a probability level of .01 is 9.21. Erler and Garstecki's (2002) observed value of 14.9 clearly exceeded the table's critical value of 9.21 needed for statistical significance. Given this result, the investigators concluded that there was a significant difference between age groups for the *married/not married* variable.

Based on what you know about Erler and Garstecki's (2002) results, answer the following questions: What age groups contained the greatest differences? Did the chi-square analysis satisfy each of the five assumptions for chi-square tests?

The chi-square test is an appropriate choice when sampling data are categorical such as in the case of count data. The chi-square test is included as an option in SPSS, Minitab, and other statistics packages. An online chi-square analysis is also available (Watkins, 2008). To use the online calculator, the observed values are simply entered into the cells. The "calculate" button completes the analysis (see Exhibit 10.8).

EFFECT-SIZE STATISTICS

Many researchers get excited because their *t*-test, ANOVA, or chi-square results are *statistically significant*. However, they may not really understand what statistical significance means. When a statistic is significant, it simply means that we are very sure the statistic is reliable. The result may not be important or may not have any *practical significance*. This important difference in meaning between "statistical significance" and "practical significance" is especially relevant in clinical studies, because a statistically significant result may have little use in real-life situations.

As an illustration, suppose we compared two treatment approaches with 1,000 participants and asked if there was a significant difference between treatment A and treatment B. The mean gain for treatment A is 19% and the mean gain for treatment B is 18%. An independent-samples *t*-test tells us that the difference is significant at the

EXHIBIT 10.7
Critical Values of Chi-Square for Significance at Various *p* Levels

df	.05	.01	.001	*df*	.05	.01	.001
	PROBABILITY LEVEL (*p*)						
1	3.84	6.64	10.83	26	38.89	45.64	54.05
2	5.99	9.21	13.82	27	40.11	46.96	55.48
3	7.82	11.35	16.27	28	41.34	48.28	56.89
4	9.49	13.28	18.47	29	42.56	49.59	58.30
5	11.07	15.09	20.52	30	43.77	50.89	59.70
6	12.59	16.81	22.46	31	44.99	52.19	61.10
7	14.07	18.48	24.32	32	46.19	53.49	62.49
8	15.51	20.09	26.13	33	47.40	54.78	63.87
9	16.92	21.67	27.88	34	48.60	56.06	65.25
10	18.31	23.21	29.59	35	49.80	57.34	66.62
11	19.68	24.73	31.26	36	51.00	58.62	67.99
12	21.03	26.22	32.91	37	52.19	59.89	69.35
13	22.36	27.69	34.53	38	53.38	61.16	70.71
14	23.69	29.14	36.12	39	54.57	62.43	72.06
15	25.00	30.58	37.70	40	55.76	63.69	73.41
16	26.30	32.00	39.25	41	56.94	64.95	74.75
17	27.59	33.41	40.79	42	58.12	66.21	76.09
18	28.87	34.81	42.31	43	59.30	67.46	77.42
19	30.14	36.19	43.82	44	60.48	68.71	78.75
20	31.41	37.57	45.32	45	61.66	69.96	80.08
21	32.67	38.93	46.80	46	62.83	71.20	81.40
22	33.92	40.29	48.27	47	64.00	72.44	82.72
23	35.17	41.64	49.73	48	65.17	73.68	84.03
24	36.42	42.98	51.18	49	66.34	74.92	85.35
25	37.65	44.31	52.62	50	67.51	76.15	86.66

.05 level, but is this a clinically important difference? The answer is most probably *no*. The 1% difference between treatments A and B is not enough to favor one treatment over the other. This scenario highlights the critical difference between statistical significance and practical significance. A statistically significant result does not necessarily mean that the result is useful in clinical situations.

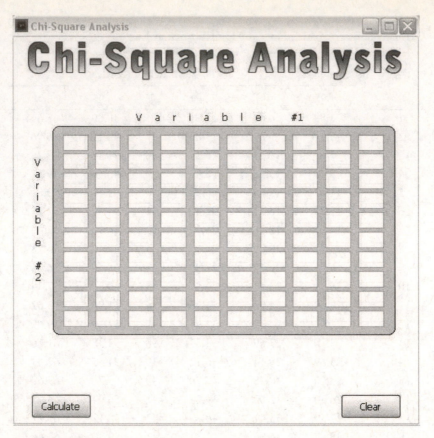

EXHIBIT 10.8
Online Program for Chi-Square Analysis

From Marley Watkins' Webpage by M. Watkins, n.d., http://www.public.asu.edu/~mwwatkin/. Reprinted with permission.

The Family of Effect-Size Statistics

The practical significance of a statistical outcome is usually expressed as an *effect size* (ES). The family of effect-size statistics provides an estimate of a treatment effect's size—small, medium, or large. In this way, researchers and clinicians are able to evaluate the importance of an effect. A "large" effect may have considerable impact in a clinician's practice, whereas a "small" effect may have none.

According to the *Publication Manual of the American Psychological Association* (2001), failing to report effect sizes is a serious defect in the design and reporting of research results. To assess the use of effect sizes in communication disorders, Meline and Schmitt (1997) surveyed ASHA journals in the 1990s and found that only 5 of 411 articles reported effect sizes. In a follow-up to the earlier survey, Meline and Wang (2004) examined research reports in five previous years and found that 120 of 433 articles reported effect sizes—a big increase in reporting effect sizes since 1997. The increase is likely due to several factors: (a) the impact of evidence-based practice on research, (b) new editorial policies that recognize the need for effect sizes, and (c) authors who understand the value of effect sizes for the interpreting their results. Reporting effect sizes is an important step toward better reporting results, but authors also need to interpret the meaning of their effect sizes. Simply reporting effect sizes without explanation is a poor practice. For example, if authors report an effect size of 0.80, what does this mean?

Meline and Wang (2004) found that only half the articles surveyed (55%) included an interpretation of their effect sizes. Authors of the other articles simply reported their effect sizes without further comment. This is a problem for consumers because the meaning of effect sizes is not always evident. Authors need to interpret the effect sizes they report, because they are in the best position to understand the intervention, target population, and outcome measures. These are the features of a study that make it unique, and effect sizes are best interpreted with these in mind.

The Simple Effect Size

There are three categories of effect size statistics. They all purport to accomplish the same goal, but some are better in certain situations. The first (and simplest) of the three categories of effect-size statistics is the *simple effect size*. As the name implies, it is simply the raw difference between treatment means. In the earlier example, the gains for treatments A and B were 19% and 18% respectively. In this case, the raw difference between treatments is 1%. Thus, the simple effect size is 1%.

Meline and Wang (2004) illustrated simple effect size in a study in which the investigators recorded reading times for five mothers who read to their children. Van Kleeck and Beckley-McCall (2002) reported average reading times in minutes and seconds for younger children (mean = 1:27) and their older siblings (mean = 5:09). It was apparent that the average reading time for mothers and their older children was substantially longer than reading times for mothers and their younger children. In this case, the simple effect size was the difference between the means (*ES* = 3 minutes, 42 seconds).

What is good about the simple effect size? It is useful when the unit of measurement is easily interpreted, but there are some problems with the simple effect size. For one, it does not account for the variability in the samples. For instance, the mothers in van Kleeck and Beckley-McCall's (2002) study varied from 0:57 to 1:50 minutes/seconds when reading to their younger children and from 3:02 to 8:17 minutes/seconds when reading to their older children. This is quite a lot of variability in time, and simple effect sizes focus entirely on the means and ignore the variability. If there were no variability, the simple effect size would be a good measure, but variability is almost always present in behavioral measurements. A second problem with simple effect size is that it rarely permits comparisons between studies, because the units of measurement usually differ. This problem is resolved by *standardizing* the unit of measurement.

The Effect-Size Correlation

A second category of effect size is the *effect-size correlation*. Effect-size correlations are the correlations between the independent variable classification and the individual scores of the dependent variable. Meline and Wang (2004) illustrated the effect-size correlation with Ingram and Morehead's (2002) analysis of data from language-impaired and typically developing children. Their independent variable was language status, either impaired or typical, and the dependent variable was the occurrence of various grammatical morphemes. Ingram and Morehead (2002) reported a *squared effect-size correlation* of 0.54 for progressive morphemes. The square of the correlation indicated the percentage of variance in progressive morphemes that could be attributed to membership in the independent variable: impaired and typically developing language. Though these authors reported the squared correlation, Rosnow and Rosenthal (2003) recommend against squaring the effect-size correlation for two reasons: (a) squared correlations lose their directionality so we do not know if the result is positive or negative, and (b) the squared correlation (r^2) may obscure the importance of an effect because it diminishes its apparent size, i.e., $0.50^2 = 0.25$ and $0.30^2 = 0.09$. Ingram and Morehead's (2002) squared correlation of 0.54 is derived from a correlation of 0.73. In most cases, there is little to be gained from squaring the effect-size correlation. It is a better practice to interpret the correlation in its raw form. This practice avoids the possibility of diminishing the importance of an effect as Rosnow and Rosenthal (2003) warned.

For researchers who prefer correlations for effect-size estimates, the correlation effect size is calculated from t values as illustrated in equation 10. For the simple ANOVA with numerator $df = 1$, we substitute the value of F for t^2.

$$r = \sqrt{\frac{t^2}{t^2 + df_{within}}}$$

and   (eq. 10)

df_{within} = the degrees of freedom for the t statistic
$N = N - 2$ in the case of two groups
N = total number of subjects in both groups

The Standardized Effect Size

The most commonly used effect-size statistic is the *standardized effect size*. The standardized effect size accounts for variability and provides a statistic that can be used for comparing the results from one study to another.

To illustrate, we can calculate a standardized effect size from the previous example with reading times for older and younger children (van Kleeck & Beckley-McCall,

2002). To do so, we find the difference between means for the two groups—just as we did when calculating the simple effect size—but we then divide that difference by the variability. This version of the standardized effect size is known as Cohen's *d*. The formula is shown in equation 11.

$$d = \frac{M_1 - M_2}{\sigma_{within}}$$

and   (eq. 11)

$$\sigma_{within} = s_{within} \sqrt{\frac{df_{within}}{N}}$$

Cohen (1988) explained that the variance in the denominator (as estimated from the standard deviation) could be derived from either group when the variances are approximately equal, but the safest approach is to use the pooled variance, which accounts for variances in both groups. For the van Kleeck and Beckley-McCall (2002) case, the standardized effect size is calculated by dividing the mean difference of 3:42 (min:sec) by the pooled standard deviation ($\sqrt{[\sigma_1^2 + \sigma_2^2 / 2]}$), which equals 1:44 (min:sec). The result is a standardized effect size of $d = 1.50$. As a convention, effect sizes are usually reported as positive when the effect is in the predicted direction and as negative when the effect is in the unpredicted direction. Van Kleeck and Beckley-McCall (2002) expected longer reading times for the older children, so the effect was in the predicted direction. The direction of the effect is an especially important consideration in clinical trials because treatments sometimes have harmful (i.e., nonbeneficial) effects.

Cohen's *d* is best used when samples are relatively large (i.e., $n > 30$). It is a biased estimator of effect size when samples are small. An alternative and better choice when samples are small is Hedge's *g*. Like Cohen's *d*, Hedge's *g* yields a standardized effect size, but it provides a correction for the small sample size. For samples that are > 30, Hedge's *g* will approximate the value of Cohen's *d*, so the choice of one or the other would not matter. The difference in calculating the two is in the denominator. Equation 12 displays the formula for Hedge's *g*.

$$g = \frac{M_1 - M_2}{s_{within}}$$

and   (eq. 12)

$$s_{within} = \sqrt{\frac{\sum (X_1 - M_1)^2 + \sum (X_2 - M_2)^2}{df_{within}}}$$

Since van Kleeck and Beckley-McCall's (2002) study included a small sample of parent-child dyads in each group ($n = 5$), the best choice for a standardized effect-size statistic is Hedge's *g*. Hedge's *g* provides a correction for error associated with the small sample size. A useful software application for calculating Hedge's *g* is Devilly's (2008) Effect Size generator (Exhibit 10.9). It calculates Cohen's *d*, Hedge's *g*, and the confidence intervals associated with these statistics. The values in Exhibit 10.9 are the decimal equivalents for van Kleeck and Beckley-McCall's (2002) measurements, which were reported in hours and minutes.

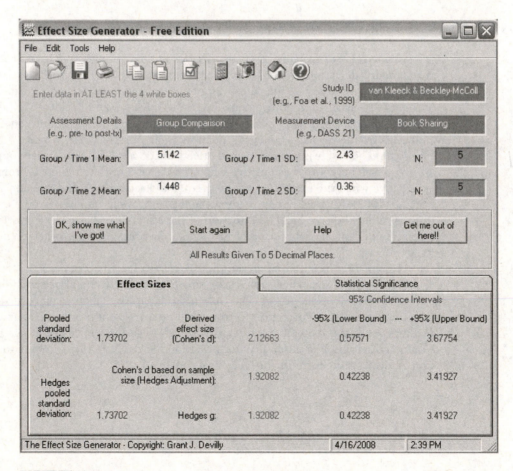

EXHIBIT 10.9
Devilly's (2008) Effect Size Generator Version 2.3.0

Data are based on van Kleeck and Beckley-McCall's (2002) results. Screen image reprinted with permission from Grant Devilly, PhD, Griffith University (Mt. Gravatt Campus), Mt. Gravatt, Queensland, Australia.

The ES values in Exhibit 10.9 are better understood if we convert them back to their original units of measurement. Once converted to hours and minutes, $d = 2{:}08$ and $g = 1{:}55$ hours/minutes. The difference between Cohen's d and Hedge's g is 13 minutes. This difference represents the downward correction in Hedge's g based on the small sample size. It is also important to examine the confidence interval that contains the effect size. Again, the confidence interval is best understood if we convert the decimal values in Exhibit 10.9 to their time equivalents. In this example, the confidence interval for Hedge's g has a lower bound of 0:25 and an upper bound of 3:25 hours/minutes. The confidence interval is wide because small samples limit the precision of an estimate. In van Kleeck and Beckley-McCall's (2002) case, the best estimate of the effect size is $g = 1{:}55$ hours/minutes, but the confidence interval tells us that the true effect size could be anywhere between 0:25 and 3:25 hours/minutes.

How Should We Interpret Effect Sizes?

A standard or some basis of comparison is needed to adequately interpret the meaning of effect-size statistics. Cohen (1988) provided operational conventions for interpreting effect-size correlations and standardized effect sizes but did so cautiously. He viewed conventional definitions as risky because they ignore the diversity of behaviors in a field like behavioral sciences. Most assuredly, some behaviors tend to produce smaller effects than others, but their importance should not be judged without due consideration to the type of intervention, the target population, and outcome measures. Most of the time, investigators adopt the operational conventions for interpreting their effect-size results. For example, in a recent research report, Eisenberg et al. (2001) chose conventional definitions to evaluate their effect sizes for noun phrase elaboration in children's spoken stories as a function of age, syntactic function, and narrative context.

The *universal conventions* that Cohen (1988) suggested for interpreting *effect-size correlations* were the following:

0.50 = large
0.30 = moderate
0.10 = small
< 0.10 = trivial

Cohen (1988) suggested the following conventions for interpreting *standardized effect sizes:*

0.80 = large
0.50 = moderate
0.20 = small
< 0.20 = trivial

Cohen's conventions have proven useful, but they should not be relied on all the time. There are other solutions that are often better for interpreting effect sizes. Hill, Bloom, Black, and Lipsey (2007) argued that universal guidelines (such as Cohen's definitions) are poor substitutes for "empirical benchmarks." According to Hill et al. (2007), we should use empirical benchmarks that reflect the nature of the intervention, its target population, and the outcome measurement. They proposed three classes of empirical benchmarks: (a) normative expectations for change over time, (b) policy-relevant gaps in achievement by demographic group or school performance, and (c) effect-size results from past research for similar interventions and target populations (Hill et al., 2007).

Hill et al.'s (2007) first empirical benchmark, *normative expectations for change over time*, refers to expectations for growth or change in the absence of an intervention. We might ask, How does the effect of an intervention compare with a typical year of growth for a target population of preschool children? Of course, the answer to this question depends on the availability of normative information about growth in preschool years. Hill et al. (2007) suggested normative samples from national standardized tests as one way to gather information about typical growth patterns. They examined tests for reading and determined that the average annual reading gain measured in effect size from grade 1 to grade 2 was 0.97 (a standardized ES) with a 95% confidence interval from 0.89 to 1.05. With information of this sort, it is relatively easy for investigators to compare the effect size from their intervention to the effect size expected to occur with one year's growth. Such a comparison provides an empirical basis for interpreting the size and importance of an intervention effect.

The second empirical benchmark proposed refers to *policy-relevant performance gaps* (Hill et al., 2007). In this case, we might ask, How does the effect of an intervention compare with existing differences among subgroups of people (e.g., students, schools, adults)? As an example, Konstantopoulus and Hedges (2005) cited the achievement gaps between ethnic groups, males and females, and rich and poor. If school reform is intended to reduce or eliminate such gaps, it makes sense to evaluate intervention effects by comparing them to the size of the existing gaps. Hill et al. (2007) illustrated such gaps with the published findings from the National Assessment of Educational Progress (NAEP). The NAEP publishes reading performance data for subgroups by race/ethnicity, income, and gender. For example, fourth-grade Hispanic students scored 0.77 standard deviations lower than white students on the reading assessment. Performance gaps such as this one can provide relevant benchmarks for effect sizes from interventions.

Hill et al.'s (2007) third empirical benchmark is observed *effect sizes for similar interventions*. Lipsey and Wilson (1993) recognized the need for an empirical benchmark for psychological, educational, and behavioral investigations. In the only large-scale effort of its kind, they collected standardized effect sizes from 302 studies and averaged the results. Exhibit 10.10 displays the distribution of mean effect sizes from these 302 studies. Lipsey and Wilson (1993) reported an average effect size of 0.50. Their average effect size ranged from 0.21 to 0.79, plus or minus one standard deviation. Thus, based on Lipsey and Wilson's (1993) results, we might expect standardized effect sizes to fall within this range most of the time.

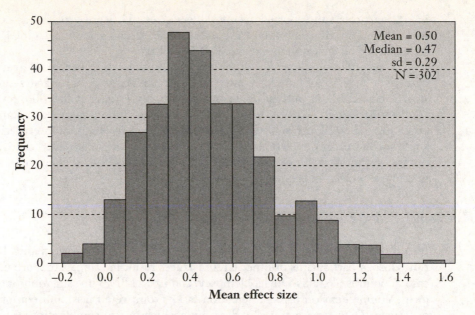

EXHIBIT 10.10
Distribution of Mean Effect Sizes from 302 Psychological, Educational, and Behavioral Treatment Studies

From "The Efficacy of Psychological, Educational, and Behavioral Treatment: Confirmation From Meta-Analysis," by M. W. Lipsey and D. B. Wilson, 1993, *American Psychologist*, *48*, p. 1193. Reproduced with permission.

Lipsey and Wilson's (1993) results are remarkably close to Cohen's (1988) conventions for interpreting standardized effect sizes. However, it may be that Lipsey and Wilson's (1993) benchmark is outdated (M.W. Lipsey, personal communication, April 3, 2008). The effect sizes from studies in the past 10 years could yield different results. Furthermore, Lipsey and Wilson's (1993) results represent many types of interventions, different target populations, and various outcome measures. As such, they should be considered as no more than general guidelines.

A better benchmark for outcomes in communication disorders is the body of research in speech, language, and hearing. When available, this research is a big help for interpreting effect sizes. For the most part, our knowledge about effect sizes comes from synthesis reviews of the research literature with meta-analysis. Meta-analysis is a method of quantifying study results in a common metric so that they can be combined. The outcome is usually an average effect size from the results of many studies.

Unfortunately, there are few reviews of this kind. However, there are reviews of child language, adult language, and stuttering. For example, Law, Garrett, and Nye (2004) reported average standardized effect sizes for receptive and expressive language interventions for children with developmental language delay/disorder. They examined 25 articles and reported average effect sizes that were grouped as combined-parent/clinician, clinician-only, and parent-only treatments. Law et al. (2004) reported standardized effect sizes ranging from –0.53 to 1.06.

A second example with a different target population reported an average standardized effect size of 0.61 for treated and untreated recoveries for acute-stage aphasics (Robey, 1998). In the case of persons who stutter, Herder et al. (2006) reviewed six studies of treated versus untreated participants and found an average standardized effect size of 0.91. The results from these reviews provide a basis for interpreting future studies with similar populations and like outcome measures. However, there are many instances when this information is not available. In these cases, effect sizes are interpreted using other benchmarks or conventions.

THE PROBLEM OF UNEQUAL SAMPLE SIZES

Ideally, the samples in research studies have equal numbers of participants, but sometimes loss of participants or other circumstances result in samples that are unequal. A case in point is Skarakis-Doyle, Dempsey, and Lee's (2008) investigation of three language comprehension tasks: a detection task, a joint retell task, and comprehension questions. Their intention was to determine which test or combination of tests could best identify children with language comprehension impairments. Their method was to compare children with typically developing language (TDL) and those with language impairment (LI), but they assigned 37 children to the TDL group and only 12 children to the LI group. This sort of imbalance between sample sizes causes a loss of power and efficiency in experimental designs because statistics generally assume that samples are equal in size. For example, an estimate of effect size with Hedge's g is derived from the observed value of t as shown in equation 13. However, Hedge's g assumes that the samples are equal in size. The effect size g is underestimated when sample sizes are unequal.

$$\text{Hedge's } g = \frac{2t}{\sqrt{N}} \qquad \text{(eq. 13)}$$

We can determine the *effect of unequal sample sizes* on the power and efficiency of a statistic by comparing the arithmetic and harmonic means of the samples. The arithmetic mean is the simple average as shown in equation 14, and the harmonic mean is the reciprocal of the arithmetic mean of the reciprocals and is calculated as shown in equation 15. The ratio of the harmonic mean sample size to the arithmetic mean sample size (equation 16) is an index of the retention of power in the unequal-n design relative to the equal-n design.

$$\text{Arithmetic Mean} = \frac{n_1 + n_2}{2} \qquad \text{(eq. 14)}$$

$$\text{Harmonic Mean} = \frac{2(n_1 n_2)}{n_1 + n_2} \qquad \text{(eq. 15)}$$

EXHIBIT 10.11
Effect of Unequal Sample Sizes on Loss of Relative Efficiency and Loss of Effective N

SIZE OF SAMPLES				LOSSES	
n_1	n_2	ARITHMETIC MEAN n	HARMONIC MEAN n	EFFICIENCY	N
25	25	25	25.00	.00	0
30	20	25	24.00	.04	2
35	15	25	21.00	.16	8
40	10	25	16.00	.36	18
45	5	25	9.00	.64	32
49	1	25	1.96	.92	46

$$\text{Loss of Relative Efficiency} = 1 - \left(\frac{harmonic\ mean}{arithmetic\ mean} \right) \qquad \text{(eq. 16)}$$

The harmonic mean sample size always equals the arithmetic mean sample size when $n_1 = n_2$. Exhibit 10.11 illustrates the loss of relative efficiency and loss of effective N for samples of various sizes. As can be seen in Exhibit 10.11, there is no loss of efficiency or loss of effective N when sample sizes are equal, but as the samples become more unequal in size the losses increase. In the case of Skarakis-Doyle et al.'s (2008) study, their loss of efficiency with unequal sample sizes ($n_1 = 12$, $n_2 = 37$) is calculated in equation 17. Their effective loss of N is calculated in equation 18.

$$\text{Loss of relative efficiency} = 1 - \left(\frac{18.12}{24.5} \right) = 0.74 \qquad \text{(eq. 17)}$$

$$\text{Effective loss of } N = \frac{N\left[1 - \left(\dfrac{n_b}{\overline{n}} \right) \right]}{49\left[1 - \left(\dfrac{18.12}{24.5} \right) \right] = 36} \qquad \text{(eq. 18)}$$

In Skarakis-Doyle et al.'s (2008) case, it is apparent that the unequal sample sizes severely affected the efficiency and power of their experimental design. The effective loss of $N = 36$ means that they would have had the same efficiency and power with equal sample sizes and $N = 13$ [49 – 36 = 13]. Investigators should aim for equal or near-equal sample sizes whenever possible. First, they should plan for equal sample sizes when designing their studies. Second, investigators should anticipate loss of participants—especially losses that affect one group of subjects more so than another group, e.g., a clinical group versus a nonclinical group.

CONCLUSION

We have seen that quantitative measurements are often used to measure the behaviors of interest in research studies. Descriptive statistics such as means, medians, and standard deviations help to explain results, but more sophisticated analyses are needed to generalize the results to the population. Quantitative analysis typically involves inferential statistics such as the *t*-test and ANOVA to test hypotheses, but effect sizes are also important to evaluate the practical significance of statistical outcomes. Throughout, we have seen the importance of sampling methods and sample characteristics. The choice of samples affects the efficiency and power of an experimental design, but the sample also determines the scope of the conclusions. In as much as no study is perfect, investigators should recognize their study's limitations and temper their conclusions based on those limitations. However, research reports sometimes contain methodological mistakes, errors in results, or conclusions that are not justified by the facts, so consumers should evaluate articles with great care.

CASE STUDIES

Case 10.1: A Quandary for Klein and Brown
Professor Klein and audiologist Brown recruited 20 older men and women to participate in an investigation of the effect of hearing-aid-adjustment instruction on user satisfaction. The dependent variable is measured on a continuous scale. Klein and Brown's research question is, Will men and women differ in their user satisfaction? The researchers are uncertain about the choice of an analysis procedure—parametric or nonparametric. As the research consultant, what questions will you ask Klein and Brown to help them choose the proper analysis procedure?

Case 10.2: Inequality Dilemma for the Chavez School Research Team
The Chavez School research team randomly selected 100 kindergarten children in their school district as participants in a study of bilingual education. They divided participants into two groups: those assigned to bilingual education classes and a control group in regular education classes. After collecting their data, the research team is uncertain about how to proceed because the standard deviations for the two groups are unequal ($SD_1 = 63.4$; $SD_2 = 72.1$). What is your advice for the Chavez School research team?

Case 10.3: Student Researchers Maria and Stephen Seek Advice
Student researchers Maria and Stephen devised a research design for a graduate course project that utilizes a survey questionnaire for gathering data. The questions in their survey instrument require yes/no answers. The independent variable is *class standing:* freshman, sophomore, junior, senior, or graduate. The researchers are uncertain about the quantitative analysis of their data. As a fellow student and ace researcher, what is your best advice? What are Maria and Stephen's options?

Case 10.4: Judging the Importance of Research Results
As his senior thesis, Ken tested the hypothesis that the Altered-Feedback Approach is better than the Contingent-Reinforcement Approach for reducing disfluencies in the speech of college students. His *t*-test results clearly identified a significant difference between the two

approaches. However, he is not sure whether the difference is one that really matters. What is your best advice for Ken? What can he do to determine whether the difference between the two approaches is important or only trivial?

Case 10.5: Beth's Dilemma

Beth's dilemma is a common one among researchers. She recruited 20 subjects for her study, but only 14 participated. Worse yet, 9 subjects are in the control group and only 5 are members of the experimental group. Given your vast knowledge of research design principles and practice, what advice should you give to Beth? What should she have done? What can she do now?

■ ■ ■ ■ ■

STUDENT EXERCISES

1. Locate a research article in a recent journal and identify the quantitative analysis procedures utilized in the study. What were the levels of measurement for dependent variables? What quantitative methods were used? What was the sample size? Did the researchers satisfy the assumptions for their quantitative analyses?

2. Identify a recent research report with analysis of variance utilized as a quantitative method. Was the ANOVA procedure one-way or multifactor? What were the independent variables? Was there an interaction effect? What post hoc tests were used?

3. Locate a research article that includes a t-*test* analysis of two means. What are the values for the means and standard deviations of the two groups (or conditions)? Is the assumption of homogeneity of variance satisfied? If not, what alternatives would you have suggested to the researchers?

4. Identify a research article that includes a survey instrument in its methods section. What were the dependent variables? What type of quantitative analysis (if any) was employed by the researchers? Did the researchers choose the proper analysis procedures? If you replicate their study, how would you improve the quantitative analysis of the data?

5. Locate a research article that includes a nonparametric procedure such as Kruskal-Wallis or Friedman tests. Why did the researchers choose a nonparametric test? Did the researchers make the proper choice?

6. Search the universe of research reports for a study that contains samples of unequal sizes, such as two samples with 10 and 12 subjects respectively. Based on the article you found, calculate the relative loss of efficiency and relative loss of power associated with this study's sample. Why did they have unequal samples? How did the unequal sample sizes affect their study?

CHAPTER 11

SYNTHESIZING RESEARCH IN COMMUNICATION DISORDERS

synthesize (sĭn′thĭ-sīz) *v.* to combine separate ideas or elements to form a coherent whole

As a whole, research in the behavioral sciences including communication disorders is poorly coordinated and sometimes disorganized. One problem is that many researchers work in relative isolation from colleagues with similar research goals. Though coordinated efforts are evidenced in urban research centers and within networks of colleagues, much research is planned and implemented by individuals or small teams of researchers who are not cognizant of ongoing research in other locales. Some disciplines have adopted *registries* of prospective and ongoing research so that research plans are openly available. Researchers are better able to plan and coordinate their own research efforts if they know what others are planning. Lyons (2004) commented on the sometimes confusing state of the research literature in the social sciences—comments equally applicable to communication disorders:

> Over the last 15 to 20 years, there has been an increased criticism of social sciences research because of the confusing state of the research literature. While one reviewer could find a set of studies that supported his viewpoint, a second reviewer commonly found several which did not support said conclusions. A common conclusion in reviews was "conflicting results in the literature, more research is needed to resolve this issue" which typically resulted in more studies which did nothing to clarify the issue.

The problem is particularly acute for *clinical-outcomes research*. *Clinical-outcomes research* is what audiologists and speech-language pathologists depend on for evidence-based practice. To encourage better organized research, Robey and Schultz (1998) proposed a universal model for researching clinical outcomes with five phases. A *phased model* is one course for organizing research outcomes into a coherent whole.

A MODEL FOR CLINICAL-OUTCOME RESEARCH

The model described by Robey and Schultz (1998) provides a conceptual framework for the progression of clinical-outcome research from the early stages that focus on exploration to the later stages that focus on refinement. Stage I research begins after the clinician-researcher formulates an idea. Robey and Schultz (1998) explained as follows:

> As an example of applying the model, consider that the genesis for an innovation in the treatment of [clients] arises from a clinical researchers' inductive reasoning based on experience and deductive reasoning based on expertise applied to observations of one or more patients. Having elaborated the initial insight to produce a basic treatment protocol, the clinician engages the model to pursue clinical-outcome research. (p. 795)

Phase I

The goal for *Phase I research* is explorative, based on a tentative treatment protocol. Phase I observations are designed to detect the presence (or absence) of a treatment effect as well as any negative consequences. The participants may not exactly represent the target population, and external controls may be lacking. Thus, Phase I studies are not rigorous experiments but are necessary to establish the ground rules for later experimentation. Typically, Phase I research is accomplished with small-group experiments (i.e., a sample size < 30), case studies, and single-case experiments such as A-B designs and their elaborations. If Phase I results show no promise of a treatment effect, researchers may discontinue this line of research. However, if Phase I results reveal the prospect of a treatment effect, researchers would be encouraged to develop Phase II research protocols.

Phase II

According to Robey and Schultz (1998), both Phase I and II are exploratory and prerequisite steps to a test of the efficacy hypothesis. *Phase II goals* differ from those of Phase I in that they aim to (a) finalize operational definitions, (b) define the exact population of interest, (c) refine methodology, and (d) explore the treatment effect's degree and permanency. Phase II research is typically implemented with case studies, small-group designs, and elaborations of single-case A-B designs.

Phase III

Based on the findings in Phase I and II studies, *Phase III clinical-outcome research* aims to test the critical hypothesis and answer the research question regarding treatment efficacy. Phase III research includes large, representative samples of subjects (i.e., a sample size > 30) and includes external controls in the form of comparison groups such as no-treatment controls. A typical Phase III design is a pretest-posttest design with the comparison group receiving a different treatment.

Phase IV

Phase IV aims to bridge the divide between research and practice, i.e., the transition from demonstrating efficacy in the laboratory to showing effectiveness in real-life settings. It is particularly important for researchers to collaborate with clinical researchers to implement Phase IV clinical-outcome research. The focus of research in Phase IV may shift to specific subpopulations or could extend the treatment protocol to different populations. For example, Phase IV research might be extended to include different ethnic groups or different clinical groups. Phase IV research typically involves large-group designs but could include rigorous single-case designs with replication.

Phase V

The focus of *Phase V clinical-outcome research* shifts to other treatment effectiveness issues, such as cost-benefit, consumer satisfaction, and quality-of-life issues. Phase V studies typically involve large-group and single-case designs but usually do not include a comparison group.

Robey and Schultz's (1998) model for clinical-outcome research provides a framework for organizing research into a more orderly process. We should recognize that it is an idealized model and as such not likely to be adopted by everyone in the research community. Nonetheless, it makes the point that research efforts can be organized into a more coherent whole.

Another means for organizing research outcomes is the *systematic review*. Systematic reviews attempt to synthesize the existing research into a coherent whole. They are particularly useful for combining the results from numerous Phase IV and Phase V studies. The systematic review method identifies studies that have a common hypothesis, combines their results, and formulates conclusions based on the sum of results. The synthesis of results in communication disorders is typically accomplished by one of the following methods: (a) narrative review, (b) quantitative review with meta-analysis, or (c) best evidence review.

THE NARRATIVE APPROACH TO SYSTEMATIC REVIEW

The traditional method for reviewing the literature and synthesizing results is the *narrative review*. Kavale (2001) defined the narrative review as "a verbal report analyzing individual studies to reach an overall conclusion" (p. 178). To be meaningful, the narrative review approach for synthesizing research requires (a) a thorough search of the pertinent literature, (b) a qualitative analysis of the results of past studies, and (c) a conclusion based on synthesis of the results.

CASE EXAMPLE

Glennen (2002) performed a narrative review of language development and delay in adopted children. According to Glennen (2002), the primary goal was to "provide speech-language pathologists with an overview of linguistic, developmental, and medical issues that can potentially affect speech and language development in internationally adopted children" (p. 338). Glennen reported that there was little objective information available, so a narrative review may have been the only available choice of methods.

Eisenberg, Fersko, and Lundgren (2001) adopted the narrative review method to examine the use of mean length of utterance (MLU) for identifying language impairment in preschool children. Based on a comprehensive review of the literature, Eisenberg et al. (2001) concluded that MLU is not the best measure of utterance length for identifying language impairment.

Narrative reviews are a valuable resource for synthesizing the existing literature on a topic, but they suffer from some serious limitations. First, narrative reviews are especially vulnerable to the effects of researcher bias. If researchers have predisposed notions regarding the review topic, personal opinions might influence the conclusions. Second, narrative reviews are prone to different interpretations by different authors. Indeed, two researchers can review the same body of literature and reach quite different conclusions.

To avoid questions of reviewer bias and the lack of reliability that accompanies traditional narrative reviews, contemporary reviewers usually adopt the systematic review approach. The *systematic review* is a summary of research that uses explicit methods to perform a thorough literature search. It also critically evaluates individual studies to identify the valid and applicable evidence. The systematic review differs from the traditional narrative review in that there is a clear and explicit protocol in place for selecting and evaluating studies before the review begins. Systematic reviews can be purely qualitative, or they may be quantitative in nature. However, in both instances, systematic reviews typically follow steps such as those prescribed by the *Cochrane Collaboration* (n.d.). The Cochrane Collaboration prescribed the following steps for reviews.

Step 1. Formulate a problem.
Step 2. Locate and select studies.
Step 3. Assess study quality.
Step 4. Collect data (qualitative or quantitative).
Step 5. Analyze and present results.
Step 6. Interpret results.

CASE EXAMPLE

The systematic review in communication disorders is exemplified in Baylor, Yorkston, Eadie, Strand, and Duffy's (2006) review of outcome measurement in unilateral vocal fold paralysis.

They recognized that there is a diversity of outcome measurements used to measure effectiveness of interventions for unilateral vocal fold paralysis. For this reason, Baylor et al. (2006) searched the literature to identify outcome measurement practices. They identified 92 studies that met their inclusion and exclusion criteria. As a result of their analysis, Baylor et al. (2006) were able to recommend improvements in the quality of measurement methods. They also observed that there were no randomized controlled trials (RCTs) among the 92 studies. One of the values of systematic reviews is to identify limitations and needs. Baylor et al. (2006) identified the need for better measurement and more controlled studies within the domain of unilateral vocal fold paralysis.

THE QUANTITATIVE APPROACH TO SYSTEMATIC REVIEWS

The earliest known *quantitative research synthesis* is attributed to Karl Pearson, circa 1904. Pearson was a founder of statistics as a field of endeavor, and is the grandfather of rigorous statistical evaluation for human behavior. Research synthesis methods have improved considerably since Pearson's early efforts.

One of the simplest methods for the quantitative synthesis of research is the *vote-counting method*. In the vote-counting method, the results of selected studies are placed into one of three categories: (a) positive findings, (b) negative findings, and (c) nonsignificant findings. The category with the largest proportion of findings is asserted to support or refute the research hypothesis. The vote-counting method is limited because it is not sensitive to sample-size effects, and it does not evaluate the size of an experimental effect in a meaningful way.

An alternative to the vote-counting method is the *combined-probability method*. According to Rosenberg, Adams, and Gurevitch (2000), combined-probability methods are the precursors to modern meta-analysis. Combined-probability methods are more powerful than vote-counting methods because they incorporate exact probabilities in the synthesis, thus they account for different sample sizes. However, combined-probability methods do not quantify the size of experimental effects, nor do they evaluate heterogeneity among the studies (Rosenberg et al., 2000). The limitations inherent in vote-counting and combined-probability methods are overcome in modern meta-analysis methods. *Modern meta-analysis* combines measures of effect size from individual studies, achieves an overall measure of effect, and tests the significance of the overall effect.

Modern Meta-Analysis

Egger, Smith, and Phillips (1997) defined *modern meta-analysis* as "a statistical procedure that interprets the results of several independent studies considered to be 'combinable'" (p. 1533). The National Library of Medicine defined meta-analysis as "a quantitative method of combining the results of independent studies (usually drawn from the published literature) and synthesizing summaries and conclusions which may be used to evaluate therapeutic effectiveness, plan new studies, etc. It is often an overview of clinical trials" (National Library of Medicine, 2004b). Robey and Dalebout (1998) explained the need for quantitative synthesis in communication disorders as follows:

> As is true of any research question, compelling evidence for scientific conclusions cannot be accomplished through a single experiment or quasi-experiment. Science requires converging evidence from all independent experiments as the basis for a compelling conclusion. (p. 1227)

An Early Review with Meta-Analysis

Andrews, Guitar, and Howie (1980) reported a very early application of meta-analysis in communication disorders. They included 42 studies in a quantitative synthesis aimed at studying the efficacy of stuttering treatment. In recent years, the numbers of meta-analytic studies in communication disorders have increased, such as Casby's (2001) meta-analysis of the effect of otitis media on language development, and Boutsen, Cannito, Taylor, and Bender's (2002) meta-analysis that focused on Botox treatment in spasmodic dysphonia. Modern meta-analysis is a powerful method for examining relationships in communication disorders, especially in clinical-outcomes research. Typically, *systematic reviews (SRs)* accomplish the following three goals:

1. SRs provide comprehensive summaries of research on a specific topic.
2. SRs provide strong evidence for clinical decision making.
3. SRs identify ideas for future research.

Synthesis by meta-analysis is based on the assumption that each study provides an independent (and different) estimate of the effect in the population. Thus, results accumulated across studies are expected to provide a better representation of the relationship between independent and dependent variables than results from individual studies can provide. In the special case of clinical-outcome research, meta-analysis has

TECHNOLOGY NOTE

MeSH (Medical Subject Headings) is the National Library of Medicine's controlled vocabulary thesaurus. The MeSH thesaurus is used by the National Library of Medicine to index articles from 4,600 journals for the MEDLINE/PubMed database. MeSH descriptors help to define searches for specific literature in communication disorders. MeSH facilitates PubMED clinical queries. The National Center for Biotechnology Information (NCBI) website includes a link to clinical queries using research filters. PubMED clinical queries can be performed with either (a) a research methodology filter or (b) a systematic review filter—at www.ncbi.nlm.nih.gov/entrez/query/static/clinical.html. The MeSH fact sheet and a downloadable electronic copy are available at the National Library of Medicine website: www.nlm.nih.gov/mesh/meshhome.html. Online tutorials for searching with the MeSH Database are available at the NCBI website.

an advantage over large controlled experiments because a synthesis of several small studies may provide equally valid conclusions in a shorter period of time at less cost.

THE BEST EVIDENCE APPROACH TO SYSTEMATIC REVIEWS

Slavin (1995) recognized the limitations inherent in both traditional and quantitative reviews and proposed an alternative, which he called the *best evidence approach*. He cited the limitations in the traditional approach as the following:

1. Traditional reviews are not exhaustive in their inclusions of studies.
2. There is review bias in selecting studies.
3. There is no systematic way to weight the evidence appropriately.

Slavin (1995) further cited what he considered the *major limitations* in quantitative reviews:

1. Quantitative reviews place too much emphasis on the whole and sacrifice the detail of individual studies.
2. It is rare for a quantitative review to describe even one study in any detail.
3. Quantitative studies usually exclude studies when an effect-size measurement is not feasible, which results in selection bias.

Clearly, the *best evidence approach* aims to combine the best aspects of both narrative and quantitative approaches to systematic reviews. Slavin (1995) described his purpose and goals in developing best evidence synthesis as follows:

> As a response to concerns about misleading conclusions from meta-analyses [quantitative reviews], I proposed an alternative procedure designed to incorporate many of the important contributions of meta-analysis but also retain many of the features of intelligent and insightful narrative reviews. I called this procedure "best-evidence synthesis," although it could just as well have been seen as a set of standards for meta-analyses designed to describe the full richness and unique contributions made by the most important studies. (p. 11)

The format for the best evidence approach to systematic reviews includes four parts:

1. The *introduction* is similar to the traditional narrative review.
2. The *method* includes a description of how studies were selected for inclusion in the review.
   (a) Best evidence criteria should describe and justify the study selection criteria employed.

    (b) Methodological adequacy criteria should focus the avoidance of systematic bias by means of random assignment, matching, sample size, and internal validity.

    (c) Reviewers should describe the set of studies that will constitute the synthesis and the characteristics of studies that are not selected for review.

3. The *literature review* should first present and discuss the study characteristics and effect sizes as well as any related issues. If the quantitative measurements are pooled, the results of the pooling should be described. Critical or exemplary studies should be described, and important conceptual and methodological issues should be explored.

4. The *conclusion* should summarize the findings from the large body of literature to give readers some indication of where the weight of evidence lies. The conclusions should be produced and defended based on the best available evidence. Alternatively, the reviewers may conclude that the available evidence does not allow for any conclusion at the present.

In summary, Slavin (1995) proposed an approach that included the best aspects of narrative reviews and quantitative reviews. An example of a recent systematic review that incorporated both qualitative and quantitative aspects is Cirrin and Gillam's (2008) review of language intervention practices with school-age children. They blended detailed descriptions of studies with quantitative analysis to form their conclusions.

STEPS IN THE SYSTEMATIC REVIEW PROCESS

Implementing the systematic review in communication disorders typically follows six steps:

1. Develop a research hypothesis and define the initial eligibility criteria for inclusion.
2. Develop a search strategy and identify the studies for inclusion and exclusion.
3. Assess the quality of included studies.
4. Collect the data. Quantitative reviews will convert the study statistics to a common effect-size metric.
5. Analyze the data and present results. Quantitative reviews will compute a summary effect.
6. Interpret the results.

Step One: Develop a Research Hypothesis and Eligibility Criteria

Initially, researchers should identify the parameters for the review, including (a) the population to be studied, (b) intervention to be examined, (c) outcomes of concern, and (d) design of studies to be reviewed, i.e., either randomized controlled experiments or quasi-experiments. Once the parameters are defined, the research hypothesis and questions to be answered should be evident.

CASE EXAMPLE

Boutsen et al. (2002) employed the systematic review method to study the effects of Botox on patients with spasmodic dysphonia. They stated the study's purpose as follows:

> The purpose of this report is to review the BT [Botulinum toxin type A] efficacy data in adductor SD [spasmodic dysphonia] to determine whether and to what extent the aforementioned issues [BT treatment in SD is safe and improves vocal quality] make it necessary to qualify the view that BT is effective. (Boutsen et al., 2002, p. 470)

From what you learned about Boutsen et al.'s (2002) statement of purpose, what parameters can be identified? What is the common hypothesis, i.e., the hypothesis shared by all the studies included in the review?

Eligibility criteria.   The criteria for including and excluding participants in a meta-analysis are known as *eligibility criteria*. The eligibility criteria are determined in the initial planning stage. They include factors such as (a) the study design, i.e., either experimental or quasi-experimental, (b) chronological window, i.e., years of publication, (c) English language used alone or with other language(s), (d) similarity of treatment, (e) completeness of information, i.e., whether summary statistics or primary statistics, (f) quality of method, and (g) combinability of subjects, treatments, and outcomes. Boutsen et al. (2002) described their study's eligibility criteria as follows:

> From the available pool of studies published between 1988 and 1999, 20 investigations were identified in which pre- and posttreatment measurements of SD speech or voice production were reported in sufficient detail to be included in a meta-analysis. These studies met the following additional criteria: (a) at least 5 SD participants sampled pre- and posttreatment, (b) the data pertained to the initial BT injection of patients who had not been treated surgically, (c) posttreatment measurements were reported short term and/or long term. (p. 477)

Based on what you have learned about Boutsen et al.'s (2002) study, answer the following questions: What were the eligibility criteria? What studies did they exclude from the meta-analysis of Botox and SD? When evaluating meta-analytic studies, the following questions should be answered:

1. Is the specific purpose of the review stated?
2. Are the hypothesis and research questions clearly and explicitly stated?
3. Are the eligibility criteria clearly and explicitly stated?

If the answers to these questions are affirmative, reviewers typically advance to the next step, which is to search the literature.

Step Two: Develop a Search Strategy and Select Studies for Inclusion

Following development of the research questions and eligibility criteria, researchers should develop a strategy to search the literature. The goal is to assemble a database

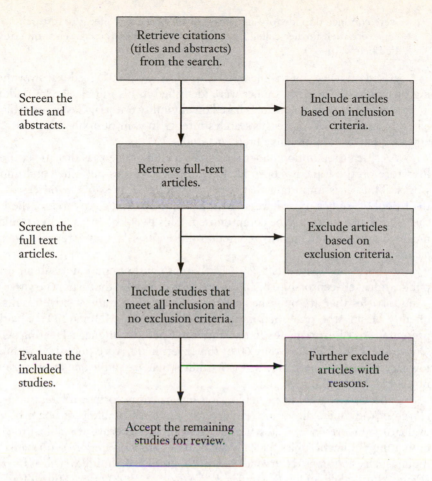

EXHIBIT 11.1
Steps in the Study Selection Process
Adapted from Meline, 2006b.

from which studies can be included or excluded based on the eligibility criteria. Exhibit 11.1 depicts the steps in the study selection process, from locating citations in the initial phase to selecting studies to be reviewed in the final phase.

The *initial pool of studies* is typically much larger than the database that will be studied. For example, Casby (2001) described his search strategy as follows:

The following electronic databases were used in a literature search of primary studies of OME [otitis media with effusion] and oral language development from the mid-1960s to the present—*ERIC, PsychINFO*, and *MEDLINE*. The keywords used in the search were *otitis media* and *language*. The noted electronic databases are considered diverse and comprehensive in their coverage of the topic of OME. A total of 61 articles were identified via *ERIC*, 66 via *PsychINFO*, and 162 through *MEDLINE*. In addition, manual searches of the citations of the primary sources and other compendiums on OME were conducted to identify and locate further potential pieces of research. All of these sets were then further culled for studies that met the project's selection criteria specified below. (p. 67)

Based on what you have learned about Casby's (2001) study, answer the following questions: How many studies were identified in his initial search? Following the inclusion and exclusion of studies based on eligibility criteria, Casby assembled a database of 32 studies. What was his search strategy? In your opinion, was the search strategy adequate for identifying all relevant studies?

A critical assumption underpinning systematic reviews is that the entire body of literature on the topic has been identified. This includes published and unpublished works. Thus, it is important that reviewers utilize all possible resources to establish their pool of studies. If reviewers do not manage an extensive search of the literature, the validity of results may be compromised. This issue concerns content validity. The most common problem with content validity in systematic reviews is known as *publication bias*.

Publication bias exists as a threat because authors may not submit articles for publication (self-censorship) or editors may reject articles that report negative findings. Thus, articles that are published are more likely to contain positive results—consequently biasing the published literature. For example, Meline (2003) identified 201 presentations of experiments in an American Speech-Language-Hearing Association Convention Program, but only 60 of the experiments were published within the following five years. There may be many studies that are published in obscure places or not published at all.

The best way to avoid publication bias is to perform a diligent and extensive search of the topical literature. However, several acceptable post hoc procedures for evaluating the presence (or absence) of publication effects are available. Procedures for evaluating publication bias typically fall into one of two categories: (a) statistical techniques such as *fail-safe* N (Orwin, 1983) or (b) graphic techniques such as the *funnel plot* (Egger, Smith, Schneider, & Minder, 1997). Robey (1998) offered the following explanation for funnel plots and their interpretation.

> Publication bias, or the file-drawer problem (i.e., negative findings tend not to be published because authors chose not to submit or editors chose not to publish), can likewise threaten the validity of a meta-analysis. A plot of sample size over effect size is one means for detecting the possibility of publication bias (e.g., Greenhouse & Iyengar, 1994). In the absence of publication bias, the plot should have the appearance of a triangle sitting on its base or an inverted funnel. That is, sampling theory would predict that (a) effect sizes derived from small sample sizes should be relatively variable compared to the more homogenous effect sizes derived from larger sample sizes, and (b) all should center around the same mean. (p. 182)

The other category of procedures for evaluating publication bias is *statistical techniques*. The most common statistical technique is known as *fail-safe* N. Robey (1998) explained his application of the fail-safe N method as follows:

> Another method for examining the validity of a meta-analysis is to calculate the number of null (i.e., [effect size] = 0.0) findings that would be necessary, if they existed, to

diminish the value of [the combined effect size] to a critically low value (Hunter & Schmidt, 1990). For the within effects, the critical value of [effect size] for treated individuals is the corresponding value of [effect size] for untreated persons. The mathematics of Hunter and Schmidt (1990, pp 512ff) indicate that a total of 9 null findings in studies (i.e., each reporting [effect size] = 0.0) of treated aphasic persons in the acute stage of recovery would be necessary to lower the treated value of [the combined effect size] = 1.15 [observed value of treated recoveries] to the untreated value of [effect size] = 0.63 [observed value of untreated recoveries]. That is an unlikely prospect. (p. 183)

To establish a database of studies, Robey (1998) conducted an extensive search that yielded 55 reports of clinical outcomes that met the eligibility criteria. Based on what you have learned about Robey's (1998) review, answer the following questions: What is the basis for his conclusion that nine null findings are an unlikely prospect? Robey (1998) used the funnel plot and fail-safe *N* as post hoc procedures. Why did he use both graphic and statistical procedures?

Search strategies usually begin with electronic databases such as PsychINFO and MEDLINE because they index a large number of journals, and they are easily accessed. However, a thorough search strategy should include as many electronic databases as possible as well as a manual search. Electronic resources such as ERIC and Dissertation Abstracts International are an integral part to search strategies because they include unpublished materials in their databases. In addition, a search strategy should include a manual search of journals, books, and monographs to locate articles that may not otherwise be identified. Reviewers should pay special attention to reference lists to locate studies.

CASE EXAMPLE

Herder et al. (2006) employed an information retrieval protocol that included both hand and electronic searches. They listed with the inclusive dates 13 relevant journals in communication sciences and disorders that they hand searched for studies to include in their initial pool of studies. Because their focus was the effectiveness of behavioral stuttering treatments, the list of journals included familiar ones such as the *Journal of Fluency Disorders* and less familiar journals such as *Behavior Therapy*. The assumption was that these 13 journals represented the periodicals that were most likely to publish articles about behavioral stuttering treatment. This information is usually gleaned from a journal's title, the journal's general information page, and common knowledge about specific journals and their publishing practices. For the electronic searches, Herder et al. (2006) chose databases that were most likely to index studies relevant to their review's focus. They chose a host of databases including PsychINFO, ERIC, MEDLINE, CINHL, C2-SPECTR, and the Cochrane Central Register of Controlled Trials and Dissertation Abstracts. The Cochrane Central Register was searched to ensure that unpublished studies were uncovered as well as published ones. To locate relevant studies in each of these databases, Herder et al. (2006) used the following search terms:

1. *Target populations:*   stutt*, stam*
2. *Interventions:*   therap*, intervene*
3. *Outcome:*   stutt*, fluen*, dysfl*, disfl*

Overall, Herder et al.'s (2006) information retrieval strategy was exemplary in its planning and execution.

Information retrieval strategies usually require more than one pass through the search protocol. Rather, the search strategy is an iterative process—one that typically requires multiple revisions. It is often the case that several trials are needed before an acceptable pool of studies is attained.

To ensure *reliability*, reviewers usually develop a standard format for recording and collecting data. Studies are subsequently selected or rejected based on the eligibility criteria incorporated in the format. If quality of the study is a factor for inclusion or exclusion, *blinding* is a necessary precaution to ensure validity and avoid experimenter bias. The best practice is to redact authors' names, institutional affiliations, journal titles (journal prestige may influence decisions), and other identifying information before studies are evaluated.

When *evaluating systematic reviews*, the following questions should be answered:

1. Were extensive search methods employed to locate studies?
2. Was an extensive search performed with appropriate databases?
3. Were other potentially important sources of studies explored?
4. Were reliability and validity issues addressed appropriately?

Step Three: Assess Study Quality

Inasmuch as studies differ in their methodological quality, systematic reviews typically incorporate some method to evaluate the quality of the studies that are selected for review. A simple strategy that is intended to ensure that only the highest quality studies are included in the review is to include randomized clinical trials (RCTs) and exclude all other research designs.

TECHNOLOGY NOTE

Meta-analysis procedures require intensive computations and complex manipulations of the data. The data collected for meta-analysis are typically entered into a spreadsheet format to facilitate analysis. There are numerous statistical software applications available for performing meta-analysis. One of the most complete applications is MetaWin 2.0 (Rosenberg, Adams, & Gurevitch, 2000). The current version is MetaWin 2.1.5. The MetaWin 2.0 package includes MetaCalc—a stand-alone program that performs statistical procedures used in meta-analysis such as converting primary statistics to effect sizes—and MetaWin, which is a comprehensive program for summarizing the results of multiple studies, calculating fixed-effects and random-effects models, and computing effect sizes and confidence intervals. *MetaWin* includes tests for heterogeneity and tests to evaluate potential publication bias. The *MetaWin* website is www.metawinsoft.com.

CASE EXAMPLE

Torgerson, Brooks, and Hall (2006) used this strategy to systematically review the research literature on the use of phonics in the teaching of reading and spelling. They reviewed 20 RCTs that focused on phonics instruction in English but did not evaluate the methodological quality of individual studies. On its face, this might seem like a good strategy because RCTs are the "gold standard" for answering cause-effect questions. However, the problem is that RCTs differ in their methodological quality: Some have much better internal validity than others. For example, Meline and Harn (2008b) examined 16 RCTs published in ASHA journals from 2003 to 2008. They found the average reporting transparency to be 71% with a range of 55% to 91%. The relatively low transparency in some reports could reflect the lesser quality of those studies, or it might simply reflect poor report writing.

Based on their review, Torgerson et al. (2006) concluded that phonics teaching was associated with better progress in reading accuracy, but there was no similar effect for reading comprehension. However, some of the 20 RCTs that they reviewed could have been methodologically sound, and others might have been methodologically weak.

If Torgerson et al. (2006) had evaluated the *methodological quality* of the individual studies and weighted the studies according to methodological strength (or weakness), their conclusions might have been different. Thus, methodological quality is an important consideration when planning a systematic review, but reviewers should not rely on type of research design alone to judge methodological quality.

Meline (2006b) argued the need for quality assessment as follows:

> Although some systematic reviewers—mostly traditionalists—dismiss quality assessment procedures as unreliable, Greenwald and Russell (1991) concluded that "investigators can be in relative agreement as to the severity and seriousness of a threat to the design quality of a study. Such threats can be reliably coded, individually, and in terms of an index of global methodological quality (p. 23). Systematic reviewers can use quality assessment a priori as eligibility criteria to select the study pool, or they may use quality assessment to weight studies for ex post facto analysis. The point to make here is that research design [methodological quality] is a critical element of the inclusion decision and must be defined at the outset of the review. (p. 24)

Once reviewers decide to evaluate the methodological quality of their studies, they face the obstacle of poor *methodological reporting*. Unfortunately, the descriptions of methodology are sometimes ambiguous or incomplete. This makes the assessment of quality difficult or sometimes impossible. The last resort is to discard what otherwise might be a relevant study because it fails to report important details such as reliability measures or steps to counter experimenter biases. Sometimes, reviewers can contact the principal researchers for additional information before deciding to exclude a study.

If sufficient information is available, reviewers can assess the methodological quality of individual studies with "quality indicators." A *quality indicator* is some characteristic that is generally agreed to be a good index of a methodologically sound study. Quality indicators are usually grouped into an evaluation instrument that could be framed as answers to questions, a binary checklist, or scales that provide quantitative estimates of overall study quality.

CASE EXAMPLES

Jadad, Moore, Carroll Jenkinson, Reynolds, Gavaghan, et al. (1996) developed a quality assessment instrument with the following questions:

1. Was the study described as randomized?
2. Was the study described as double blind?
3. Was there a description of withdrawals and dropouts?
4. Were the objectives of the study defined?
5. Were the outcome measures defined clearly?
6. Was there a clear description of the inclusion and exclusion criteria?
7. Was the sample size justified (e.g., power calculation)?
8. Was there a clear description of the intervention?
9. Was there at least one control (comparison) group?
10. Was the method used to assess adverse effects described?
11. Were the methods of statistical analysis described? (p. 7)

Bothe, Davidow, Bramlett, and Ingham (2006) adopted five methodological criteria to judge quality in their review of behavioral approaches to stuttering treatment. Their criteria for quality were as follows:

1. A basic design of random assignment to groups or single-subject design with ABA or multiple baselines and a stable baseline rate;
2. The use of blind or independent observers with interjudge agreement of at least 80%;
3. The availability of both pre- and post-test data;
4. The availability of beyond-clinic [natural environment] data;
5. The presence of controls for measures of speech rate, speech naturalness, and judge agreement. (p. 325)

Based on what you have learned about Bothe et al.'s (2006) systematic review, what do you think their rationale was for each of the quality criteria? In your opinion, were these quality indicators likely to include quality studies and exclude poor quality studies? In what way would you have changed their criteria?

There are two general approaches used to assess the quality of studies for systematic reviews: (a) the *threshold approach*, and (b) the *quality-weighting approach*.

The threshold approach.   The first approach, the threshold approach, is the least inclusive of the two approaches. In other words, it tends to exclude more studies from the systematic review because it sets an absolute threshold for each study to meet. If the study meets the threshold, it is included. If it does not meet the threshold, it is excluded. This was the approach that Bothe et al. (2006) used to select studies for review based on their quality indicators. For example, they required studies to have blind observers. If a study had blind (or independent) observers, the study was included.

If a study did not have blind observers, it was summarily excluded. This illustrates the threshold approach for quality assessment.

In principle, the threshold approach assures a minimum level of quality when selecting studies for systematic review. However, the decision to include or exclude a study based on threshold criteria is not always easy. In reality, some studies may clearly exceed the threshold while others may be questionable. As an answer to this dilemma, Abrami et al. (1988) proposed a continuum of confidence from *obviously meets* to *obviously fails to meet* the criterion. Based on their ratings along this continuum of confidence, Abrami, Cohen, and d'Apollonia al. (1988) included the studies that reasonably met the criteria.

The quality-weighting approach.   The *quality-weighting approach* is more inclusive than the threshold approach because it includes most studies but weighs them according to their quality. In this way, the better quality studies weigh more heavily in the conclusions than the poorer quality studies. For example, reviewers who adopt the quality-weighting approach might use a predetermined instrument to assess the quality of each study on an ordinal scale from 1 (lowest quality) to 5 (highest quality). The quality-weighting approach diminishes the likelihood of selection biases, which is a potential problem with the threshold approach. Overall, the quality-weighting approach has at least three clear advantages: (a) It provides a larger pool of studies, (b) the larger pool of studies better represents the available research on the topic, and (c) it enables the reviewers to examine the relationship between methodology and study outcomes. In regard to the last advantage, the reviewers can answer the question, Does the quality of studies affect the intervention outcome? This is an important question because smaller, less methodologically rigorous studies sometimes report positive outcomes, but later and more rigorous studies often report negative outcomes. However, the reverse is also possible, though less often seen in the research literature.

The most prominent threat to the review's internal validity that the quality-weighting approach raises is the potential for bias in assigning the quality weights to individual studies. However, this threat is alleviated by (a) ensuring the reliability of the instrument used to assess quality and (b) utilizing blind observers or independent judges to assign quality weights.

Step Four: Collect Data and Convert Study Statistics to a Common Metric

Once the pool of studies is set, the goal for quantitative reviews is to convert statistics from each study into a *common metric*. In this way, the outcomes from each study can be combined into an omnibus statistic. The common metric is typically an effect size. In the case of qualitative reviews, reviewers look for common themes across studies. Qualitative reviewers typically organize outcomes from their studies in tables so that similarities and differences among studies are evident.

For quantitative reviews, effect sizes are calculated. This is dependent on the availability of data in the primary studies. There are three categories of primary data: (a) summary statistics such as means, standard deviations, and sample size, (b) count data, e.g., two-by-two contingency tables, and (c) F, t, and χ^2 statistics. If summary statistics are available, there are several alternatives for converting them into effect sizes. For example, a common effect-size metric is Cohen's d, expressed mathematically in equation 1.

$$d_{Cohen} = \frac{mean^E - mean^C}{\sigma}$$

$$\sigma = \sqrt{\frac{N^E - 1)(s^E)^2 + (N^C - 1)(s^C)^2}{N^E + N^C}}$$

(eq. 1)

To *compute Cohen's* d, subtract the mean of the control group (C) from the mean of the experimental group (E) and divide by the pooled standard deviation (σ). The result is a standardized effect size that is interpreted like other standardized scores; i.e., an effect size of 1.00 is one standard deviation above the mean, an effect size of 2.00 is two standard deviations above the mean, and so on.

An alternative to Cohen's d is the effect-size statistic known as the *response ratio*. The response ratio (R) is the ratio of the experimental group's outcome to the control group's outcome. The response ratio quantifies the proportionate change that results from an experimental manipulation (Hedges, Gurevitch, & Curtis, 1999). It is expressed mathematically in equation 2.

$$R = \ln\frac{mean^E}{mean^C}$$

(eq. 2)

According to Rosenberg, Adams, and Gurevitch (2000) the *natural log of the response ratio* (ln R) has "preferable statistical properties," so it may be best to transform R before interpreting its meaning. In any case, the response ratio is easily interpreted. A value of zero indicates no difference in effects between experimental and treatment groups. Negative values indicate that control group effects exceed treatment group effects, and positive values indicate that experimental group effects exceed control group effects.

CASE EXAMPLE

Robey (1998) reported that the average effect size for treated individuals with aphasia was 1.83 times greater than that for untreated individuals with aphasia. Based on this information, how would you interpret Robey's (1998) result in the context of treatment and no-treatment conditions? Was it a negative or positive outcome? Finally, how does this result relate to clinical practice?

A second category of primary data found in communication disorders studies is the count data presented in two-by-two contingency tables. In this case, there are two groups (i.e., experimental and control) and two outcomes (i.e., response and no response). Exhibit 11.2 displays a two-by-two contingency table with fictitious data.

EXHIBIT 11.2
A Two-by-Two Contingency Table

	TREATMENT	CONTROL	TOTAL
Response	8*	2	10
No Response	2	8	10
Total	10	10	20

*Number of observations

There are several effect-size metrics appropriate for contingency tables, but a simple one that is easily interpreted is *relative rate* (RR)—the rate of the experimental group relative to the control group. Based on the data in Exhibit 11.2:

$$RR = P_T / P_C = 0.8 / 0.2 = 4.00$$

The interpretation of relative rate is straightforward. No difference between experimental and control groups is represented by 1.00. Values greater than 1.00 indicate positive trials where treatment effects are observed to exceed control effects. Values less than 1.00 indicate negative trials, i.e., control effects exceed treatment effects. The following criteria are general rules for evaluating the importance of the relative-rate metric:

1.0 **trivial** RR effect
1.9 **moderate** RR effect
3.0 **large** RR effect
5.7 **very large** RR effect

A third category of primary data commonly found in studies of communication disorders is *primary statistics*, including F, t, and χ^2. If summary statistics are not available to calculate Cohen's d or an alternative effect-size metric, primary test statistics such as F may be converted to effect-size metrics in two steps: (a) convert the primary statistic to a correlation, and (b) convert the correlation to a z-score. The conversion of primary test statistics to correlations is accomplished as shown in the following equations (eqs. 3–6).

$$F \text{ statistic: } r(eta) = \sqrt{\frac{F}{F + df_{ERROR}}} \qquad \text{(eq. 3)}$$

$$X^2 \text{ statistic: } r(phi) = \sqrt{\frac{x^2}{N}} \qquad df = 1 \qquad \text{(eq. 4)}$$

$$X^2 \text{ statistic: } r = \sqrt{\frac{\chi^2}{\chi^2 + N}} \quad df > 1 \hspace{2cm} \text{(eq. 5)}$$

$$t \text{ statistic: } r = \sqrt{\frac{t^2}{t^2 + df}} \quad df = N - 2 \hspace{2cm} \text{(eq. 6)}$$

The general rules for evaluating the importance of the correlation coefficients are as follows:

< 0.1   **trivial** correlation effect
0.3–0.5   **moderate** correlation effect
0.5–0.7   **large** correlation effect
0.7–0.9   **very large** correlation effect

Equation 7 is *Fisher's z-transform*, which is used to convert correlation coefficients to standard effect-size metrics.

$$z = \frac{1}{2}\ln\left\{\frac{1 + r}{1 - r}\right\} \hspace{2cm} \text{(eq. 7)}$$

When evaluating quantitative studies, the following questions should be answered:

1. Were study statistics converted to a common metric?
2. Was the method for converting study statistics clear and explicit?
3. Were appropriate procedures used for converting study statistics to effect-size metrics?

Once study statistics are converted to common effect-size metrics, they are combined to form a *cumulative effect size*. Calculating a cumulative effect size is the last of the four basic steps for quantitative analysis.

Step Five: Analyze and Present Results

The fifth step for quantitative synthesis involves *computing* a cumulative effect and interpreting its meaning. This step is unique to quantitative reviews. The most common statistic for measuring a cumulative effect is the average or mean. However, quantitative data typically include a mix of studies that are diverse in their settings, subject characteristics, and sample sizes. In addition, the overall quality of individual studies affects the aggregate result.

In general, large samples (i.e., $n > 30$) have smaller variances, and smaller samples (i.e., $n < 30$) have larger variances, but the mean statistic does not account for the differences in variation. The average of the cumulative result should give more weight to larger studies and less weight to smaller studies. According to Robey and Dalebout (1998), each effect size is weighted by its sample size so that the effects from small samples do not unduly bias the calculated value of the average. Thus, the individual results from studies are computed as the product of each effect size and its corresponding weight. The cumulative effect is calculated as the average of the weighted effect sizes. However, a credible interpretation of the weighted cumulative average is not possible without examining the *heterogeneity* of the database in some detail.

The results of individual studies may be mathematically incompatible with the results of other studies in the database (Greenhalgh, 1997b). This phenomenon is known as *heterogeneity*. Some heterogeneity between studies is unavoidable given the diversity of studies typically included in synthesis studies, but a significant degree of heterogeneity between studies may seriously undermine the interpretation of the cumulative effect.

Measuring heterogeneity.   There are several procedures for measuring the *degree of heterogeneity* present in a sample of studies. A simple method is to visually inspect the data. For example, Egger et al. (1997) recommended a graphic display of individual study results that includes means, standard deviations, and confidence intervals. However, visual inspection of the individual study results is not a definitive test for heterogeneity.

A definitive test for heterogeneity may be computed as the Q-*statistic* (Hedges & Olkin, 1985), but there are other procedures available for testing heterogeneity. A significant Q-statistic indicates that the variance among effect sizes is greater than expected by sampling error alone (sampling or measurement errors). In this case, variance is due to sampling error and the presence of confounding variables such as experimental biases or other threats to internal validity. If the Q-statistic is not significant, researchers may assume that the sample of studies is homogeneous, and the variance is attributable mostly to sampling error. If there is a significant degree of heterogeneity, researchers may examine their database more closely for the possibility of one or more moderator variables.

A *moderator variable* is an independent variable other than the treatment variable that explains a significant amount of the variance between studies. Robey and Dalebout (1998) explained moderator variables in the following fashion:

> Because one or more sources of variation (e.g., severity of disorder, duration of disorder, age) influence the outcomes of primary studies, the average effect for all studies contributing to a synthesis is often a moderately sized effect with a broad confidence interval. A stratified analysis, separate analyses for each level (or class or category) of a theory-driven explanatory variable, may result in understandably different average effect sizes. Such a categorical independent variable (or one that can be made categorical) is termed a moderator variable. (p. 1231)

The presence of one or more moderator variables can significantly enhance the interpretation of meta-analysis findings.

■ ■ ■ ■ ■ ━━━━━━━━━━━━━━━━━━━━━━━━━━━━━━━━━━━━━━━

CASE EXAMPLE

Robey (1998) synthesized aphasia treatment outcomes from various studies. The cumulative effect for all studies was a moderate effect with a wide confidence interval. A further examination of Robey's (1998) data disclosed the presence of a moderator variable: *time post-onset for treatment*. Based on evidence for a moderator variable, Robey (1998) concluded that patients who were treated early (1 month post-ictus) demonstrated larger gains than patients who were treated late (12 months post-ictus). An analysis of the data is important for identifying possible moderator variables, but the analysis is limited by the number of studies included in a meta-analysis (Robey & Dalebout, 1998). Thus, researchers cannot inspect the data for moderator variables when the number of studies is small.

Statistical models.   Researchers typically adopt one of two statistical models to represent the data, based on the results of heterogeneity tests. The two general models are known as (a) the fixed-effects model, and (b) the random-effects model. The *fixed-effects model* assumes that the variability of results between studies is attributable to random variation alone, which is more typical in randomized controlled experiments.

Alternatively, the *random-effects model* assumes that the variability of results between studies is attributable to random variation plus the effects of confounding variables, such as experimental biases and other threats to internal validity. The random-effects model more often fits the data accumulated from quasi-experimental studies. The fixed-effects model is the more powerful model but not appropriate if the data are heterogeneous. Researchers may assign one or the other model to their aggregate data based on the results of heterogeneity tests.

The interpretation of the cumulative effect of synthesis by meta-analysis depends on the validity of the database, the calculation of cumulative effects, the presence or absence of moderator variables, and other factors. When evaluating quantitative reviews, the following questions should be answered:

1. Was the method for accumulating results from individual studies clear and explicit?
2. Were the methods for combining study effects appropriate?
3. Were the data tested for heterogeneity and an appropriate statistic model utilized for the analysis?
4. Were the data inspected for possible moderator variables?
5. Were interpretations and conclusions consistent with the results?
6. Were results discussed in relation to evidence-based practice?
7. Were implications for future research discussed?

Step Six: Interpret the Results

Reviewers depend on the synthesis of results for their interpretation. To this end, Nye and Harvey (2006) offered advice for interpreting and maintaining evidence from systematic reviews. They advised reviewers to update reviews as often as needed.

The decision to reject or adopt a specific intervention is not the sole purpose of a systematic review, meta-analysis, or the effect size data. The collection, summary, analysis, and interpretation of intervention effects are all important and necessary functions of developing an evidence-based portfolio of research that can guide the practice of speech-language pathologists [and audiologists]. It would, however, be a mistake to think of this as a one-shot solution to meeting the need for EBP. Current research and practice should be a cumulative process of building a knowledge base from past research. In order to maintain a viable and useful EBP, a commitment also has to be made to continually update the portfolio. The need for a review of systematic reviews and meta-analyses on a regular basis will be critical to improving the delivery of clinical services as well as the communication skills of individuals being treated for communication disorders. As new research is made available, those data need to be included in existing reviews and analyses and the results reinterpreted if necessary. It is certainly possible that with more evidence in a given area, the strength and direction of intervention could be altered. (Nye & Harvey, 2006, p. 59)

THE EPIDEMIOLOGY OF SYSTEMATIC REVIEWS

In an effort to describe the status quo in regard to systematic reviews, Moher, Tetzlaff, Tricco, Sampson, and Altman (2007) set out to examine a sample of systematic reviews as published in the medical literature. Thus, they searched the MEDLINE database for relevant systematic reviews. Systematic reviews are very popular in medicine because they are the basis for the majority of evidence-based practice decisions.

Based on their search and analysis of systematic reviews, Moher et al. (2007) estimated the annual frequency of systematic reviews published at 2,500 as indexed in MEDLINE. They further estimated that about 20% of these reviews could be attributed to the Cochrane Collaboration. The remaining 80% were non-Cochrane reviews attributed to various authors. The United States contributes about 23% of the total number of systematic reviews. The remaining 77% were attributed to the United Kingdom and reviewers in other countries. They reported that the focus of reviews was overwhelmingly treatment issues (71%), and nearly half of the total number of reviews (47%) focused on pharmacological treatments. Furthermore, about one-half of all reviews combined their results statistically; most reviews failed to assess or consider publication bias; and Cochrane reviews were superior in quality to non-Cochrane reviews. Moher et al. (2007) explained the difference between Cochrane and non-Cochrane reviews as follows:

> for therapeutic reviews our comparison of Cochrane and non-Cochrane reviews provides the most discouraging results and suggests little improvement in the quality of reporting of non-Cochrane reviews over time. The Cochrane Collaboration has a strict set of policies and guidance as to how systematic reviews] should be conducted and reported. (p. 0451)

It is clear that consumers should be aware that systematic reviews are unequal in their quality. However, it is equally clear that consumers are more likely to find competent reviews in the Cochrane Collaboration's database than elsewhere. Moher et al. (2007) also reported that they found few updates of past systematic reviews. A critical need in evidence-based medicine as well as in the evidence-based practices of audiologists and speech-language pathologists is for up-to-date systematic reviews. Unfortunately, few reviewers choose to update reviews in a timely manner.

WHEN IS A SYSTEMATIC REVIEW OUT-OF-DATE?

Shojania, Sampson, Ansari, Ji, Doucette, and Moher (2007) have addressed relevancy of systematic reviews in regard to their currency. They utilized a survival analysis to examine 100 quantitative reviews. Eligible reviews included those that evaluated the benefit or harm of a specific drug, class of drug, device, or procedure and included randomized and quasi-randomized controlled trials. A *survival analysis* is a study of the birth and death (i.e., lifetime) of a system or entity—in this case the useful life of a systematic review. However, for a survival analysis to be meaningful, the analyst must define both birth and death in operational terms. In the case of systematic reviews, the definition of *birth* is relatively easy. Shojania et al. (2007) defined it as the date that the review was first published. They defined *death* as the occurrence of one or more signals for the need to update the review. Exhibit 11.3 lists the signals to observe. If one or more of these signals is noted, the present review is out of date, and an update is justified.

What Is the Life of a Systematic Review?

Shojania et al. (2007) found the median length of time free of a signal for updating to be 5.5 years (CI, 4.6–7.6 years). However, a signal for updating occurred within two years for 23% of the reviews that they examined, and within one year for 15% of the reviews. In as much as Shojania et al.'s (2007) analysis focused on medical interventions, it may or may not be applicable to interventions in communication disorders. However,

---

EXHIBIT 11.3
Signals for the Need to Update Systematic Reviews

Goal: To detect a potential change in the evidence that warrants a formal update.

QUANTITATIVE SIGNALS

✓ Be alert to a relative change in effect size of 50% or more in the primary outcome.

✓ Ignore trivial changes in effect size.

QUALITATIVE SIGNALS

✓ Be alert to new information about harm or benefit that may affect clinical decisions.

✓ Be alert to important caveats to the original results.

✓ Be alert to the emergence of superior alternative treatments.

✓ Be alert to important changes in the certainty or direction of the effect.

Adapted from Shojania et al., 2007.

the life of a systematic review depends largely on the availability of new research outcomes and new developments. In as much as advancements occur frequently in many areas of communication disorders, the lifetime of reviews may be similar to Shojania et al.'s (2007) findings.

THE REALIST REVIEW METHOD

Pawson, Greenhalgh, Harvey, and Walshe (2005) proposed a model of research synthesis based on the realist approach to evaluation. It is especially appropriate when a rich, detailed and highly practical understanding of complex social interactions is needed such as when planning and implementing programs at local, state, and national levels. For example, health initiatives are programs that are typically adopted at local, state, or national levels. According to Pawson et al. (2005), the aim is to help decision-makers to better understand an intervention and how it can be made to work most effectively. The steps in the realist review framework are sometimes overlapping and often iterative. The key steps in the realist review method are as follows:

Step 1. **Clarify the scope** by identifying the review question, refining the purpose of the review, and articulating key theories to be explored. What are the underlying theories about how the intervention is meant to work? What impacts are expected from its implementation?

Step 2. **Search for evidence.** First conduct an exploratory search. Second, progressively focus on key program theories. Utilize purposeful sampling to test a defined subset of these theories. Finally, extract data from different studies to populate the evaluative framework with evidence.

Step 3. **Appraise the primary studies** for relevance and rigor and extract data.

Step 4. **Synthesize the evidence** to achieve refinement of the program theory and draw conclusions.

Step 5. **Disseminate, implement, and evaluate.**

On the surface, the *realist review* looks very similar to other forms of systematic reviews. However, the realist review focuses on the theory or theories underlying an intervention to a greater extent than other review methods. According to Pawson et al. (2005), "Research is unlikely to produce the facts that change the course of policy-making. Rather, policies are born out of a clash and compromise of ideas, and the key to enlightenment is to insinuate research results into this reckoning" (p. 33). Thus, the realist review method focuses on theories and ideas, which policy-makers are more likely to understand than data alone.

CONCLUSION

It should be clear that synthesis plays a major role in the advancement of science, especially in the applied sciences. The best evidence for making clinical practice decisions comes from systematic reviews of the available evidence, but EBP also depends on updated reviews as new information becomes available. It is also clear that consumers should not blindly rely on systematic reviews to inform their practices, because the quality of reviews varies considerably. One of the problems for EBP is that systematic reviews are not possible when there are few or no relevant studies to review. In communication disorders, the availability of studies for systematic review is uneven across the many special interest areas. As Baylor et al.'s (2006) review of unilateral vocal fold paralysis revealed, some specialty areas have no evidence from RCTs. In another case, Helm-Estabrooks, Hanson, Yorkston, and Beukelman (2004) reviewed 25 years of research for speech supplementation techniques for dysarthria, and they found only 19 studies to include in their review.

Though we could despair from the paucity of available research, systematic reviews serve the important purpose of identifying research needs and pointing out deficiencies in past research so that methods can be improved. We should expect the numbers of systematic reviews in communication disorders to increase dramatically over the next 10 years as new studies are added to the research base and new interventions are introduced. For example, in pharmacology and stuttering, the pharmacological agents tested thus far are less than acceptable due largely to adverse side effects, but the success of one new drug could change the outlook for future treatment (Meline & Harn, 2008a). In any case, the systematic review is an important means for integrating research findings, though not a perfect one.

CASE STUDIES

Case 11.1: Database Dilemmas
A team of researchers that includes an academic researcher and clinical researchers identified an initial database of 60 studies based on multiple searches in MEDLINE and PsychINFO databases. They consulted you to help determine whether the database is adequate for analysis. What advice will you offer to the research team? Once they have exhausted the search for topical literature, how should they proceed? What is the next step?

Case 11.2: More or Less for Professor Moore and Associates
Professor Moore and associates accumulated a database for analysis, and they tested it for heterogeneity. The result was a significant test for heterogeneity. They have considered adopting a random-effects model and analyzing the data accordingly. In as much as you are the expert in meta-analysis, they consulted you for an alternative course of action. What is an alternative to accepting the random-effects model? Is a reexamination of the studies in their database possible? What can Professor Moore and associates do to improve their database?

Case 11.3: A Problem of Incompatibility
Professor Tolkien and SLP Mathers have undertaken a meta-analysis of clinical outcomes for phonologically impaired children. They successfully established a database of 40 studies, but they are not sure how to convert the individual study results to a common metric. Some of the study results are expressed as means, standard deviations, and sample sizes alone. Other study results are expressed as *F* or *t* statistics with no means or standard deviations available. As a

research consultant, what course of action do you recommend to Tolkien and Mathers? Can they find a common metric for the studies in their database?

Case 11.4: A Question of Need
Rebecca and Carly are not sure whether a systematic review of neuromuscular electrical stimulation for swallow is feasible. They are seeking your best advice. What can you tell them about determining the need and feasibility for a systematic review? What guidelines should they apply?

Case 11.5: A Stodgy Professor
Professor McGonagall is a somewhat stuffy, dull, and unimaginative professor but your thesis advisor. Your idea is to explore the need for a systematic review as a thesis project, but the professor says that is not good science. How can you convince the professor that systematic reviews are an important methodology for the advancement of science (and particularly for practices)? What are the points that you will make to convince the professor that a systematic review is a good idea for a thesis project?

STUDENT EXERCISES

1. Search the current journals in communication disorders for a narrative synthesis. What is the researchers' rationale for selecting the narrative research method? Could they have performed a quantitative analysis of the data?
2. The Q statistic is one procedure for determining the heterogeneity of a sample of studies. What other techniques are available for testing heterogeneity? What are their applications and limitations?
3. Search the current journals in communication disorders and identify a synthesis review with meta-analysis. What was the researchers' search strategy? How did they evaluate their database for a possible publication bias effect?
4. Identify a systematic review with meta-analysis in communication disorders journals. What is the authors' interpretation of the data and their conclusions? Evaluate their conclusions for consistency with results and completeness. Did the researchers recommend future courses for studying the problem?
5. Identify a systematic review in the communication disorders literature and evaluate its methodology. How did the researchers aggregate the outcomes from individual studies? How would you improve their method of study? Did they cite any limitations?
6. Utilizing one or more databases for your search (PubMed, MEDLINE), locate as many reviews (e.g., narrative, systematic, meta-analyses) as possible that were published over the course of the past 10 years. What is the trend? Are there more reviews in later years? Based on whatever trend you identify, project the number of reviews that will be published in the next 10 years.

PART IV

APPLIED RESEARCH FOR AUDIOLOGISTS AND SPEECH-LANGUAGE PATHOLOGISTS

CHAPTER 12

EVALUATING RESEARCH FOR PRACTICE IN COMMUNICATION DISORDERS

evaluate (ĭ-văl′yŏŏ āt′) *v.* to examine and judge carefully; appraise the value or worth of something

The ability to access vast amounts of information in the 21st century is unparalleled in history, but not all information is created equal, and not all information is good, according to the National Information Center on Health Services Research and Health Care Technology (National Library of Medicine, 2004b). For these reasons, *information literacy* has emerged as an important goal for educators, students, researchers, and practitioners. The Association of College and Research Libraries (ACRL, 2000) issued information-literacy competency standards for higher education that provided a framework for assessing information literacy in individuals. The ACRL (2000) published a definition of *information literacy* and emphasized the challenges that information literacy poses for society:

Information literacy is a set of abilities requiring individuals to "recognize when information is needed and have the ability to locate, evaluate, and use effectively the needed information." Information literacy also is increasingly important in the contemporary environment of rapid technological change and proliferating information resources. Because of the escalating complexity of this environment, individuals are faced with diverse, abundant information choices—in their academic studies, in the workplace, and in their personal lives. Information is available through libraries, community resources, special interest organizations, media, and the Internet—and increasingly, information comes to individuals in unfiltered formats, raising questions about its authenticity, validity, and reliability. In addition, information is available through multiple media, including graphical, aural, and textual, and these pose new challenges for individuals in evaluating and understanding it. The uncertain quality and expanding quantity of information pose large challenges for society. (pp. 2–3)

The ACRL (2000) prescribed standards of information literacy for the following:

1. Determining the nature and extent of information needed
2. Accessing needed information effectively and efficiently
3. Evaluating information and its sources critically and incorporating selected information into one's personal knowledge base and value system
4. Using the information effectively to accomplish a specific purpose
5. Understanding the economic, legal, and social issues surrounding the use of information—accessing and using the information ethically and legally

In regard to literacy and evidence-based practice, Nail-Chiwetalu and Bernstein Ratner (2003) remarked:

[There are] direct parallels between evidence-based practice as endorsed by the [Certificates of Clinical Competence] and the information literacy competency standards. Importantly, it is difficult to achieve the goals of [evidence-based practice] if one cannot obtain and interpret the evidence appropriately. (pp. 166–167)

According to Law's (2000) scheme, evidence-based practice involves the systematic use of best evidence for solving clinical problems and includes eight steps for achieving evidence-based practice. The eight steps are:

1. Clearly identify the clinical problem.
2. Gather information from research studies about this problem.
3. Ensure that you have adequate knowledge to read and critically analyze research studies.
4. Decide if a research article or review is relevant to your clinical problem.
5. Summarize the information so that it can be easily used in your practice.
6. Define the expected outcomes for the children [or adults] and their families.
7. Provide education and training to implement the suggested change in practice.
8. Evaluate the practice change and modify (if necessary). (Law, 2000, pp. 33–34)

To gather information about the problem, consumers need to know what resources are available. There are two broad sources of information for evidence-based practice: (a) *raw evidence*—information that has not been subjected to expert review—and (b) *pre-filtered evidence*—information that has been reviewed by experts, as is the case for articles in peer-reviewed journals. However, regarding pre-filtered evidence, Beeman (2002) warned that research published in scientific journals gives the readers some confidence in the scientific credibility of research findings, but scientific credibility does not necessarily mean that the findings represent the truth. Both pre-filtered and raw evidence types require careful evaluation by consumers.

After identifying a clinical problem, researchers, students, and practitioners usually search electronic databases for pertinent information. The alternative is to hand search selected journals, but hand searches are slow and subject to human error. Hand searches are sometimes used to supplement electronic searches.

Modern technology provides computerized search engines that facilitate searching the databases with keywords. *Keywords* are index terms or descriptors used in information retrieval systems. They are intended to capture the essence of a topic. Keywords are important because they are used to retrieve documents or other sources of information in an information system's database. Keywords are stored in the system's search index. To increase efficiency, common words such as articles and conjunctions are not treated as keywords. Each information retrieval system has its unique characteristics, so users should acquaint themselves with the features of the system they are using. For example, the Google search engine has the following features:

1. A Google search is not case sensitive. The keywords *dYsPHagIa* and *dysphagia* retrieve the same information.
2. Google returns only pages that include all of your search terms. If you search with keywords *tinnitus* and *cause*, you will retrieve only pages with both terms included.
3. Common words (i.e., stopwords) are usually dropped from the search, so if you search for *apraxia and swallow*, the conjunction is dropped.
4. Google requires keywords to be enclosed in quotes for phrase searches, such as "aphasia treatment." In this case, the search engine looks for phrases that are exact matches.
5. Google uses the minus symbol (–) as a limiter. For example, *dysphonia–neurological* searches for *dysphonia* but excludes pages that contain *neurological*.

Nail-Chiwetalu and Bernstein Ratner (2003) described their experience using different search engines to gather evidence about stuttering treatment:

> In our next search, we simulated the task of a student who wanted to know about treatment of stuttering using altered auditory feedback. Once again, we went first to Google. What we got here was a true mix, the kind that bedevils many professors attempting to mark papers. Of the 2,000 Web sites that were identified, a large proportion of the top listed sites on the first few pages were commercial ventures selling auditory aids for people who stutter. A few were sites featuring publicized aids on shows such as *Oprah* and *Today*. A few were unpublished conference papers. A few were chat rooms discussing personal experiences and devices. Taken together, they provided a relatively poor mix of resources for a student to determine whether or not auditory aids were appropriate treatment options for people who stutter. Next, we went to the database, Academic Search Premiere, and include[d] ERIC, MEDLINE, PsychInfo, and other major health-related databases in its search scope. We retrieved far fewer items, but the articles did tend to address whether or not auditory feedback affected stuttering frequency and severity. (pp. 176–177)

Locke, Silverman, and Spirduso (2004) adopted *five basic questions* as a guide for evaluating research reports, and their questions are a useful guide to evaluate research for practice in communication disorders. Greenhalgh and Taylor (1997c, pp. 741–742) proposed an *alternative set of questions* that specifically target the evaluation of qualita-

TECHNOLOGY NOTE

The Internet permits easy access to vast amounts of information, but Internet-based information exists along a continuum of quality and reliability. An important goal for students and practitioners is to efficiently track down the best evidence with which to answer focused questions (Kuster, 2002). Kuster's (2002) tutorial on web-based information resources for evidence-based practice in speech-language pathology is a starting point for developing information literacy skills. An Internet-based interactive source for acquiring information literacy skills is the *Terrapin Information Literacy Tutorial* (TILT)—developed by the University of Texas System Digital Library. The TILT interactive experience includes an introduction, three learning modules, and a follow-up component. The TILT helps users acquire abilities for locating, evaluating, and effectively using information. The Terrapin Information Literacy Tutorial is accessed via http://tilt.lib.utsystem.edu/.

tive (as opposed to quantitative) research. Greenhalgh and Taylor's (1997c) questions for evaluating qualitative research studies were:

1. Did the paper describe an important problem addressed via clearly formulated questions?
2. Was a qualitative approach appropriate?
3. How were the setting and the subjects selected?
4. What was the researchers' perspective, and has this been taken into account?
5. What methods did the researcher use for collecting data—and are these described in enough detail?
6. What methods did the researcher use to analyze the data—and what quality control measures were implemented?
7. Are the results credible, and if so, are they clinically important?
8. What conclusions were drawn, and are they justified by the results?

The Locke, Silverman, and Spirduso (2004) taxonomy included five basic questions that are applicable to both quantitative and qualitative research. Locke et al.'s (2004) questions were (a) What is the report about? (b) How does the study fit into what is already known? (c) How was the study done? (d) What was found? (e) What do the results mean?

WHAT IS THE REPORT ABOUT?

What is the report about? An answer is found in an article's *title*, *keywords*, *abstract*, and *statement of purpose*. The *Publication Manual of the American Psychological Association* (APA, 2001) recommended: "A title should summarize the main idea of the paper simply and with style," and "A title should be fully explanatory when standing alone" (pp. 10–11).

CASE EXAMPLE

Ingham, Fox, Ingham, Xiong, Zamarripa, Hardies, and Lancaster's (2004) article was titled: "Brain Correlates of Stuttering and Syllable Production: Gender Comparison and Replication." What does this title tell you about the article, and what does it not tell you? The *keywords* associated with Ingham et al.'s article (2004) were *stuttering*, *brain imaging*, and *gender differences*.

Titles and keywords are especially important because these terms are typically used to index articles in the repositories of major databases such as MEDLINE, ERIC, and PsychINFO. Daniels, Corey, Hodskey, Legendre, Priestly, Rosenbeck, and Foundas (2004) chose the title *Mechanism of Sequential Swallowing During Straw Drinking in Healthy Young and Older Adults* for their research report. What does the title tell you about their study? Who were the participants? What were the experimental variables? What was the purpose of their study?

It is important that researchers state the *purpose* of their study in clear and concise words.

■ ■ ■ ■ ■

CASE EXAMPLE

Jupiter and Palagonia's (2001) article investigated the use of the *Hearing Handicap Inventory* with elderly Chinese Americans. In this case, the authors addressed the purpose of their study in the first line of their abstract as follows: "The purpose of this study was to determine whether the *Hearing Handicap Inventory for the Elderly* (HHIE) screening version translated into Chinese can be used as a valid screening instrument for the identification of hearing impairment in Chinese-speaking elderly persons" (p. 99). Given what you know about Jupiter and Palagonia's (2001) study, answer the following questions: Was their purpose stated clearly and concisely? Do you understand the purpose of their study based on the statement in the abstract?

An article's *abstract* is a brief and comprehensive summary of the article. A good abstract is (a) accurate, (b) self-contained, (c) concise and specific, (d) nonevaluative, and (e) coherent and readable (APA, 2001). Ingham et al. (2004) wrote the following abstract for their article titled "Brain Correlates of Stuttering and Syllable Production: Gender Comparison and Replication":

This article reports a gender replication study of P. T. Fox et al. (2000) performance correlation analysis of neural systems that distinguish between normal and stuttered speech in adult males. Positron-emission tomographic (PET) images of cerebral blood flow (CBF) were correlated with speech behavior scores obtained during PET imaging for 10 dextral female stuttering speakers and 10 dextral, age- and sex-matched normally fluent controls. Gender comparisons were made between the total number of vowels per region significantly correlated with speech performance (as in P. T. Fox et al., 2000) plus total vowels per region that were significantly correlated with stutter rate and *not* with syllable rate. Stutter-rate regional correlates were generally right-sided in males, but bilateral in the females. For both sexes the positive regional correlates for stuttering were in right (R) anterior insula and the negative correlates were in R Brodmann area 21/22 and an area within left (L) inferior frontal gyrus. The female stuttering speakers displayed additional positive correlates in L anterior insula and in basal ganglia (L globus pallidus, R caudate), plus extensive right hemisphere negative correlates in the prefrontal area and the limbic and parietal lobes. The male stuttering speakers were distinguished by positive correlates in L medial occipital lobe and R medial cerebellum. Regions that positively correlated with syllable rate (essentially stutter-free speech) in stuttering speakers and controls were very similar for both sexes. The findings strengthen claims that chronic developmental stuttering is functionally related to abnormal speech-motor and auditory region interactions. The gender differences may be related to differences between the genders with respect to susceptibility (males predominate) and recovery from chronic stuttering (females show higher recovery rates during childhood). (p. 321)

Based on your reading of Ingham et al.'s (2004) abstract, answer the following questions: What is your evaluation of their abstract given the APA *Publication Manual's* criteria? Is the abstract accurate, self-contained, concise and specific, nonevaluative, and coherent and readable? Rate the abstract for each of these five criteria along a continuum from poor (1) to good (5). Ingham et al.'s (2004) *statement of purpose* was written in the following paragraph from the article's introductory section.

The present study replicates the Fox et al. (2000) procedure by comparing adult female stuttering speakers and normally fluent controls with previously studied male counterparts so as to (a) identify regions functionally related to stuttering across genders, and (b) determine the extent to which the regional effects associated with stuttering are gender-specific (p. 323).

After examining an article's *title*, *keywords*, and *abstract*, consumers should know if the article's content is relevant to their focus of interest.

HOW DOES THE STUDY FIT INTO WHAT IS ALREADY KNOWN?

The answer to this question is found in the introductory pages of an article in what is known as the "Review of Literature." The APA's *Publication Manual* (2001) recommends (a) introducing the problem, (b) developing the background, and (c) stating the purpose and rationale in an article's introductory section. The literature review should describe past research results that are relevant to the problem at hand. The literature review is usually limited to current research but may include one or more classic studies if they are relevant. The literature review sometimes ends with a statement that addresses the relevancy of the current study. For example, Alt, Plante, and Creusere (2004) concluded their article's introductory section with a statement of how their study differed from previous studies and how their study was likely to contribute to the research literature:

Thus far, the literature has mostly provided information on how many words a child with [specific language impairment] can learn and how quickly he or she can learn them.

Clearly, word knowledge is a process more involved than simply recognizing or producing a label. ... This study addresses word learning in terms of (a) fast-mapping the phonetic strings that represent novel lexical labels, (b) fast-mapping semantic features associated with objects and actions represented by the novel lexical labels, and (c) the relative difficulty of mapping phonetic and semantic features for objects (nouns) and actions (verbs). (pp. 410–411)

When evaluating the introductory section of a research article, consumers should ask questions such as those proposed by Beeman (2002). Beeman (2002) asked the following questions: "Does the study provide new knowledge? Does it test a new program? Does it contribute to what we know and don't know?" (p. 3). What are some other questions that you might ask to evaluate the content of an article's introductory section?

HOW WAS THE STUDY DONE?

The answer to this question is found in the "Methods" section of a research article. The APA's *Publication Manual* (APA, 2001) explained the methods section as follows:

The Methods section describes in detail how the study was conducted. Such a description enables the reader to evaluate the appropriateness of your methods and the reliability and the validity of your results. It also permits experienced investigators to replicate the study if they so desire. (p. 17)

The *Methods* section typically contains three subsections, with detailed descriptions of (a) participants or subjects, (b) apparatus and materials, and (c) procedure—the step-by-step execution of the research plan.

Description of Participants or Subjects

A detailed description of subjects in research reports is critical for both the advancement of science and the advancement of practice in communication disorders. A detailed description of subjects permits a credible evaluation of results and allows practitioners to judge the transferability of results to their clinical settings. It also permits other researchers to replicate the study for confirmation of the results or to combine the results in the form of a *synthesis review*. A synthesis review is a study that aims to examine the results of similar studies to form a conclusion based on the collective results. A detailed description of subjects also permits other researchers to perform secondary data analysis. If the description of participants or subjects in a study is lacking, none of these goals can be successfully accomplished. Though each study is unique, the following questions represent the types of questions that consumers should ask:

1. What was the procedure for selecting subjects? Were subjects randomly selected? Did subjects volunteer to participate?
2. What was the procedure for assigning subjects to groups?

3. Is the control group equivalent to the treatment group?
4. Were subjects paid to participate in the study?
5. What are the demographic characteristics of participants—such as age, gender, and ethnicity?
6. Was there subject attrition during the course of the study?
7. What was the sample size? How many subjects completed the experiment? Is the sample size adequate for making meaningful conclusions?

The demographic characteristics of subjects are particularly important when they constitute experimental variables such as *clinical status*, *disability*, *socioeconomic status*, or *sexual orientation*. When animals are experimental subjects, researchers should report characteristics such as genus, species, sex, age, weight, and physical condition. In all cases, researchers should provide enough detail for other researchers to successfully replicate the study and sufficient detail for generalizing results to clinical settings when the study has clinical relevance.

CASE EXAMPLE

Daniels et al. (2004) described participants in their study of sequential swallowing during straw drinking as follows:

> Thirty-eight healthy adults were studied, including 20 right-handed young males between the ages of 25 and 35 years and 18 right-handed older males above the age of 60 years (range = 60–83). Fourteen young participants tested in a previous study (Daniels & Foundas, 2001) were included in the present study. Previous deglutition research has identified large effects (range = 0.90–2.0) when comparing the delay in onset of the pharyngeal swallow in older and young participants (Tracy et al., 1989). Power analysis revealed that an effect size greater than .89 would be detected with power equal to .80 with a sample size of 20 (α = .05), suggesting adequate power with the present sample. Exclusion criteria included a history of dysphagia, neurological disorders, chronic obstructive pulmonary disease, oropharyngeal structural damage, and a family history of dementia or Parkinson's disease. The study protocol was approved by the Institutional Review Boards at the Tulane University Health Sciences Center and the Veterans Affairs Medical Center in New Orleans. Informed consent was obtained from each participant. (p. 34)

Based on what you know about Daniels et al.'s (2004) study, answer the following questions: How would you evaluate their description of subjects? Are you satisfied with the demographic information that they provided? Why did they exclude participants with a history of dysphagia, dementia, or Parkinson's disease?

Daniels et al. (2004) provided a rationale for the number of subjects included in their study, but many researchers do not. Small numbers of subjects are especially problematic for group research designs because with very small samples it is easy for coincidental relationships to emerge (Almer, 2000). Furthermore, Almer (2000) pointed out that a conclusion based on a very small sample with no basis in logic or theory is suspect. Very small samples are also problematic because real treatment effects may be obscured by the failure to reach statistically significant levels, such as the .05 confidence level. This scenario is possible because statistical significance is dependent on sample size. With smaller samples, the likelihood of identifying statistical significant effects is less.

Description of the Apparatus and Material

The apparatus and material subsection in the methods section provides a brief description of whatever apparatus and material are used in the study. There is no need for detailed descriptions of standard equipment that is familiar to most consumers. On the other hand, the apparatus and material should be described in detail if it is not commonly known. Though each study's apparatus and material are unique, the following questions represent the types of questions that consumers should ask:

1. Are the stimuli that were presented to the subjects clearly described?
2. Can you clearly visualize the physical layout of the situation?
3. Is each instrument or material clearly described?
4. Is enough detail provided to determine whether the instruments are reliable and valid?

CASE EXAMPLE

Justice, Weber, Ezell, and Bakeman (2002) described the materials used in their study in the following paragraph:

> Materials included audiovisual equipment, one children's picture book, and a videotape for parent instruction. Reading sessions were recorded using two Panasonic VHS camcorders. To ensure that each dyad's book-reading behaviors were adequately captured during filming, one camcorder recorded a front view of the dyad and a second recorded a close-up of the open book. One children's picture book was used for all the reading sessions. *This Is the Bear* (Hayes, 1986) is a rhyming book that contains 24 pages, large narrative print, colorful illustrations, and numerous instances of contextualized print embedded within the pictures. The typical page contains between 8 and 10 words in the narrative and one or two instances of contextualized print in the illustration (e.g., in one illustration, a boy is waving down a truck by yelling "Stop! Stop!"). This combination of features was considered important for enhancing children's enjoyment of the activity and for providing ample opportunity for interactions regarding print. (pp. 32–33)

Given what you know about Justice et al.'s (2002) study, answer the following questions: How would you evaluate their description of materials? Why did they describe the children's picture book in detail? What apparatus or material in the study is assumed to be standard equipment—familiar to everyone, and what apparatus or material in the study is assumed to be unusual or unique to the study?

Description of the Procedure

The *procedure subsection* of the methods section describes what was done and how it was done. The procedure should be described in sufficient detail for replication by others and for transfer to clinical settings if the research has clinical application. The procedure subsection should (a) summarize each step in the execution of the study, (b) describe instructions to the subjects, and (c) describe specific experimental manipulations. It should also include descriptions of control features that the researchers employed, such as randomization or counterbalancing techniques. There is no need to provide detailed descriptions of commercial tests or standard testing procedures that should be familiar to consumers. If a language other than English is used, the language should be specified. Though each study's procedures are unique, consumers typically ask the following questions:

1. Are the instructions to subjects clearly described?
2. Is it clear how the dependent variable was measured?
3. Is the timeline for collecting data clearly described?
4. Are the manipulations of the independent variable(s) clearly described?
5. Are operational definitions for the experimental variables provided?
6. Are procedures free of the influence of extraneous variables?

Justice et al. (2002) described the *general procedures* in their study as follows:

Eligibility sessions took place in children's homes or on the university campus, based on parental preference. After eligibility was established, an individual data collection session was scheduled for each dyad on campus. This session consisted of the following. Parents first were asked to view the brief video training tape that demonstrated the use of print-referencing strategies. The children were engaged in an art activity in the same room while their parents were occupied. After viewing the video, print-referencing strategies were briefly reviewed by the examiner (the first author) using the picture book *This Is the Bear* (Hayes, 1986). To this end, each strategy was described again for the parents and two to three examples of each were demonstrated. Parents then were asked to use these print-referencing strategies while reading with their children. Parents were provided the book *This Is the Bear* and a set of written instructions that asked them to read with a normal volume and to keep the book flat on the table, both for video-recording purposes. This reading session was videotaped in its entirety and served as the basis for the analysis of shared book-reading interactions that occurred in this investigation. (p. 33)

Based on what you know about their study, answer the following questions: What is your evaluation of Justice et al.'s (2002) description of general procedures? Did they describe the procedure in enough detail to replicate the procedure in another research facility or within a clinical setting?

WHAT WAS FOUND?

The answer to this question should be in the "Results" section of a research report. The APA's *Publication Manual* (2001) described the results section as follows: "The results section summarizes the data collected and the statistical or data analytic treatment used. Report the data in sufficient detail to justify the conclusion" (p. 20). Researchers typically use tables, figures, photos, or other graphical means to enhance the readability and clarity of their presentation of results. The APA's *Publication Manual* also recommended *confidence intervals* as the best strategy for reporting statistical results. Confidence intervals are an alternative to traditional statistical significance tests of the null hypothesis (Guyatt, Jaeschke, Heddle, Cook, Shannon, & Walter, 1995). Though each study's procedures are unique, consumers typically ask the following questions:

1. Is there a clear presentation of the results in tabular or graphical form?
2. Is there a verbal description of results such as a statement of the difference between pre- and posttest treatments or a statement of the difference between experimental and control groups?
3. Are the correct statistical tests used? Do the researchers use distribution-free (nonparametric) tests when appropriate?
4. Are descriptive statistics appropriate for the dependent variable's level of measurement?
5. Are results reported in sufficient detail to answer each of the research questions?
6. Are the statistical analyses sufficient to address questions of *practical significance* and *clinical importance?*

The last question is especially important for consumers to ask, because the answer is critical for evidence-based practice.

Do Results Address Practical Significance and Clinical Importance?

In order to evaluate research for practice in communication disorders, it is important to recognize the difference between the terms "efficacy" and "effectiveness." Greenhalgh (1998) explained:

> There is a huge difference between efficacy (how well something works in the laboratory or controlled environment of the clinical research trial) and effectiveness (how well it works in the "real world" of the hospital ward, the clinic, the home and the community). (p. 1716)

Though researchers may report significant statistical findings in their results section, the results are not necessarily *clinically important.* Furthermore, the results may not be as effective in a clinical milieu—or may not be effective at all.

■ ■ ■ ■ ■ ▬▬▬▬▬▬▬▬▬▬▬▬▬▬▬▬▬▬▬▬▬▬▬▬▬▬▬▬▬

CASE EXAMPLE

Bender, Cannita, Murry, and Woodson (2004) studied speech intelligibility in severe adductor spasmodic dysphonia (ADSD). Bender et al. (2004) described their study's purpose in the final paragraph of the "Introduction" section as follows:

Thus, the purpose of the current study was to investigate speech intelligibility in severe ADSD before and after Botox injection. We hypothesized that (a) intelligibility of speakers with ADSD before Botox injection would be significantly poorer than that of normal speakers, (b) following Botox injection, intelligibility of ADSD speech would significantly improve, and (c) intelligibility in ADSD would remain poorer than normal at 3–6 weeks following injection. (p. 23)

Bender et al. (2004) adopted a pretest-posttest design with Botox injection as the intervening treatment. As a control measure, the researchers included an age- and gender-matched comparison group. After describing their methods in detail, the researchers reported results with verbal descriptions and in tabular and graphical forms. Bender et al.'s (2004) primary result was their finding that the post-Botox condition was significantly greater (in speech intelligibility) than the pre-Botox condition ($p < .01$). The mean difference in speech intelligibility between pre- and posttest conditions was about 10% (the percentages for speech intelligibility reported here are rounded to whole numbers). Based on this result alone, it seems that Botox may be an effective treatment for improving the speech intelligibility of ADSD speakers—or is it? Bender et al. (2004) did not report a confidence interval (CI) for the mean difference nor did they report an effect size.

Effect size is a measure of practical significance (Meline & Paradiso, 2003). The *confidence interval* measures the precision of a statistical estimate, such as the estimated mean difference between pre-Botox and post-Botox conditions reported in Bender et al.'s (2004) article.

If sufficient data are reported in the results section of a research article, consumers can perform secondary statistical analyses. In the Bender et al. (2004) case, the researchers presented sufficient data to construct a confidence interval. The resulting 95% CI was 4% to 17%.

How Is the Confidence Interval Interpreted?

First, the most likely value for the difference between pre-Botox and post-Botox conditions is about 10%—the mean difference reported by Bender et al. (2004). However, the true difference may be as large as 17% or as small as 4%. Values further away from 10% are increasingly improbable.

A verbal description of the CI result is written as "ADSD patients who choose Botox treatment most likely (but not certainly) will experience improved speech intelligibility, but the size of the improvement in intelligibility may be small or large." The 95% confidence level means that there is a 95% percent probability that the true difference between means lies somewhere between the upper and lower boundaries of the confidence interval. In the Bender et al. (2004) case, the lower limit of the confidence interval is greater than zero, so their result is interpreted as a *positive trial*. If a confidence interval includes zero (i.e., the lower limit is zero or a negative value), the result is interpreted as a *negative trial*.

Another secondary statistical analysis that provides useful information for evaluating research for practice in communication disorders is the effect size. *Effect size (ES) measures* are indicators of the "practical significance" associated with an experimental outcome. In the case of Bender et al.'s (2004) outcome, an effect size is calculated as the difference between the means divided by the pooled variance. Bender et al. (2004)

reported the pre-Botox mean (*SD*) as 79.43 (12.27), and the post-Botox mean (*SD*) as 89.86 (5.28). Given these values, the effect size (*d*) is calculated as follows:

$$d = M_1 - M_2 \text{ / pooled variance} = -1.10$$

where pooled variance $= \sqrt{[\sigma_1^2 + \sigma_1^2]} \, / \, 2$

In this case, the ES statistic is Cohen's *d*, which is a standardized effect size. The values of *d* are reported in standard units of measurement. Thus, a *d* value of 1.00 is equivalent to one standard deviation from the mean. The resulting effect size for the Bender et al. (2004) result is *d* = –1.10. The negative sign indicates the direction of the outcome—the difference between the mean percentages for speech intelligibility in the pre-Botox and post-Botox conditions. In this case, the magnitude of the experimental effect is slightly more than one standard deviation unit below the mean.

CASE EXAMPLE
A Small Sample

Bender et al.'s (2004) study included 10 participants in an experimental group and 10 participants in a control group—a relatively small sample. When sample size is small, *Hedge's* g is best for calculating effect size. Hedge's *g* corrects for small sample size, so the result is an effect size that is slightly smaller than Cohen's *d*. Hedge's *g* can be calculated in various ways. It is derived from Cohen's *d* as follows:

$$\text{Hedge's } g = d \left\{ 1 - \frac{3}{4(n_1 + n_2) - 9} \right\}$$

In Bender et al.'s (2004) case, Hedge's *g* equals –1.05. The ES value of ± 1.05 is usually evaluated as a large effect, but it is better understood by considering the alternative interpretations in Exhibit 12.1.

Exhibit 12.1 includes four columns of numbers with effect sizes from 0.0 to 2.0 in the leftmost column. The second column displays the percentile standings associated with the effect sizes in column one. Thus, an effect size of 1.0 is associated with the 84th percentile. The third column displays the percentages of overlap associated with the effect sizes in column one. For example, an effect size of 1.0 is associated with a 45% overlap (55% nonoverlap). *Degree of overlap* refers to the amount of variation shared by two variables, conditions, or treatments. Less overlap means a greater difference between treatments. Thus, effect size and degree of overlap are inversely related. The final column displays the probability of guessing group membership (such as experimental vs. control groups) from a single subject's score, rating, or performance—whatever value is assigned to the dependent variable.

In the Bender et al. (2004) study, the effect size that described the magnitude of the experimental effect between pre-Botox and post-Botox conditions was 1.05 after a correction for sample size. This value is equivalent to the 85th percentile and represents a 43% overlap (57% nonoverlap). In terms of guessing whether a single subject belongs to the pre-Botox condition or to the post-Botox condition, the probability of guessing correctly is about 70% (7 out of 10 times).

EXHIBIT 12.1
Interpreting Standardized Effect-Size Statistics: (a) Percentile Standing, (b) Percentage Overlap, and (c) Probability of Guessing Group Membership

EFFECT SIZE	(A) PERCENTAGE OF SUBJECTS IN THE CONTROL GROUP BELOW AVERAGE SUBJECT IN THE TREATED GROUP	(B) DEGREE OF OVERLAP	(C) PROBABILITY OF GUESSING GROUP MEMBERSHIP FROM A SINGLE SUBJECT'S SCORE
0.0	50%	100%	50%
0.2	58	85	54
0.4	66	73	58
0.6	73	62	62
0.8	79	53	66
1.0	84	45	69
1.2	88	38	73
1.4	92	32	76
1.6	95	27	79
1.8	96	23	82
2.0	98	19	84

Adapted from "Evidence-Based Practice in Schools: Evaluating Research and Reducing Barriers," by T. Meline and T. Paradiso, 2003, *Language, Speech, and Hearing Services in Schools, 34,* p. 278, Table 1.

WHAT DO THE RESULTS MEAN?

If researchers report results and analyses in sufficient detail, the conclusion to the research article is typically straightforward. However, if the results and analyses are not reported in sufficient detail, the research conclusions and associated clinical implications may be tenuous. The final section of the research report is known as the "Discussion" section. At this point in the presentation, researchers aim to examine, interpret, qualify, and draw inferences from their results. The conclusions should be logical, and they should be consistent with the reported results. The APA *Publication Manual* (2001) explained as follows:

After presenting the results, you are in a position to evaluate and interpret their implications, especially with respect to your original hypothesis. [...] Open the Discussion sec-

TECHNOLOGY NOTE

A recent survey found that effect-size (ES) statistics were included in less than half the articles published in ASHA journals, and only about half of those articles included interpretations of effect sizes (Meline & Wang, 2004). Thus, consumers may be left to evaluate the practical significance of research results on their own. In the case of treatment and comparison groups where means and standard deviations are reported, a standardized effect size can be estimated as the difference between the means divided by the standard deviation of the control group. In other cases, effect sizes may have to be computed from omnibus statistics—such as F or t statistics, which are frequently, reported in research results. Online calculators for ES are available at http://www.lyonsmorris.com/MetaA/contents.cfm/ *and* http://web.uccs.edu/becker/Psy590/escalc3.htm/.

tion with a clear statement of the support or nonsupport for your original hypothesis. (APA, p. 26)

A factor that sometimes interferes with the formulation of meaningful conclusions is known as *confounding*. *Confounding* is a scientific term that refers to research studies in which there are two or more explanations for a given outcome (Almer, 2000). To illustrate, some patients complain of swallowing problems in the days and weeks immediately following onset of a stroke, but their dysphagic symptoms disappear after a short course of therapy. Based on these observations, should we conclude that the therapy alone is responsible for the improvement in swallow function, or is there a plausible alternative explanation? Though each study's procedures are unique, consumers typically ask the following questions:

1. Do the researchers discuss the importance of their findings, and are their claims consistent with the results?
2. Do the researchers discuss unexpected results and explain their meaning?
3. Do the researchers explain how their results fit with existing theories and how they are consistent (or inconsistent) with related studies?
4. Do the conclusions match the findings reported in the results section?
5. Do the researchers discuss *cautions* or *limitations* in regard to findings?
6. Do the researchers discuss *clinical implications*, and are their conclusions valid?
7. Do the researchers recommend directions for further research?

In regard to the Bender et al. (2004) study, the authors concluded, "It is clear from these results that intelligibility is impaired in speakers with severe ADSD and that pharmacological therapy such as Botox injection provides a significant improvement in speech intelligibility" (p. 29). Given what you have learned about Bender et al.'s (2004) study, answer the following questions: How would you evaluate this statement? Does Botox provide a significant improvement in speech intelligibility?

For consumers who are evaluating research outcomes for evidence-based practice, a critical question is, What is a clinically important change? Bender et al. (2004) reported a 10% improvement in speech intelligibility following Botox treatment. However, the true improvement in speech intelligibility is probably somewhere between 4% and 17%. What is a clinically important change? Is it 5%, 10%, 20%, or none of these values? A second question that is critical for consumers who are evaluating research for evidence-based practice concerns clinical economics: Is the benefit of the change cost effective, or is there an alternative treatment that may provide a similar benefit at a lower cost? In regard to the efficacy and cost of Botox treatment, Bender et al. (2004) commented, "In the present push for treatment efficacy data, functional outcomes such as speech intelligibility can provide the justification for continued treatment via Botox, a very expensive form of treatment" (p. 29).

In this case, an important question is, How much change in speech intelligibility is needed to justify the high cost of the Botox treatment? When evaluating research for practice in communication disorders, it is especially important to ask: (a) Is the treatment transferable to my clinical setting? (b) How effective is the treatment likely to be in my clinical setting? (c) What are the economic considerations for my clinical setting?

CONCLUSION

The need for critical evaluation of research outcomes for practice in communication disorders is evident (Reilly, Douglas, & Oates, 2004). To this end, there are many resources available to speech-language pathologists and audiologists that assist the process of transferring research results to practice. One such resource is in the form of a checklist. In as much as *evidence grading* is an important aspect of evaluating research for practice, checklists are a means for grading the ability of research to predict the effectiveness of clinical practice.

Exhibit 12.2 is a checklist for evaluating the *introduction, methods, results,* and *discussion* sections of research articles in communication disorders. Alternative checklists are available at the Evidence-Based Medicine Tool Kit website: http://www.ebm. med.ualberta.ca/. The *EBM Toolkit* includes worksheets for evaluating articles about therapy and/or diagnostic tests.

More than 300 medical and public health journals, including those published by the American Speech-Language-Hearing Association, have endorsed the *CONSORT* and *TREND statements.* The Consolidated Standards of Reporting Trials (CONSORT) includes 22 criteria that are critical for ensuring that the reports of randomized clinical trials (RCTs) are complete and transparent. For nonrandomized research designs, the Transparent Reporting of Evaluations with Nonrandomized Designs (TREND) is the appropriate standard. The TREND and CONSORT statements are intended to guide authors in reporting their studies. However, they also are a useful means to assess the transparency of published reports. Research reports with high levels of transparency are easily understood, fairly evaluated, and useful for clinical decision making. Reports with low transparency are not fully understood, difficult to evaluate, and usually constitute poor evidence for clinical decision making.

EXHIBIT 12.2
Checklist for Evaluating Research in the Practices of Audiology and Speech-Language Pathology

Introduction Section: Review of the Literature and Purpose

1. Is the problem clearly identified at the beginning?   ☐ Yes   ☐ No   ☐ N/A

2. Is the review of literature selective, current, and critical?   ☐ Yes   ☐ No   ☐ N/A

3. Does the literature review focus on research findings rather than opinion?   ☐ Yes   ☐ No   ☐ N/A

4. Does the purpose, research questions, and hypothesis flow logically from the introduction?   ☐ Yes   ☐ No   ☐ N/A

5. Are the research questions clearly written and operational?   ☐ Yes   ☐ No   ☐ N/A

Methods Section: Materials, Procedures, and Participants

6. Are materials and any apparatus described in detail?   ☐ Yes   ☐ No   ☐ N/A

7. Are instruments properly calibrated and reliable?   ☐ Yes   ☐ No   ☐ N/A

8. Are human observers (judges) properly trained and reliable?   ☐ Yes   ☐ No   ☐ N/A

9. Are samples of questions or directions provided?   ☐ Yes   ☐ No   ☐ N/A

10. Is there evidence of informed consent?   ☐ Yes   ☐ No   ☐ N/A

11. Are procedures described in detail?   ☐ Yes   ☐ No   ☐ N/A

12. Are treatments described in detail?   ☐ Yes   ☐ No   ☐ N/A

13. Were blinding procedures used?   ☐ Yes   ☐ No   ☐ N/A

14. Is the experimental setting described in detail?   ☐ Yes   ☐ No   ☐ N/A

15. Were subjects randomly assigned to groups or matched on critical variables?   ☐ Yes   ☐ No   ☐ N/A

16. Is the sampling procedure described in detail?   ☐ Yes   ☐ No   ☐ N/A

17. Were subjects randomly selected from the population?   ☐ Yes   ☐ No   ☐ N/A

18. Is the sample adequate for generalizing results to others?   ☐ Yes   ☐ No   ☐ N/A

19. Is the sample size adequate for the research purpose?   ☐ Yes   ☐ No   ☐ N/A

20. Are participants described in detail?   ☐ Yes   ☐ No   ☐ N/A

Results Section: Statistics, Interpretation, and Presentation

21. Are results clearly stated?   ☐ Yes   ☐ No   ☐ N/A

22. Are results adequately interpreted?   ☐ Yes   ☐ No   ☐ N/A

23. Are the statistical tests appropriate?   ☐ Yes   ☐ No   ☐ N/A

24. Are effect sizes included with interpretation?   ☐ Yes   ☐ No   ☐ N/A

25. Do the results directly relate to the research questions?   ☐ Yes   ☐ No   ☐ N/A

(Continued)

EXHIBIT 12.2
(Continued)

Discussion/Conclusion Section: Limitations and Clinical Implications

26. Are the purpose and research questions restated?   ☐ Yes   ☐ No   ☐ N/A
27. Are limitations of the research design discussed?   ☐ Yes   ☐ No   ☐ N/A
28. Are results related to the review of literature?   ☐ Yes   ☐ No   ☐ N/A
29. Are clinical implications of results discussed?   ☐ Yes   ☐ No   ☐ N/A
30. Are future research needs discussed?   ☐ Yes   ☐ No   ☐ N/A

CASE STUDIES

Case 12.1: Professor Matlin's Dilemma
Professor Matlin and two clinical assistants completed an investigation to identify which of two treatments is the better one for improving speech fluency. Based on their pretest-posttest results, treatment B had an 18% improvement overall, and treatment A resulted in a 14% improvement. Which is the more efficacious treatment? What other considerations should be taken into account in their discussion of clinical implications?

Case 12.2: Collaborating for Reading Fluency
Dr. Gary and SLP Ruth are collaborating in a research project designed to identify the best protocol for improving third-grade children's reading fluency. Both of the treatments (*modeling* and *unison reading*) resulted in statistically significant improvements in reading fluency. As a research consultant, you are asked to help them with the interpretation of results. What is your advice for Dr. Gary and SLP Ruth?

Case 12.3: Implications for Evidence-Based Practice?
As an expert reviewer for the journal *Language, Speech, and Hearing Services in Schools*, you are asked to critically review the manuscript for a research report. The manuscript's authors found a 10% difference between their pretest and posttest conditions and concluded that the treatment is an effective one that should be utilized by practitioners, but the justification for their conclusions is weak. What can you recommend to the authors to improve the reporting of results and improve their discussion of clinical implications?

12.4: Clinically Significant?
Karen and Max are assigned to find a study with a pretest/posttest design and calculate effect size. They also must interpret its meaning for clinical application. Karen and Max locate an appropriate article with the following descriptive statistics reported:

> Pretest and posttest means are 71 and 89.
> Standard deviations are 9.6 and 10.9.
> Experimental and control groups have 10 subjects each.

Because you are the expert, help Karen and Max by calculating the effect size and interpreting its meaning.

12.5: Efrain's Dilemma

Efrain has an assignment due in two days. His graduate course requires an evaluation of a research article for its clinical relevance. Efrain has no notion how to get started with this project. What advice can you give Efrain to help him evaluate the research article? Where should he begin?

STUDENT EXERCISES

1. Develop a *checklist* for evaluating the content of a quantitative research report, a qualitative research report, or both.
2. Select a journal issue, such as the April issue of *Language, Speech, and Hearing Services in Schools*, and evaluate the title of each article included in the issue. For titles that you evaluate as "poor," revise the titles so that they better satisfy the APA *Publication Manual's* criteria.
3. Select a journal issue, such as the fall issue of *Contemporary Issues in Communication Science and Disorders* (i.e., the National Student Speech-Language-Hearing Association journal), choose a research article, and evaluate its abstract. How would you rewrite the article's abstract to improve it?
4. Select a journal issue, such as the May issue of the *American Journal of Speech-Language Pathology*, choose an article, and evaluate its introductory section. Do the authors address the relevancy of their research? Does their literature review provide an adequate background for the focus of the study?
5. Select a journal issue, such as the August issue of the *Journal of Speech, Language, and Hearing Research*, and evaluate the researchers' conclusions. Did the researchers answer all of the research questions posed in the introductory section? Are the conclusions supported by the results of the study?
6. To practice search strategies, try several searches on a popular search engine such as Google, MEDLINE, ERIC, or another search engine that is available on your library's webpage. Use at least two words as keywords, and then try searching with the same words as a phrase. Compare the number of "hits." How can you make your search strategy more effective?

CHAPTER 13

WRITING FOR RESEARCH IN COMMUNICATION DISORDERS

disseminate (dĭ-sĕm′ə-nāt′) *v.* to spread widely; to diffuse; to promulgate

The research process involves planning, implementing, and dissemination. *Dissemination* is the act of sharing research methods, results, and conclusions with colleagues, the public, and others. Whereas the planning and implementation phases of research are relatively private enterprises, writing is a social enterprise and "a bold attempt to be part of our discourse community" (Academic Writing for Publication, 2002). The "discourse community" in communication disorders consists of academic teachers, scientists, practitioners, and students. These individuals comprise the audience for listening, reading, and evaluating research in communication disorders.

Researchers disseminate their research products for one or more reasons: (a) to contribute to the scientific foundations of communication disorders, (b) to stimulate further research in their area of study, or (c) to test their results and conclusions within the discourse community. The members of the discourse community—teachers, scientists, practitioners, students—ultimately determine the worth of a research product. For example, some employ citation rates to measure researchers' success. *Citation rate* is the number of times members of the discourse community reference a particular research product. Another measure of success is the use of the research product in speech-language pathology and audiology practices.

Citation rates and use in practice are fair measures of success, but no measure of a product's value is obtainable when researchers do not publish or otherwise disseminate their results. When this happens, members of the discourse community have no opportunity to review the results. For example, widely circulated journals publish less than half of the research presented at professional conventions (Meline, 2003). Thus, many

TECHNOLOGY NOTE

The thesis is a special case of writing in communication disorders. Waddell (2004) offered a metaphoric connection between thesis and Theseus—the mystical hero of ancient Greece who traversed the Cretan Labyrinth by following a thread. Like the labyrinth of old, the thesis is a labyrinth of ideas connected by a thread of thought that permits writers and readers to find the way. A thesis is a well-written analytical essay that addresses a research topic. A good thesis is (a) clearly defined, (b) adequately focused, (c) well supported, and (d) high in the orders of knowledge (Waddell, 2004). Many Internet resources are available to help thesis writers. For example, MIT's web site advised thesis writers to think of the thesis as a series of small and related tasks: http://web.mit.edu/Writing_Types/writingthesis.html. Thesis writing resources are also available at the KU Writing Center: http://www.writing.ku.edu/students/docs/thesis.html, and the UW-Madison's Writing Center, http://www.wisc.edu/writing/Handbook/Thesis.html.

research findings go unreported for one reason or another. The reason is typically one of the following: (a) editorial rejections, (b) editorial censorship, or (c) self-censorship.

According to McGue (2000), *editorial rejections* most often happen due to lack of theoretical significance or some serious limitation in a study's methodology. A second reason for rejection is *editorial censorship*, which may be due to controversial issues. Finally, *self-censorship* occurs when researchers choose not to report their otherwise publishable findings. Self-censorship is especially troublesome because it raises ethical concerns. McGue (2000) commented on the ethics dilemma surrounding self-censorship:

> For example, some individuals agree to participate in a research investigation only because they believe doing so contributes to a larger societal good. Failure to publish denies them the opportunity to fulfill that intention. Most significant, censoring certain research findings has the effect of producing biases and distortions in the research record. (p. 87)

Those persons engaged in research have a duty to report their results in some form or fashion if feasible. Not reporting research findings is harmful in that it prevents evaluation of the results.

PLANNING, EXECUTING, AND WRITING IN RESEARCH

Planning and executing a research study are usually exciting and challenging endeavors, but many researchers dread writing results. They may view writing as tedious and dull. Sternberg (1993) observed this phenomenon with students who were completing research projects:

Many students lose interest in their research projects as soon as the time comes to write about them. Their interest is in planning for and making new discoveries, not in communicating their discoveries to others. A widely believed fallacy underlies their attitudes. The fallacy is that the discovery process ends when the communication process begins. Although the major purpose of writing a paper is to communicate your thoughts to others, another important purpose is to help you form and organize your thoughts. (p. 5)

Clearly, the process of writing is more than just a means to disseminate research products to the discourse community. Rather, writing is a recursive process that helps researchers generate new ideas and rethink old notions as they write. The general goal for writing and presenting research in communication disorders is to publish or disseminate research products for review by the discourse community. However, writing has four specific goals:

1. To inform—present the relevant facts.
2. To explain the relevant facts.
3. To connect the relevant facts—past and present.
4. To persuade the audience that the authors' explanation is the best explanation from among the plausible alternative explanations.

Each of these four goals is equally important for successfully disseminating research products to the discourse community in communication disorders.

MODELS OF THE WRITING PROCESS

Writing is a creative process, but *instruction and practice* help to teach the mechanics of writing as well as the nuances of style. The writing process is not a linear process from beginning to end but is a recursive process with endless loops (Emig, 1971). Experts have described the writing process in one of two ways: (a) in simple linear stages of activities or (b) as a complex interplay of thinking activities.

The *stage-process model* depicted in Exhibit 13.1 is simple and somewhat superficial, but it is a useful guide because it delineates writing activities. The *cognitive-process model* depicted in Exhibit 13.2 is more complex in its interactions. It is especially useful because it informs us as to the mental strategies of good and poor writers. For example, good writers are extra sensitive to the task environment, i.e., topic and audience. Furthermore, good writers typically write for the widest possible audience, and they appreciate that anyone would want to read their work. Both *stage-process* and *cognitive-process models* are iterative in as much as they depict movements back and forth between modes. The models are valuable in that they help to increase awareness of the writing process and its complexities. In addition, the models raise appreciation for the writing process and its demands.

A question for successful writers is, What makes you a good writer? Some of the most successful writers have answered this question. Exhibit 13.3 is a synopsis of the personal reflections volunteered by Nobel laureates and other successful writers. The

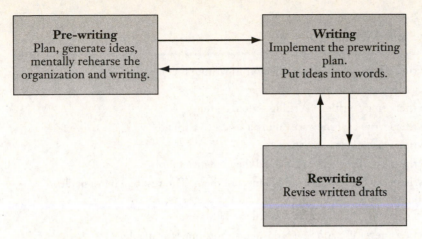

EXHIBIT 13.1
A Stage-Process Model for Writing

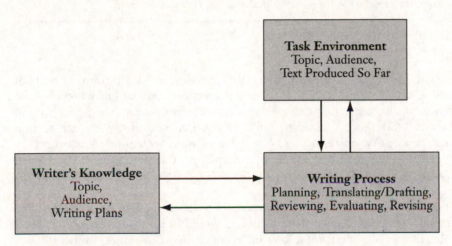

EXHIBIT 13.2
A Cognitive-Process Model for Writing

common themes are (a) good writers are concise, (b) good writers avoid complex language, and (c) good writers enjoy what they do.

THE IMPORTANCE OF READER EXPECTATIONS

Gopen and Swan (1990) pointed out that readers do more than simply read written words—rather, they interpret what they read. Thus, 10 readers might interpret the same piece of prose in 10 different ways. Typically, readers have certain expectations about the substance and structure of prose, and these expectations shape their inter-

EXHIBIT 13.3
What Makes a Good Writer?

1. Good writers write with vigor, and vigorous writing is concise.
2. A good writer reads a lot.
3. Good writers enjoy writing. Writing should be fun.
4. Good writers write as if they are telling a secret to a friend.
5. Good writers have their heart in it.
6. Good writers practice their writing and then practice more.
7. Good writers catch adjectives and kill most of them. The rest will be valuable (according to Mark Twain).
8. A good writer gets rid of the fancy words and phrases.
9. Good writers never use a long word when a short one is available.
10. Good writers simplify and then simplify more.
11. Good writers pay attention to the world around them.
12. Good writers read what they write aloud and ask, *How does it sound?*

Advice is attributed to Nobel laureates and others.

pretations. According to Gopen and Swan (1990), good writers are intuitively aware of their readers' expectations. Reader expectations are most apparent at the level of the largest units of discourse. For example, readers of scientific reports expect to find "Introduction," "Methods," "Results," and "Discussion" sections, with each section true to its purpose. When results and discussion sections are confused or others are intermingled, readers may have difficulty interpreting the substance of the report. Readers also expect smaller units of discourse, such as sentences or paragraphs, to follow the conventions of discourse.

Exhibit 13.4 presents six writing principles based on reader expectations. The first principle maintains, "Grammatical subjects should be as close as possible to their verbs." Readers usually interpret a long interruption between subject and verb as of minor importance, so they may pay little attention to its substance. According to Gopen and Swan (1990), the arrival of the verb fulfills the reader's need for syntactic resolution. The reader does not know what the subject is doing, or what the sentence is about until he or she reaches the verb. Separating of subjects from verbs is a common structural problem in professional writing. Instances of subject–verb separations appear in most professional writing.

CASE EXAMPLE

An example of subject–verb separation in communication disorders reporting is a sentence in the discussion section of a report in the *Journal of Speech-Language-Hearing Research*. In this instance, a rather long interruption (22 words) separated the subject noun from its verb.

EXHIBIT 13.4
Writing Principles Based on Reader Expectations

1. Grammatical subjects should be as close as possible to their verbs. This is a common structural defect in professional writing.

2. Every unit of discourse, small or large, should serve a single function or make a single point.

3. Save the most important information for last—information for emphasis should appear at points of syntactic closure.

4. Place information in the topic position (beginning of the discourse unit) that establishes a perspective from which the reader can view the whole.

5. Place "old" information in the topic position and "new" information in the emphasis position. This helps readers to backward-link new information to old. The opposite arrangement is a serious problem in American professional writing.

6. Link sentences and avoid logical gaps so that each sentence proceeds logically from the last. When old information is missing, readers have to construct the logical link by themselves.

Adapted from Gopen and Swan, 1990.

A **factor** of potential interest for the question of why not all adolescents with MMHL show significant critical period effects in their language performance **concerns** the length of the period of unaided HL. (emphasis added; Delage & Tuller, 2007, p. 1310)

The *problem with this sentence* is that it ignores a reader's need for syntactic resolution. As a result, readers may pay little attention to the substance of the material that intervenes between the subject and verb. Delage and Tuller (2007) are not the only authors who have made the mistake of separating a subject from its verb. A close look at reports in any professional journal reveals examples of subject–verb separation.

The following *revision* of the Delage and Tuller (2007) sentence resolves the subject–verb separation problem, but only Deluge and Tuller can judge whether it accurately reflects their intentions.

Not all adolescents with MMHL show significant critical period effects in their language performance. The length of the period of unaided HL is a factor of potential interest.

Although subject–verb separation is an especially common problem, all the principles in Exhibit 13.4 are important. Prospective writers should understand the reader expectations for their audience. Writers who are intuitively aware of reader expectations are able to communicate more effectively.

The writing process divides into five stages of activities for the convenience of discussion. The *five stages* are (a) prewriting, (b) writing and drafting, (c) rewriting and revision, (d) editing, and (e) publication and presentation. A description of each of the five stages follows.

THE PREWRITING AND PLANNING STAGE

Bem (2004) posed the rhetorical question: "For whom should you write?" According to Bem's (2004) philosophy, good writing is good teaching. Bem (2004) advised authors as follows:

> Direct your research writing to the student in Psychology 101, your colleague in the Art History Department, and your grandmother. No matter how technical or abstruse your article is in its particulars, intelligent non-[researchers] with no expertise in statistics or experimental design should be able to comprehend the broad outlines of what you did and why. (p. 189)

Clearly, the broad discourse community is the preferred target audience for writing level and style—not colleagues in the sciences. It also benefits evidence-based practice if researchers write papers to satisfy the needs of practitioners as well as academics (Meline & Paradiso, 2003).

The prewriting/planning stage is a time to generate ideas and mentally rehearse the organization and writing of the research product. Sternberg (1993) posited what he considered *eight common misconceptions* about research papers as follows:

Misconception 1. *Writing the [research] paper is the most routine, least creative aspect of the scientific enterprise, requiring much time but little imagination.*

Misconception 2. *The important thing is what you say, not how you say it.*

Misconception 3. *Longer papers are better papers, and more papers are better yet.*

Misconception 4. *The main purpose of a [research] paper is the presentation of facts, whether newly established (as in reports of experiments) or well established (as in literature reviews).*

Misconception 5. *The distinction between scientific writing, on the one hand, and advertising or propaganda, on the other hand, is that the purpose of scientific writing is to inform whereas the purpose of advertising or propaganda is to persuade.*

Misconception 6. *A good way to gain acceptance of your theory is by refuting someone else's theory.*

Misconception 7. *Negative results that fail to support the researcher's hypothesis are every bit as valuable as positive results that do not support the researcher's hypothesis.*

Misconception 8. *The logical development of ideas in a [research] paper reflects the historical development of ideas in the [researcher's] head.* (Sternberg, 1993, pp. 5–13)

Given what you know about Sternberg's misconceptions, answer the following questions: In what way is each of Sternberg's eight statements a misconception? After answering, compare your answers to Sternberg's (1993) comments regarding each of the eight misconceptions.

The journals published by the American Speech-Language-Hearing Association and most behavioral and social science periodicals expect contributors to adopt the style prescribed in the *Publication Manual of the American Psychological Association* (APA, 2001). According to the APA *Publication Manual's* guidelines, research papers should include (a) an *introduction*, (b) a *method section*, (c) a *results section*, (d) a *discussion section*, (e) an *abstract*, (f) a *title*, and (g) a list of *references*. However, Sternberg (1993) pointed

TECHNOLOGY NOTE

The Internet includes many instructional aids for writing and presenting research in communication disorders. The KU Medical Center offers online tutorials for developing effective oral presentations, designing visual aids, and creating posters: www.kumc.edu/SAH/OTEd/jradel/effective.html. An American Speech-Language-Hearing Association *page* (www.asha.org/about/events/convention/papers) provides "tip sheets" for all types of presentations. Online instructional aids are also available at the Purdue University Online Writing Lab (OWL): http://owl.english.purdue.edu/ and the University of Missouri Online Writery: www.missouri.edu/~writery. The Online Writery provides an evaluation of writing samples with interactive feedback.

out that the steps followed in planning and carrying out research do not neatly correspond to the successive sections of the research paper. Rather, authors may write one or another section first (or last) depending on their personal style—though writing a section such as the results clearly facilitates writing subsequent sections of the research paper such as the discussion. There is no preset length of time prescribed for prewriting and planning activities, but the better the plan, the easier the task of writing and drafting the research product. The *writing/drafting stage* follows the prewriting and planning activities in the first stage of writing research in communication disorders.

THE WRITING AND DRAFTING STAGE

Most important to achieving good scientific writing are accuracy and clarity according to Bem (2004). To write clearly, authors should first organize their research product and then adopt a simple and direct writing style (Bem, 2004). Sternberg (1992) offered 21 tips for better writing, including seven tips that specifically addressed the content of a research paper:

1. Start strong.
2. Tell readers why they should be interested.
3. Make sure that the article does what it says it will do.
4. Make sure that the literature review is focused, reasonably complete, and balanced.
5. Always explain what your results mean—don't force the reader to decipher them.
6. Be sure to consider alternative interpretations of the data.
7. End strongly and state a clear take-home message. (p. 13)

The Possibility of Plagiarism

Authors should also be alert to the possibility of plagiarism. According to McGue (2000), *plagiarism* occurs when writers take the words, ideas, or contributions of others (or themselves) from speech or writing without proper citation or other acknowledgment. Authors are expected to properly cite their own work as well as others' works. Otherwise, authors are guilty of *self-plagiarism* and possibly copyright infringement. Writers should seek a copyright release to reproduce large amounts of material from published sources, such as tables, figures, or long quotes from books, monographs, and articles. The American Psychological Association grants "limited permission" automatically and free of charge for the reuse of certain APA book or journal materials (APA, 2008). However, authors must obtain permission from one author and include a credit line. Other publishers have different policies, so prospective authors should check with the publisher of the material that they want to reuse. The APA grants limited permission to reuse the following materials:

1. Authors can reuse a maximum of three figures or tables from one APA journal article or book chapter.
2. Authors can reuse single text extracts of less than 400 words.
3. Authors can reuse a series of text extracts that total less than 800 words.

Writing the Introduction

According to the APA *Publication Manual* (APA, 2001), the introduction of a research paper should (a) introduce the problem, (b) develop the background, and (c) state the purpose and rationale. If the research method is qualitative, Pyrczak and Bruce (2003) suggested that authors consider discussing their choice of a qualitative design over a quantitative design in their introduction.

To strengthen the opening, Bem (2004) suggested that authors open with a statement about people or animals, rather than open with statements about speech-language pathologists, audiologists, or their research. Furthermore, Sternberg (1992) recommended that authors open their research paper by telling readers what the article is about in a provocative way that catches their attention. Sternberg (1992) suggested a strong start that asks a question or states a problem pertinent to the theme of the article. Williams (2000) provided an example of a strong opening paragraph with a series of questions in her research paper, including the following question: "Is one intervention approach suited for children of varying degrees of phonological impairment?" (p. 289). In similar fashion, Kamhi (2004) opened his article with a series of questions, such as "Why do some terms, labels, ideas, and constructs prevail where others fail to gain acceptance?" (p. 105).

Walters and Chapman (2000) illustrated a strong start of a different kind. They opened their research paper with the following information:

> Comprehension monitoring (Markman, 1977) is a necessary language skill in the classroom, as it is important for children to assess their own understanding of task instructions and teaching content (Paul, 1995). This metacognitive skill of monitoring comprehension is made up of two parts: Detecting a comprehension problem and indicating the problem to the speaker (Dollaghan, 1987). Dollaghan and Kaston (1986) propose[d] a comprehension monitoring intervention program for first-graders with specific language impairment that sequences the goals of monitoring acoustic distortions, inadequate content, and excessively lengthy and complex commands. This study

examines whether Dollaghan and Kaston's (1986) sequence of goals corresponds to a developmental effect measures at ages three, six, and nine. (Walters & Chapman, 2000, p. 48)

Walters and Chapman's (2000) opening paragraph was strong in that it clearly informed readers about the research purpose. Asking questions, telling the reader what the paper is about, and stating the problem in the opening paragraph are writing techniques that help to get readers' attention. The introduction of the research paper continues beyond the opening paragraph with a review of the pertinent literature (background) and a statement of the research purpose and rationale. Authors should demonstrate some logical connection between the previous literature and the present work. The introduction typically ends with a statement of the hypothesis or a list of the questions that the researchers expect to answer.

Writing the Research Method

The *method* includes a description of the participants, the apparatus and materials used, and the procedures followed to collect data. Sufficient detail in descriptions of participants/subjects is required to permit others to replicate the study. Thus, it is important to describe the participants' ethnicity, gender, age, intelligence, socioeconomic status, and other characteristics—especially those that may interact with the experimental variables. Researchers should describe in detail the apparatus and materials used in the study—if atypical. If the apparatus and materials are common enough to be familiar to most communication disorders professionals, there is no need to describe them in detail. Finally, authors should describe the execution of the research step by step. It is necessary to describe the procedure in sufficient detail to permit others to replicate the method.

■ ■ ■ ■ ■

CASE EXAMPLE

Jarvis, Merriman, Barnett, Hanba, and Van Haitsma (2004) reported three experiments in one paper, and they described the participants in one of their experiments as follows:

> Participants were 60 preschoolers and kindergartners ($M = 4;9$, range = 3;10-6;4, all but 2 were 4 or 5 years old; PPVT-R $M = 94$, $SD = 14$) from predominately middle- to upper-middle-class families. Ten boys and 10 girls were assigned to each condition. (p. 400)

Based on what you know about Jarvis et al.'s (2004) study, answer the following questions: Did Jarvis and fellow researchers describe subjects in sufficient detail for a systematic replication of the experiment? What details, if any, are lacking in their description of participants?

Writing the Research Results

The APA *Publication Manual* (APA, 2001) specifies that the results section should summarize the data collected and the statistics or data analysis used. In addition, authors should include *tables* and *figures* to display results. According to the APA *Publication Manual*, authors should also report statistical significance, confidence intervals, and effect size.

Researchers should not wait until the discussion section to explain their results. Rather, they should interpret the results as they present them in the results section of the research paper. Bem (2004) argued that descriptive results are more important than statistical results. He also recommended that researchers first state a result and then give its statistical significance, and in no case should the statistical test stand alone without a thorough interpretation. Readers should not be left to interpret statistical results without the guidance of authors.

Furthermore, Bem (2004) recommended a description of individual participants as follows:

> After you have presented your quantitative results, it is often useful to become more informal and briefly to describe the behavior of particular individuals in your study. Again, the point is not to prove something, but to add richness to your findings, to share with readers the feel of the behavior. (p. 201)

In addition, descriptions of individual participants are helpful for transferring research to evidence-based practices. Meline and Paradiso (2003) explained the importance of individual participant descriptions to evidence-based practice in the following way.

> For example, if a researcher reports a large change (for the better) between pre- and posttest means for a group of 20 subjects, does that mean that all 20 subjects improved? In reality, 10 subjects may have improved dramatically, while the remaining 10 subjects may have failed to improve at all. Thus, it is important that researchers report and interpret individual outcomes along with group results. (p. 280)

Reynolds, Callihan, and Browning (2003) asked the question, Do lessons have a significant effect on young children's rhyming skills? Reynolds et al. (2003) authored the report of an experiment that included 3- and 4-year-old children as participants. The researchers used a pretest/posttest design with participants randomly assigned to treatment and nontreatment conditions. Reynolds et al.'s (2003) research team introduced their results section as follows:

> An alpha level of .05 was used for all statistical tests. Results indicated a significant main effect for time; $F(1, 14) = 35.773$, $p < .05$, indicating that rhyming skills improved for all children between the pretest and the posttest. This result was qualified, however, by a significant time by group interaction, $F(1, 14) = 14.21$, $p < .05$. Examination of the mean differences in improvement for each group showed that rhyming scores improved significantly more for the experimental group (Pretest $M = 4.63$, $SD = 3.66$; Posttest $M = 16.75$, $SD = 7.68$) than they did for the control group (Pretest $M = 8.88$, $SD = 6.42$; Posttest $M = 11.63$, $SD = 8.55$). These results can be seen in Figure 1 [a line graph of pretest and posttest means]. (p. 44)

Based on what you know about Reynolds et al.'s (2003) study, answer the following questions: What is your evaluation of the Reynolds et al. (2003) results section? What information about results was included in the research report? What information is missing? How would you revise their results section?

Writing the Discussion

The *discussion section* is a place to evaluate and interpret the implications of the results. The APA *Publication Manual* recommends that authors open the discussion with a statement of support or nonsupport for their research hypothesis. The discussion section is also the place to comment on the importance of the findings. How do the results affect current theory? How do the results impact current practices in speech-language pathology or audiology?

Sternberg (1992) recommended that authors end the article strongly and state a clear "take-home message" for readers. Alt, Plante, and Creusere (2004) ended their *Discussion* section with the following paragraph:

> The established difficulty of children with SLI in learning labels for words is paralleled in the fast-mapping of semantic features. As such, limited encoding by children with SLI has an impact on their ability to add lexical labels to their corpus of vocabulary and may lead to an impoverished understanding of the meanings conveyed by those labels acquired. Collectively, in this field, we face the challenge of discovering the exact nature of the relationship between learning lexical labels. If we are able to help children with SLI become better word learners, we need to address all components of word learning. (p. 418)

Based on what you know about Alt et al.'s (2004) study, answer the following questions: What is your evaluation of their ending paragraph? What was their take-home message? In your opinion, was it a strong message?

Writing the Title and Abstract

It is usually best to write the *title* and *abstract* after writing the introduction, method, results, and discussion sections. A title should summarize the main idea of the paper simply and with style (APA, 2001). The title should (a) name the variables, if possible, (b) be concise (the APA *Publication Manual* suggests 10–12 words), (c) indicate what was studied but not results or conclusions, (d) mention the population of interest if possible, and (e) use subtitles to designate the type of research—pilot study, qualitative study, or meta-analysis/synthesis study. Pyrczak and Bruce (2003) suggested including *qualitative* in the title or abstract when the study's design is qualitative. For example, Culatta, Kovarsky, Theodore, Franklin, and Timler (2003) chose the title: "Quantitative and Qualitative Documentation of Early Literacy Instruction." They also included the term *qualitative* in their abstract.

Southwood and Russell (2004) chose "Comparison of Conversation, Freeplay, and Story Generation as Methods of Language Sample Elicitation" as their research report's title. What information does the title provide? What was their research pur-

TECHNOLOGY NOTE

The Internet offers opportunities for information sharing—good and bad. Because it allows access to vast archives of materials, papers, and articles, the potential for *plagiarism* is great. Examples of plagiarism are given on Princeton University's Academic Integrity site (www.princeton.edu/pr/pub/integrity/pages/plagiarism.html). The University of Puget Sound's website—*Academic Honesty and Intellectual Ownership*—includes guidelines for academic honesty in writing and exercises for properly citing sources. To thwart plagiarism, plagiarism detection tools are available online, though they are limited. *WCopyfind* is plagiarism detection freeware that compares written papers but only files stored on local hard drives (http://plagiarism.phys.virginia.edu/Wsoftware.html). Another plagiarism detection tool, *Eve*, allows online comparisons with content published on the Internet—but not in local archives (www.canexus.com/eve/index.shtml). *Turnitin.com* permits comparisons with content on the Internet and archived in the Turnitin.com database (www.turnitin.com). *SafeAssign* is a plagiarism prevention service offered by Blackboard (www.safeassign.com).

pose? What were their experimental variables? What information is missing from the Southwood and Russell (2004) title?

Titles sometimes ask a question, though questions in titles are uncommon. Walters and Chapman (2000) asked a question in their title: "Comprehension Monitoring: A Developmental Effect?" How would you judge Walters and Chapman's title? What information does the title provide? What information is missing?

Abstracts are brief, concise, and comprehensive summaries of research. The APA *Publication Manual* specifies a length of 120 words or less for abstracts. It also says that the abstract should be accurate, self-contained, nonevaluative, coherent, and readable. Furthermore, a good abstract should (a) specify the research hypothesis, purpose, or questions, (b) provide highlights of the methodology, (c) provide highlights of the results, (d) be short, and (e) name the theory—if integral to the research.

CASE EXAMPLE

The abstract accompanying Burk and Wiley's (2004) article titled "Continuous Versus Pulsed Tones in Audiometry" is as follows:

The purpose of this study was to compare auditory thresholds obtained for continuous and pulsed tones in listeners with normal hearing. Auditory thresholds, test-retest reliability, false-positive responses, and listener preference were compared for both signals. Hearing thresholds and test-retest reliability were comparable for the 2 signals, and there were no significant differences in the number of false positives or the number of presentations required to reach threshold. Listener preference, however, indicated that pulsed tones were preferred over continuous tones by 67% of the listeners when listening to low-level or high-frequency tones. These findings, coupled with previous reports demonstrating the benefits of using automatically pulsed tones in threshold assessment for listeners with tinnitus, support the general use of pulsed tones in clinical audiometry. (p. 54)

What is your evaluation of Burk and Wiley's (2004) abstract? Does it specify the purpose? Does it provide highlights of the methodology and results? Is the abstract brief, concise, and generally readable?

Writing References and Appendixes

References appear in a list at the end of a research paper. References should account for every citation that appears in the body of the paper, including the narrative, tables, and figures. References and citations are a common source of errors in every professional paper. Authors should check and recheck references and citations for their accuracy.

The style for writing references should follow the form specified in the APA *Publication Manual* (APA, 2001) unless the journal's "Information for Authors" page indicates otherwise. Guidance for writing electronic citations and references is available at the American Psychological Association's webpage: http://apastyle.apa.org.

Appendixes are an optional part of the research paper but an important one. As a rule, the appendix includes critical material that does not fit into the body of the research paper, such as samples of narratives, raw subject data, or stimulus materials.

Once a draft of the research paper is complete, the rewriting/revision stage begins. However, because the writing process is recursive and because each writer has a unique style, rewriting/revision may begin at any point in the writing/drafting stage. For example, writers may choose to write their introduction and revise it before beginning the method section.

THE REWRITING AND REVISION STAGE

The first draft of a research paper never achieves perfection. Authors typically encounter some serious revisions following their initial writing and first draft. Bem (2004) suggested that rewriting is especially demanding because of the following: (a) your own writing is difficult to edit, (b) rewriting requires a high degree of compulsiveness and attention to detail, and (c) substantial restructuring of the paper is usually

TECHNOLOGY NOTE

The American Psychological Association's *Style Helper 5.1* automatically formats documents in compliance with APA guidelines. Style Helper is a software program that works with Microsoft Word. While working in Style Helper, a special task bar provides access to its features, which include an organizer tool, context-sensitive help, and citation and reference handling tools. Consumers may download and purchase a single user license at the APA's website: www.apa.org/software.

necessary. In the latter case, rewriting typically requires authors to discard whole sections and add new ones. Some questions to consider when revising one or more sections of the research paper are as follows:

1. Is your writing sufficient in detail for a systematic replication of the study?
2. Is your writing redundant? Did you repeat unnecessary information?
3. Is your writing accurate in fact?
4. Have you cited sources of information properly?
5. Is your writing logically organized?
6. Is your interpretation of results adequate and meaningful for clinical practice?
7. Do the method and results support your conclusions?
8. Is your writing clear, brief, and precise?

If the answers to the preceding questions are affirmative, it is time to proceed to the editing stage. If not, authors should consider setting the paper aside for a few days or longer and returning to it later with a fresh perspective. A short break from the writing process is often helpful and usually rejuvenating.

THE EDITING STAGE

The *editing stage* typically follows rewriting and revision, but, because the writing process is recursive, editing may happen at any point in time. The use of word processors with automatic spelling and grammar checkers permits editing as writing proceeds. The editing stage has more to do with the mechanics of writing (i.e., form) and less to do with what is said (i.e., content). This is a time to make cosmetic improvements in the research paper—to correct errors in spelling, punctuation, and grammar. Bem (2004) recommended the following ways to improve writing style:

1. Omit needless words.
2. Avoid meta-comments on the writing. For example, do not say, *Now that we have discussed the psychoanalytic theory of stuttering, we will explain the purpose of our experiment.*
3. Avoid jargon except when the jargon term makes an important conceptual distinction not apprehended by lay terminology.
4. Use the active voice unless content dictates otherwise.
5. Use the past tense when reporting the previous research of others.
6. Avoid language bias for gender, race, sexual orientation, disabilities, and ethnicity. Guidance for removing bias in language is available at the American Psychological Association's web page: http://apastyle.apa.org.
7. Avoid common errors of grammar and usage. For example, the word *data* is plural, the word *none* is singular, and *that* is usually the correct relative pronoun—not *which*.

The *editing stage* is also a time to ensure the paper complies with writing style (usually APA) as well as other instructions found on the journal's "Information for

TECHNOLOGY NOTE

Spell checkers, and grammar and style-checking tools are useful in the editing phase of the writing process. Microsoft Word includes spelling and grammar checking options on its Tools menu, and WordPerfect incorporates the *Grammatik* utility for grammar checking. The use of spell checkers is relatively free from debate; however, grammar and style-checking tools are more controversial. Some English mavens warn that grammar checkers dampen creativity—students may rely on them and fail to acquire good grammar habits. Other experts argue that grammar checkers help to focus attention on sentences and constructions that may benefit from a rewrite. Clearly, grammar- and style-checking tools do not substitute for good writing skills, but they do help with basic writing devices such as active/passive voice, subject/verb agreement, and punctuation.

Authors" page Failure to account for all the citations in the body of the research paper is a common error. The editing stage is a time for checking each citation in the body of the paper to ensure there is a corresponding reference. Furthermore, references typically contain errors of accuracy and style, so authors should carefully check references for spelling, punctuation, and form.

THE PUBLICATION AND PRESENTATION STAGE

Writing, rewriting, and editing tasks conclude (at least for the moment) when authors submit the research product for publication or presentation. Reviewers typically reject research papers and proposals because of one or more of the following reasons: (a) bad writing, (b) serious methodological flaws, or (c) lack of theoretical importance. The authors' diligence in rewriting and editing the paper for clarity and precision should avoid rejection because of *bad writing*.

The most accomplished writers (and the less accomplished) benefit from the advice of colleagues. Before submitting the research paper or a proposal for a research paper, authors should ask colleagues to critically read the paper and provide constructive comments. If the intended audience includes practitioners, authors should ask speech-language pathologists or audiologists to read the paper and share their perspectives. With colleagues' comments in hand, authors can revise the research product accordingly and submit the paper for review when they are satisfied the paper is ready.

No research product passes review without revisions. If editors do not summarily reject the paper, authors will have an opportunity to revise it. To facilitate publication, authors should carefully address reviewers' comments. Authors should submit a cover letter with the revised paper that explains how the revision incorporates the reviewers' suggestions. If authors choose not to incorporate suggestions, they should explain their rationale. The editorial process continues until editors and authors agree that the research paper is ready for publication.

TECHNOLOGY NOTE

Successful writing requires feedback from peers before dissemination of a paper or submission for publication. A model for online writing help is *The Forum for Writing in Communication Sciences and Disorders*—an online writers' forum established on the University of Florida's website: www.clas.ufl.edu/boards/owl/csd/. The Forum for Writing in Communication Sciences and Disorders permits online comments from peers and teachers. It also allows answers to questions regarding drafts of writing assignments. Students submit their questions or writing samples and receive feedback online. The submissions to the Forum for Writing include literature reviews, bibliographies, resumes, and SOAP (Subjective, Objective, Assessment, and Plan) notes. To ensure privacy and adhere to ethical principles, writers must redact the personal identifying information of clients, research subjects, or others before submitting written drafts for public review.

WRITING THE THESIS

The *thesis* is a challenging and rewarding endeavor for college seniors and graduates. It is challenging because it is often the author's first experience writing a scientific report. The thesis combines expository writing with a scientific writing style. It follows a set of rules that the student's college or school typically prescribes. Most theses in communication disorders follow the style dictated by the American Psychological Association, but there are exceptions. Prospective thesis writers should determine the exact requirements before they begin writing.

Thesis writing is a specialized type of scientific writing, but the same principles of good writing apply to theses that apply to all professional writing endeavors. Thesis writing is an excellent way to develop a foundation for good writing. Some establish bad writing habits early on, but the thesis project is an opportunity to develop the best writing habits early in the professional career.

Wegman (2008) provided some helpful tips for prospective thesis writers. Exhibit 13.5 summarizes some of Wegman's tips. Another help for thesis writers is Easterbrook's (n.d.) "How Theses Get Written: Some Cool Tips." For authors who have completed their theses (or dissertations), the APA (2007) offered guidelines to help convert the thesis into a journal article. They recommended the following points as guidelines for writing the journal article:

1. Theses are typically very long, so the author must reduce a document of 100-plus pages to a compact 20- to 25-page manuscript for publication. The author aims to preserve the substance while cutting the irrelevant details. However, the author should not just "cut and paste" but should select relevant material and rewrite.
2. In theses, authors tend to say everything about the research problem. The author may be able to narrow the focus to a specific topic. Typically, theses include more

EXHIBIT 13.5
Tips for Thesis Writing in Communication Disorders

1. Choose your thesis topic early.

2. Choose a topic that is interesting enough to keep your attention for a year or more. Also, choose a very specific topic. Whatever topic you choose, you will soon realize that the topic is much bigger than originally thought.

3. Find an advisor who is compatible with you and your topic.

4. Begin the research as soon as possible.

5. Take detailed notes, organize them, outline the articles that you review, and do not throw anything away.

6. Establish a time table with a deadline for each step.

7. Refer back constantly to the original sources that prompted your thesis. This will remind you of the themes that you intended to follow in the beginning.

8. Build your reference list as you go. Whenever you cite something, immediately record the full citation in your reference list.

9. Ask your friends to read sections as you finish them and give you feedback.

10. Know when to let go. The thesis is just another paper—albeit a very big paper. You need to leave it alone at times, regain your perspective, and return to it with renewed energy.

Adapted from Wegman, 2008.

results than are needed for a journal article. Try to select the most important results. Theses and dissertations usually include more references than needed for a journal article. The author should select the most important and necessary references to cite.

3. Theses do not necessarily follow APA writing style. The author should follow APA writing style, include relevant sections, and exclude material that was necessary for the thesis but not needed for the journal article. Be aware of the quality of your expository writing. Thesis writing tends to overuse passive voice and often contains other stylistic problems that are less acceptable in journal articles. Take special care to observe good writing habits in preparing the journal article.

4. Thesis writers often overinterpret their data. Be aware that all research endeavors have limitations, so be prepared to face them when writing your journal article. Authors should exercise restraint in forming their conclusions.

CONCLUSION

Good writing places many demands on writers. Professional writing should inform, explain, combine relevant facts, and persuade. Good writers are aware of readers' expectations, so they are better able to communicate their true intentions to readers. Most writing is skill based, and writers can acquire new skills. However, new habits must replace old habits before effective writing is a reality. An adherence to good writing practices and recognition of readers' needs are a sound basis for writing. *Good writing practices* will especially benefit college seniors and graduates who will communicate with written reports, professional correspondence, and publications throughout their careers.

In a recent study, Gregg, Coleman, Stennett, and Davis (2002) compared the discourse complexity of various college writers. They compared expository writing samples from persons without disability to persons with learning disabilities or attention-deficit/hyperactivity disorder (ADHD). The most noteworthy differences between groups were diversity of words, total word counts, and the use of hedges. *Hedges* are devices used to lessen the impact of an utterance—typically an adjective or adverb—such as:

He is a **slightly** stupid person.
She is **somewhat** spoiled.
There were **few** significant problems.

Gregg et al. (2002) reported that nondisabled writers used significantly fewer hedges. The nondisabled writers also used a greater diversity of words and more total words in their writing. These features are usually associated with good writing practices. Every college writer, with or without disability, can improve his or her writing products by paying attention to what he or she writes, practicing good writing habits, and seeking advice from friends and fellow writers. The perspectives of others are especially important. Most important, enjoy what you write.

CASE STUDIES

Case 13.1: Plan for Collaborative Writing?
Dr. Kroner and Ms. Parker collaborated in a research project to evaluate the efficacy of electrotherapy for treating oral/pharyngeal dysphagia. They shared equally in the planning and execution stages of the research, but Kroner and Parker are not sure who should write the research paper. They asked you for advice. What is your plan to help Kroner and Parker write their research paper?

Case 13.2: Will Julie and Eddie Avoid Plagiarism?
Julie and Eddie are students who are writing their senior theses in communication disorders. They have written their initial drafts and included content from several sources including books, journal articles, class notes, and interviews with professors. Julie and Eddie want to avoid plagiarism, but they are not sure what content is attributable to its source and what content does not need to be attributed to its source. They asked you for some guidance. What guidelines will you provide for Julie and Eddie?

Case 13.3: Ana and Jose Need Advice
Speech-language pathologists, Ana and Jose, are writing their research method section, but they are not sure what to include or how much detail to include. Their study included 16 adults as participants, several commercial tests, and a set of picture cards that they designed. As the research consultant, what is your advice for Ana and Jose?

Case 13.4: Writing Cramps

Vanessa is writing her proposal for a senior thesis, but after many rewrites, it is a mess. She is not sure if she has organized it properly. Furthermore, it does not say what she wants it to say. Though otherwise highly motivated, Vanessa is seriously considering telling her advisor that she cannot do this project because she cannot write. What advice will you give to Vanessa? What steps should she follow? Is there a chance that she can complete her senior thesis successfully?

Case 13.5: Clarissa Is Reluctant

Clarissa has a great idea for a thesis, but she is reluctant to commit to the thesis project—especially because it is a year-long project. What advice would you give Clarissa to encourage her to do the thesis project? What are some early steps she can take to make the thesis project easier?

STUDENT EXERCISES

1. Locate a journal article with an interesting title. Read the *abstract*, evaluate its content, and identify shortcomings. Rewrite the abstract to improve its clarity and to satisfy the requirements specified in the APA *Publication Manual* (2001).

2. Choose a research article from a communication disorders journal and evaluate its *title* for content and form. Does the title meet the standards for good writing? Rewrite the title, and compare your revision with the authors' title.

3. Reynolds et al. (2003) reported a pretest mean and standard deviation of 4.63 (3.66) and a posttest mean and standard deviation of 16.75 (7.68). What is the effect size for their pretest/posttest results? How would you interpret the effect size?

4. Choose an article from a communication disorders journal and evaluate the *introduction's* opening paragraph. Is the opening paragraph strong enough to interest readers? Does it open with a statement about people? animals? Does it include a description of the research problem? Rewrite the opening paragraph to make it stronger. HINT: Try rewriting the opening paragraph with one or more questions.

5. Choose a research report from a communication disorders journal. Evaluate the *discussion* section's closing paragraph. Is the closing paragraph clear and precise? What is the authors' message in the closing paragraph? How would you rewrite the closing paragraph to improve its quality?

6. Randomly or not so randomly, choose an article written for a professional journal in audiology or speech-language pathology. Look the article over carefully, and identify one or more violations of the principles of reader expectations. How would you improve the discourse? Try rewriting the offending material to make it a better product.

REFERENCES

Abelson, R., & Friquegnon, M. (1991). *Ethics for modern life* (6th ed.). New York: Bedford/St. Martin's.

Abrami, P.C., Cohen, P.A., & d'Apollonia, S. (1988). Implementation problems in meta-analysis. *Review of Educational Research, 58,* 151–179.

All My Children. (2005). *Tuesday, November 15, 2005.* Retrieved December 28, 2008, from http://www.soapoperadigest.com

AllPsych ONLINE (2004). *The virtual psychology classroom.* Retrieved June 5, 2008, from http://allpsych.com

Almer, E. C. (2000). *Statistical tricks and traps: An illustrated guide to the misuses of statistics.* Los Angeles: Pyrczak Publishing.

Alt, M., Plante, E., & Creusere, M. (2004). Semantic features in fast-mapping: Performance of preschoolers with specific language impairment versus preschoolers with normal language. *Journal of Speech-Language-Hearing Research, 47,* 407–420.

Altman, D. G., & Bland, J. M. (1999). Statistics notes: How to randomize. *British Medical Journal, 319,* 703–704.

Ambrose, N. G., & Yairi, E. (2002). The Tudor study: Data and ethics. *American Journal of Speech-Language Pathology, 11,* 190–203.

American Academy of Audiology. (2006). *The clinical practice guidelines development process.* Retrieved April 17, 2009, from http://www.audiology.org/resources/documentlibrary/Pages/ClinicalPracticeGuidelines.aspx

American Academy of Audiology. (2007). *Code of ethics.* Retrieved December 28, 2007, from http://www.audiology.org/publications/documents/ethics/

American Academy of Audiology. (2008). *Publications.* Retrieved June 9, 2008, from http://www.audiology.org/publications/jaaa/

American Academy of Family Physicians. (2004). Clinical practice guidelines: Diagnosis and management of acute otitis media. Retrieved December 18, 2007, from http://www.aafp.org/online/en/home/clinicalrecs/aom.html

American Psychological Association. (2001). *Publication manual of the American psychological association.* Washington: Author.

American Psychological Association. (2002). *Ethical principles of psychologists and code of conduct.* Retrieved August 26, 2004, from http://www.apa.org/ethics/code2002.html

American Psychological Association. (2007). *Converting the dissertation into a journal article.* Retrieved April 18, 2009, from http://www.apa.org/journals/authors/guide.html#dissertation

American Psychological Association. (2008). *Converting the dissertation into a journal article.* Retrieved April 8, 2008, from http://www.apa.org/journals/authors/guide.html

American Speech-Language-Hearing Association. (1994, March). The role of research and the state of research training within communication sciences and disorders. *Asha, 36*(Suppl. 12), 21–23.

American Speech-Language-Hearing Association. (2003). Code of ethics (revised). *ASHA Supplement, 23,* 13–15.

American Speech-Language-Hearing Association. (2005). *Evidence-based practice in communication disorders [Position Statement].* Retrieved April 17, 2009, from http://www.asha.org/docs/html/PS2005-00221.html

American Speech-Language-Hearing Association. (2007). *Guidelines for the responsible conduct of research: Ethics and the publication process*. Retrieved April 11, 2009, from http://www.asha.org/policy

American Speech-Language-Hearing Association. (2008). *ASHA publications*. Retrieved June 9, 2008, from http://www.asha.org/about/publications

Amlani, A. M. (2001). Efficacy of directional microphone hearing aids: A meta-analytic perspective. *Journal of the American Academy of Audiology, 12,* 202–214.

Andrews, G., Guitar, B., & Howie, P. (1980). Meta-analysis of the effects of stuttering treatment. *Journal of Speech and Hearing Disorders, 45,* 287–307.

Anthony, J. P., Allen, D. B., Trabulsky, P. P., Mahdavian, M., & Mathes, S. J. (1995). Canine laryngeal transplantation: Preliminary studies and a new heterotopic allotransplantation model. *European Archives of Oto-Rhino-Laryngology, 252,* 197–205.

Associated Press. (2007, May 21). *UNM criticized over use of mice in study*. Retrieved June 9, 2008, from http://www.boston.com/news/science/articles/2007/05/21/unm_criticized_over_use_of_mice_in_study/

Association of College and Research Libraries (2000). *ACRL information literacy web site*. Retrieved August 27, 2004, from http://www.ala.org

ATLAS.ti (2008). *Atlas.ti*. Retrieved June 9, 2008, from http://www.atlasti.com

Bartholomew, M. (2002). James Lind's treatise of the scurvy (1753). *Postgraduate Medicine Journal, 78,* 695–696.

Baylor, C. R., Yorkston, K. M., Eadie, T. L., Strand, E. A., & Duffy, J. (2006). A systematic review of outcome measurement in unilateral vocal fold paralysis. *Journal of Medical Speech-Language Pathology, 14,* xxvii–lvii.

Beach, M. C. (2005). *Commentary: Evidence-based medicine and ethics*. Retrieved December 3, 2007, from http://www.unitedhealthfoundation.org/download/ebm-eth.pdf

Beach, M. C., & Faden, R. (2005). *Commentary: Evidence-based medicine and ethics. Clinical evidence*. Retrieved April 17, 2009, from http://clinicalevidence.bmj.com

Beeman, S. K. (2002). *Evaluating violence against women research reports*. Applied Research Forum: National Electronic NetWork on Violence Against Women. Retrieved August 27, 2004, from http://www.vawnet.org/DomesticViolence/Research/vawnetDocs/AR_evalresearch.PDF

Bem, D. J. (2004). Writing the empirical article. In J. M. Darley, M. P. Zanna, & H. L. Roediger III (Eds.), *The compleat academic: A career guide* (pp. 185–219). Washington, DC: American Psychological Association.

Bender, B. K., Cannito, M. P., Murray, T., & Woodson, G. E. (2004). Speech intelligibility in severe adductor spasmodic dysphonia. *Journal of Speech-Language-Hearing Research, 47,* 21–32.

Berlin, J. A., Laird, N. M., Sacks, H. S., & Chalmers, T. C. (1989). A comparison of statistical methods for combining event rates from clinical trials. *Statistics in Medicine, 8,* 141–151.

Bernard, C. (1957). *An introduction to the study of experimental medicine* (H.C. Greene, Trans.). New York: Dover. (Original work published in 1865)

Bernstein Ratner, N. (2006). Evidence-based practice: An examination of its ramifications for the practice of speech-language pathology. *Language, Speech, and Hearing Services in Schools, 37,* 257–267.

Bess, F. H. (1995). Evidence-based audiology. *American Journal of Audiology, 4,* 5.

Birchall, M. A., Lorenz, R. R., Berke, G. S., Genden, E. M., Haughey, B. H., Siemionow, M., & Stroms, M. (2006). Laryngeal transplantation in 2005: A review. *American Journal of Transplantation, 6,* 20–26.

Black, N. (1996). Why we need observational studies to evaluate the effectiveness of health care. *British Medical Journal, 312*, 1215–1218.

Bloom, L. (1970). *Language development: Form and function in emerging grammars*. Cambridge, MA: The MIT Press.

Blood, G. W., Ridenour, J. S., Thomas, E. A., Qualls, C. D., & Hammer, C. S. (2002). Predicting job satisfaction among speech-language pathologists working in public schools. *Language, Speech, and Hearing Services in Schools, 33*, 282–290.

Bloom, A. (1995). Letter to the editor. *American Journal of Audiology, 4*, 88–89.

Bok, S. (1999). *Lying: Moral choice in public and private life*. New York: Vintage Books.

Borden, G. J., Harris, K. S., & Raphael, L. J. (2002). *Speech science primer: Physiology, acoustics, and perception of speech*. New York: Lippincott Williams & Wilkins.

Bothe, A. K., Davidow, J. H., Bramlett, R. E., & Ingham, R. J. (2006). Stuttering treatment research 1970–2005: I. Systematic review incorporating trial quality assessment of behavioral, cognitive, and related approaches. *American Journal of Speech-Language Pathology, 15*, 321–341.

Boutsen, F., Cannito, M. P., Taylor, M., & Bender, B. (2002). Botox treatment in adductor spasmodic dysphonia: A meta-analysis. *Journal of Speech-Language-Hearing Research, 45*, 469–481.

Bracht, G. H., & Glass, G. V. (1968). The external validity of experiments. *American Educational Research Journal, 5*, 437–474.

Brobeck, T. C., & Lubinsky, J. (2003). Using single-subject designs in speech-language pathology practicum. *Contemporary Issues in Communication Science and Disorders, 30*, 101–106.

Brookshire, R. H. (1983). Subject description and generality of results in experiments with aphasic adults. *Journal of Speech and Hearing Disorders, 48*, 342–346.

Burk, M. H., & Wiley, T. L. (2004). Continuous versus pulsed tomes in audiometry. *American Journal of Audiology, 13*, 54–61.

California Employment Development Department. (1995). *California occupational guide number 453*. Retrieved August 26, 2004, from http://www/calmis.cahwnet.gov/file/occguide/SPEECHPA.HTM

Campbell, D. T. (1957). Factors relevant to the validity of experiments in social settings. *Psychological Bulletin, 54*, 297–312.

Campbell, D. T., & Stanley, J. C. (1963). Experimental and quasi-experimental designs for research or teaching. In N. L. Gage (Ed.), *Handbook of research on teaching* (pp. 171–246). Chicago: Rand McNally.

Campbell, J. P. (1982). Editorial: Some remarks from the outgoing editor. *Journal of Applied Psychology, 67*, 691–700.

Cannito, M. P., & Kondraske, G. V. (1990). Rapid manual abilities in spasmodic dysphonic and normal female subjects. *Journal of Speech and Hearing Research, 33*, 123–133.

Carr, J. E., & Burkholder, E. O. (1998). Creating single-subject design graphs with Microsoft EXCEL. *Journal of Applied Behavior Analysis, 31*, 245–251.

Carrow-Woolfolk, E. (1999). *Test for auditory comprehension of language (TACL 3)*. Circle Pines, MN: AGS Publishing.

Casby, M. W. (2001). Otitis media and language development: A meta-analysis. *American Journal of Speech-Language Pathology, 10*, 65–80.

Catts, H. W., Fey, M. E., Tomblin, J. B., & Zhang, X. (2002). A longitudinal investigation of reading outcomes in children with language impairments. *Journal of Speech-Language-Hearing Research, 45*, 1142–1157.

Centers for Disease Control and Prevention. (2008). *Qualitative methods in health research: Opportunities and considerations in application and review.* Retrieved February, 18, 2008, from http://obssr.od.nih.gov/Documents/Publications/Qualitative.PDF

Centre for Reviews and Dissemination. (1999). *Getting evidence into practice.* Retrieved December 10, 2007, from http://www.york.ac.uk/inst/crd/ehc51.pdf

Centre for Reviews and Dissemination. (2001, March). *CRD Report 4* (2nd ed.). Retrieved December 11, 2007, from http:www.york.ac.uk/inst/crd/report4.htm

Chalmers, I. (2007). Why fair tests are needed: A brief history. *Evidence-Based Nursing, 10,* 4–5.

Chambers, J. M., Cleveland, W. S., Kleiner, B., & Tukey, P. A. (1983). *Graphical methods for data analysis.* Belmont, CA: Wadsworth.

Cirrin, F. M., & Gillam, R. B. (2008). Language intervention practices for school-age children with spoken language disorders: A systematic review. *Language, Speech, and Hearing Service in Schools, 39,* 110–137.

Cochrane, A. L. (1979). 1931–1971: A critical review, with particular reference to the medical profession. In G. Feeling-Smith & N. Wells (Eds.), *Medicines for the year 2000* (pp. 1–11). London: Office of Health Economics.

The Cochrane Collaboration. (n.d.). Retrieved April 8, 2009, from http://www.cochrane.org

Cohen, J. (1988). *Statistical power analysis for the behavioral sciences* (2nd ed.). Hillsdale, NJ: Erlbaum.

Collins, C. R., & Blood, G. W. (1990). Acknowledgement and severity of stuttering as factors influencing nonstutterers' perceptions of stutterers. *Journal of Speech and Hearing Disorders, 55,* 75–81.

Condouris, K., Meyer, E., & Tager-Flusberg, H. (2003). The relationship between standardized measures of language and measures of spontaneous speech in children with autism. *American Journal of Speech-Language Pathology, 13,* 349–358.

Cooper, H. (2003). Editorial. *Psychological Bulletin, 129,* 3–9.

Cooper, H. M., & Rosenthal, R. (1980). Statistical versus traditional procedures for summarizing research findings. *Psychological Bulletin, 87,* 442–449.

Court of Appeals of Maryland. (2001). *Ericka Grimes v. Kennedy Krieger Institute, Inc. (No. 128) case number 24-C-99-000925.* Retrieved August 27, 2004, from http://www.courts.state.md.us/opinions/coa/2001/128a00.pdf

Cox, L. R., Cooper, W. A., & McDade, H. L. (1989). Teachers' perceptions of adolescent girls who wear hearing aids. *Language, Speech, and Hearing Services in Schools, 20,* 372–380.

Cox, K. M., Lee, D. J., Carey, J. P., & Minor, L. B. (2003). Dehiscence of bone overlying the superior semicircular canal as a cause of an air-bone gap on audiometry: A case study. *American Journal of Audiology, 12,* 11–16.

Cream, A., Onslow, M., Packman, A., & Llewellyn, G. (2003). Protection from harm: The experience of adults after therapy with prolonged speech. *International Journal of Language and Communication Disorders, 38,* 379–395.

Creative Research Systems. (2008). *The Survey System.* Retrieved June 9, 2008, from http://www.surveysystem.com

Crombie, I. K. (1990). *Pocket guide to critical appraisal.* London: BMJ Books.

Crosbie, J. (1993). Interrupted time-series analysis with brief single-subject data. *Journal of Consulting and Clinical Psychology, 61,* 966–974.

Culatta, B., Kovarsky, D., Theodore, G., Franklin, A., & Timler, G. (2003). Quantitative and qualitative documentation of early literacy instruction. *American Journal of Speech-Language Pathology, 12,* 172–188.

Damico, J. S., & Simmons-Mackie, N. N. (2003). Qualitative research and speech-language pathology: A tutorial for the clinical realm. *American Journal of Speech-Language Pathology*, *12*, 131–143.

Daniels, S. K., Corey, O. M., Hodskey, L. D., Legendre, C., Priestly, D. H., Rosenbeck, J. C., & Foundas, A. L. (2004). Mechanism of sequential swallowing during straw drinking in healthy young and older adults. *Journal of Speech-Language-Hearing Research*, *47*, 33–45.

Davis, B., Qiu, W., & Hamernik, R. P. (2005). Sensitivity of distortion product otoacoustic emissions in noise-exposed chinchillas. *Journal of the American Academy of Audiology*, *16*, 69–78.

Dekroon, D. M. A., Kyle, C. S., & Johnson, C. J. (2002). Partner influences on the social pretend play of children with language impairments. *Language, Speech, and Hearing Services in Schools*, *33*, 253–267.

Delage, H., & Tuller, L. (2007). Language development and mild-to-moderate hearing loss: Does language normalize with age? *Journal of Speech, Language, and Hearing Research*, *50*, 1300–1313.

Dennis, J., & Abbott, J. (2006). Information retrieval: Where's your evidence? *Contemporary Issues in Communication Science and Disorders*, *33*, 11–20.

Denzin, N. K. (1978). *The research act: A theoretical introduction to sociological methods* (2nd ed.). New York: McGraw-Hill.

DePaul, R., & Kent, R. D. (2000). A longitudinal case study of ALS: Effects of listener familiarity and proficiency on intelligibility judgments. *American Journal of Speech-Language Pathology*, *9*, 230–240.

Deutsch, L. J. (1995). Letter to the editor. *American Journal of Audiology*, *4*, 89–90.

Devilly, G. J. (2008). *Effect Size Generator—Free Edition* [Computer software]. Retrieved June 7, 2008, from http://devilly.org/ClinTools/clintools.html

Dewar, J. A. (1998). *The information age and the printing press: Looking backward to see ahead* (Document No. P-8014). Santa Monica, CA: Rand.

Diener, E., & Eid, M. (2006). The finale: Take-home messages from the editors. In M. Eid & E. Diener (Eds.), *Handbook of measurement in psychology* (pp. 457–463). Washington, DC: American Psychological Association.

Digital Era Copyright Enhancement Act of 1999, H.R. 3048, 105th Cong. (1999). Retrieved August 26, 2004, from http://www.copyright.gov

Dillman, D. A. (2007). *Mail and Internet surveys* (2nd ed.). Hoboken, NJ: Wiley.

Dunn, L. M., & Dunn, L. M. (1997). *Peabody picture vocabulary test (PPVT 3)*. Circle Pines, MN: AGS Publishing.

Eadie, P. A., Fey, M. E., Douglas, J. M., & Parsons, C. L. (2002). Profiles of grammatical morphology and sentence imitation in children with specific language impairment and Down syndrome. *Journal of Speech-Language-Hearing Research*, *45*, 720–732.

Easterbrook, S. (n.d.). *How theses get written: Some cool tips*. Retrieved April 18, 2009, from http://www.cs.toronto.edu/~sme/presentations/thesiswriting.pdf

Edwards, P. J., Roberts I. G., Clarke M. J., DiGuiseppi C., Wentz R., Kwan I., Cooper R., Felix L., & Pratap S. (2003). Methods to increase response rates to postal questionnaires. *Cochrane Database of Systematic Reviews*, 4. Art. No.: MR000008. DOI: 10.1002/14651858.MR000008.pub3

Egger, M., Schneider, M., & Smith, G. D. (1998). Meta-analysis: Spurious precision? Meta-analysis of observational studies. *British Medical Journal*, *316*, 140–144.

Egger, M., & Smith, G. D. (1997). Meta-analysis: Potentials and promise. *British Medical Journal*, *315*, 1371–1374.

Egger, M., Smith, G. D., & Phillips, A. N. (1997). Meta-analysis: Principles and procedures. *British Medical Journal, 315,* 1533–1537.

Egger, M., Smith, G. D., Schneider, M., & Minder, C. (1997). Bias in meta-analysis detected by a simple graphical test. *British Medical Journal, 315,* 629–634.

Eisenberg, S. L., Fersko, T. M., & Lundgren, C. (2001). The use of MLU for identifying language impairment in preschool children: A review. *American Journal of Speech-Language Pathology, 10,* 323–342.

Ekman, P., & Friesen, W. V. (1969). The repertoire of nonverbal behavior: Categories, origins, usage, and coding. *Semiotica, 1,* 49–98.

Emanuel, D. C. (2002). The auditory processing battery: Survey of common practices. *Journal of the American Academy of Audiology, 13,* 93–117.

Emig, J. A. (1971). *The composing processes of twelfth graders.* Urbana, IL: The National Council of Teachers of English.

Erler, S. F., & Garstecki, D. C. (2002). Hearing loss– and hearing aid–related stigma: Perceptions of women with age-normal hearing. *American Journal of Audiology, 11,* 83–91.

Ethics Board, American Speech-Language-Hearing Association. (2002). *Ethics in research and professional practice.* Retrieved August 27, 2004, from http://www.asha.org/NR/rdonlyres/750A8380-D6CD-4591-97E7-C4E794A665DB/0/18792_1.pdf

Eysenbach, G., & Till, J. E. (2001). Ethical issues in qualitative research on internet communities. *British Medical Journal, 323,* 1103–1105.

Faith, M. S. Allison, D. B., & Gorman, B. S. (1997). Meta-analysis of single-case research. In R. D. Franklin, D. B. Allison & B. S. Gorman (Eds.), *Design and analysis of single-case research* (pp. 245–277). Mahwah, NJ: Erlbaum.

Finn, P., Bothe, A. K., & Bramlett, R. E. (2005). Science and pseudoscience in communication disorders: Criteria and applications. *American Journal of Speech-Language Pathology, 14,* 172–186.

Fitzgibbon, B. (1995). Letter to the editor. *American Journal of Audiology, 4,* 89.

Flores, G., Lee, M., Bauchner, H., & Kastner, B. (2000). Pediatricians' attitudes, beliefs, and practices regarding clinical practice guidelines: A national survey. *Pediatrics, 105,* 496–501.

Flower, L., & Hayes, J. R. (1981). A cognitive process theory of writing. *College Composition and Communication, 32,* 365–387.

Franklin, R. D., Allison, D. B., & Gorman, B. S. (1997). *Design and analysis of single-case research.* Mahwah, NJ: Erlbaum.

Frazek, M. (2003). Ethics vs. legal jurisdiction. *ASHA LeaderOnline.* Retrieved August 29, 2004, from http://www.asha.org/about/ethics/ethics-jurisdiction.htm

Freund, J. E. (1988). *Modern elementary statistics.* Englewood Cliffs, NJ: Prentice Hall.

Friedman, M. I. (1953). *Essays in positive economics.* Chicago: University of Chicago Press.

Friedman, H. H., Herskowitz, P. J., & Pollack, S. (1993). The biasing effects of scale-checking styles on response to a Likert scale. *Proceedings of the American Statistical Association Annual Conference: Survey Research Methods,* 792–795.

Gartlehner, G., Hansen, R. A., Nissman, D., Lohr, K. N., & Carey, T. S. (2006). *Criteria for distinguishing effectiveness from efficacy trials in systematic reviews.* Retrieved April 30, 2007, from Agency for Healthcare Research and Quality website: http://www.ahrq.gov/downloads/pub/evidence/pdf/efftrials.pdf

Gelfand, S. A., Schwander, T., & Silman, S. (1990). Acoustic reflex thresholds in normal and cochlear-impaired ears: Effects of no-response rates on 90th percentiles in a large sample. *Journal of Speech and Hearing Disorders, 55,* 198–205.

Gibbs, G. R., Friese, S., & Mangabeira, W. C. (2002, May). The use of new technology in qualitative research. *Using Technology in the Qualitative Research Process, 3*(2). Retrieved August 27, 2004, from http://www.qualitative-research.net/fqs-texte/2-02/2-02hrsg-e.htm

Gillon, G. T. (2000). The efficacy of phonological awareness intervention for children with spoken language impairment. *Language Speech and Hearing Services in Schools, 31*, 126–141.

Girden, E. R. (1996). *Evaluating research articles from start to finish*. Thousand Oaks, CA: Sage.

Glass, G. V. (2000). *Meta-analysis at 25*. Retrieved June 9, 2008, from http://glass.ed.asu.edu/gene/papers/meta25.html

Glennen, S. (2002). Language development and delay in internationally adopted infants and toddlers: A review. *American Journal of Speech-Language Pathology, 11*, 333–339.

Goldstein, B., & Washington, P. S. (2001). An initial investigation of phonological patterns in typically developing 4-year-old Spanish-English bilingual children. *Language, Speech, and Hearing Services in Schools, 32*, 153–164.

Golper, L. A. C., Wertz, R. T., Frattali, C. M., Yorkston, K., Myers, P., Katz, R. et al. (2001). *Evidence-based practice guidelines for the management of communication disorders in neurologically impaired individuals: Project introduction*. Retrieved April 17, 2009, from http://www.ancds.org/pdf/PracticeGuidelines.pdf

Gopen, G. D., & Swan, J. A. (1990). The science of scientific writing. *American Scientist, 78*, 550–558.

GraphPad Quick Calcs. (2004). *Free online calculators for scientists*. Retrieved August 26, 2004, from http://www.graphpad.com

Green, J., & Britten, N. (1998). Qualitative research and evidence based medicine. *British Medical Journal, 316*, 1230–1232.

Greg, N., Coleman, C., Stennett, R. B., & Davis, M. (2002). Discourse complexity of college writers with and without disabilities: A multidimensional analysis. *Journal of Learning Disabilities, 35*, 23–38, 56.

Greenhalgh, T. (1997a). How to read a paper: The Medline database. *British Medical Journal, 315*, 180–183.

Greenhalgh, T. (1997b). How to read a paper: Papers that summarize other papers (systematic reviews and meta-analyses). *British Medical Journal, 315*, 672–675.

Greenhalgh, T. (1998). Outside the ivory towers: Evidence based medicine in the real world. *The British Journal of General Medicine, 48*, 1716–1717.

Greenhalgh, T. (2001). *How to read a paper: The basics of evidence based medicine*. London: BMJ Books.

Greenhalgh, T., & Taylor, R. (1997c). Papers that go beyond numbers (qualitative research). *British Medical Journal, 315*, 740–743.

Grose, J. H., Hall III, J. W., & Bass, E. (2004). Duration discrimination in listeners with cochlear hearing loss: Effects of stimulus type and frequency. *Journal of Speech-Language-Hearing Research, 47*, 5–12.

Guitar, B., & Marchinkoski, L. (2001). Influence of mothers' slower speech on their children's speech rate. *Journal of Speech-Language-Hearing Research, 44*, 853–861.

Guttman, L. (1968). A general nonmetric technique for finding the smallest coordinate space for a configuration of points. *Psychometrika, 33*, 469–506.

Guttman, L. (1977). What is not what in statistics? *Statistician, 26*, 81–107.

Guyatt, G. H. (1991). Evidence-based medicine. *ACP Journal Club, 114*, A-16.

Guyatt, G., Jaeschke, R., Heddle, N., Cook, D., Shannon, H., & Walter, S. (1995). Basic statistics for clinicians 1: Hypothesis testing. *Canadian Medical Association Journal, 152*, 27–32.

Halloran, P. F., Reeve, J., & Kaplan, B. (2006). Lies, damn lies, and statistics: The perils of the p value. *American Journal of Transplantation, 6,* 10–11.

Hedges, L. V., Gurevitch, J., & Curtis, P. S. (1999). The meta-analysis of response ratios in experimental ecology: Meta-analysis in ecology. *Ecology, 80,* 1150–1156.

Hedges, L. V., & Olkin, I. (1985). *Statistical methods for meta-analysis.* San Diego, CA: Academic Press.

Helm-Estabrooks, N., Hanson, E. K., Yorkston, K. M., & Beukelman, D. R. (2004). Speech supplementation techniques for dysarthria: A systematic review. *Journal of Medical Speech-Language Pathology, 12,* ix–xxix.

Herbert, R. D., Sherrington, C., Maher, C., & Moseley, A. M. (2001). Evidence-based practice—Imperfect but necessary. *Physiotherapy Theory and Practice, 17,* 201–211.

Herder, C., Howard, C., Nye, C., & Vanryckeghem, M. (2006). Effectiveness of behavioral stuttering treatment: A systematic review and meta-analysis. *Contemporary Issues in Communication Science and Disorders, 33,* 61–73.

Hersen, M., & Barlow, D. H. (1976). *Single case experimental designs: Strategies for studying behavior change.* New York: Pergamon Press.

Hetzroni, O. E., Quist, R. W., & Lloyd, L. L. (2002). Translucency and complexity: Effects on Blissymbol learning using computer and teacher presentations. *Language, Speech, and Hearing Services in Schools, 33,* 291–303.

Hill, C. J., Bloom, H. S., Rebeck Black, A., & Lipsey, M. W. (2007, July). *Empirical benchmarks for interpreting effect sizes in research.* MDRC Working Papers in Research Methodology, New York, NY.

Hinkle, D. E., Wiersma, W., & Jurs, S. G. (1988). *Applied statistics for the behavioral sciences.* Boston: Houghton Mifflin.

Hoaglin, D. C. (1988). Transformations in everyday experience, *Chance, 1,* 40–45.

Hoff, C. (2003). Immoral and moral uses of animals. In R. Abelson & M.-L. Friquenon (Eds.), *Ethics for modern life* (6th ed., pp. 472–484). Boston: Bedford/St. Martin's.

Hoffman, V., & Gillam, R. B. (2004). Verbal and spatial information processing constraints in children with specific language impairment. *Journal of Speech-Language-Hearing Research, 47,* 114–125.

Holcomb, Z. C. (2004). *Interpreting basic statistics.* Glendale, CA: Pyrczak Publishing.

Hong Kong Polytechnic University. (2002). *Academic writing for publication.* Retrieved June 5, 2008, from http://www.engl.polyu.edu.hk/EECTR/awphandbook/AWP.htm

Hopper, T., Bayles, K. A., Harris, F. P., & Holland, A. (2001). The relationship between minimum data set ratings and scores on measures of communication and hearing among nursing home residents with dementia. *American Journal of Speech-Language Pathology, 10,* 370–381.

Hubbard, C. P. (1998). Stuttering, stressed syllables, and word onsets. *Journal of Speech-Language-Hearing Research, 41,* 802–808.

Huer, M. B., & Saenz, T. I. (2003). Challenges and strategies for conducting survey and focus group research with culturally diverse groups. *American Journal of Speech-Language Pathology, 12,* 209–220.

Huff, D. (1982). *How to lie with statistics.* New York: W. W. Norton.

Ingham, R. J., Fox, P. T., Ingham, J. C., Xiong, J., Zamarripa, F., Hardies, L. J., & Lancaster, J. L. (2004). Brain correlates of stuttering and syllable production: Gender comparison and replication. *Journal of Speech-Language-Hearing Research, 47,* 321–341.

Ingram, D., & Morehead, D. (2002). The development of base syntax revisited. *Journal of Speech-Language-Hearing Science, 45,* 559–563.

Institute für Experimentelle Psychologie (2008). *G*Power 3*. Retrieved June 9, 2008, from http://www.psycho.uni-duesseldorf.de/abteilungen/aap/gpower3/

Institute of Medicine. (1990). *Clinical practice guidelines: Directions for a new program*. Washington, DC: National Academy Press.

Jadad, A. R., Moore, R. A., Carroll, D., Jenkinson, C., Reynolds, D. J., Gavaghan, D. J., et al. (1996). Assessing the quality of randomized trials: Is blinding necessary? *Controlled Clinical Trials*, *17*, 1–12.

Jarvis, L. H., Merriman, W. E., Barnett, M., Hanba, J., & Van Haitsma, K. S. (2004). Input that contradicts young children's strategy for mapping novel words affects their phonological and semantic interpretation of other novel words. *Journal of Speech-Language-Hearing Research*, *47*, 392–406.

Jennions, M. D., & Møller, A. P. (2003). A survey of the statistical power of research in behavioral ecology and animal behavior. *Behavioral Ecology*, *14*, 438–445.

Jupiter, T., & Palagonia, C. L. (2001). The hearing handicap inventory for the elderly screening version adapted for use with elderly Chinese American individuals. *American Journal of Audiology*, *10*, 99–103.

Justice, L. M., Chow, S., Capellini, C., Flanigan, K., & Colton, S. (2003). Emergent literacy intervention for vulnerable preschoolers: Relative effects of two approaches. *American Journal of Speech-Language Pathology*, *12*, 320–332.

Justice, L. M., Weber, S. E., Ezell, H. K., & Bakeman, R. (2002). A sequential analysis of children's responsiveness to parental print references during shared book-reading interactions. *American Journal of Speech-Language Pathology*, *11*, 30–40.

Kamhi, A. G. (2004). A meme's eye view of speech-language pathology. *Language Speech and Hearing Service in Schools*, *35*, 105–111.

Kamhi, A. G., Masterson, J. J., & Apel, K. (Eds.). (2007). *Clinical decision making in developmental language disorders*. Baltimore: Paul H. Brookes.

Kavale, K. A. (2001). Meta-analysis: A primer. *Exceptionality*, *9*, 177–183.

Kazdin, A. E. (1982). Single-case experimental designs. In P. C. Kendall & J. N. Butler (Eds.), *Handbook of research methods in clinical psychology* (pp. 461–490). Hoboken, NJ: Wiley & Sons.

Kazdin, A. E. (2001). Almost clinically significant (p < .10): Current measures may only approach clinical significance. *Clinical Psychology: Science and Practice*, *8*, 455–462.

Kent, R. D. (1997). The perceptual sensorimotor examination for motor speech disorders. In M. R. McNeil (Ed.), *Clinical management of sensorimotor disorders* (p. 46). New York: Thieme.

Kerlinger, F. N. (1973). *Foundations of behavioral research*. New York: Holt, Rinehart and Winston.

Kerlinger, F. N. (1979). *Behavioral research: A conceptual approach*. New York: Holt, Rinehart and Winston.

Kerridge, I., Lowe, M., & Henry, D. (1998). Ethics and evidence based medicine. *British Medical Journal*, *316*, 1151–1153.

Keselman, H. J., Huberty, C. J., Lix, L. M., Olejnik, S., Cribbie, R. A., Donahue, B., Kowalchak, R. K., Lowaman, L. L., Petoskey, M. D., & Keselman, J. C. (1998). Statistical practices of educational researchers: An analysis of their ANOVA, MANOVA, and ANCOVA analyses. *Review of Educational Research*, *68*, 350–386.

Kimmel, A. J. (1991). Predictable biases in the ethical decision making of American psychologists. *American Psychologist*, *46*, 786–788.

Kiran, S. (2008). Typicality of inanimate category exemplars in aphasia treatment: Further evidence for semantic complexity. *Journal of Speech, Language, and Hearing Research*, *51*, 1550–1568.

Kiran, S., & Thompson, C. K. (2003). The role of semantic complexity in treatment of naming deficits: Training semantic categories in fluent aphasia by controlling exemplar typicality. *Journal of Speech-Language-Hearing Research*, *46*, 608–622.

Konstantopoulos, S., & Hedges, L. V. (2005). *How large an effect can we expect from school reforms?* Working Paper 05–04. Evanston, IL: Northwestern University, Institute for Policy Research. Retrieved June 7, 2008, from http://www.northwestern.edu/ipr/publications/papers/2005/WP-05-04.pdf

Korchin, S. J., & Cowan, P. A. (1982). Ethical perspectives in clinical research. In P. C. Kendall & J. N. Butcher (Eds.), *Handbook of research methods in clinical psychology* (pp. 59–94). New York: Wiley & Sons.

Kratochwill, T. R. (1978). *Single subject research: Strategies for evaluating change*. New York: Academic Press.

Kritikos, E. P. (2003). Speech-language pathologists' beliefs about bilingual/bicultural individuals. *American Journal of Speech-Language Pathology*, *12*, 73–91.

Kuster, J. M. (2002). Web-based information resources for evidence-based practice in speech-language pathology, *Perspectives on Language Learning and Education*, *6*, 6–14.

Labott, S. M., & Johnson, T. P. (2004). Psychological and social risks of behavioral research. *IRB: Ethics & Human Research*, *26*, 11–15.

Lachin, J. M. (1988). Properties of simple randomization. *Controlled Clinical Trials*, *9*, 312–326.

Lachin, J. M., Matts, J. P., & Wei, L. J. (1988). Randomization in clinical trials: Conclusions and recommendations. *Controlled Clinical Trials*, *9*, 365–376.

Language Analysis Lab. (2009). *Salt software*. Retrieved April 17, 2009, from http://www.languageanalysislab.com

LaPointe, L. (1985). Aphasia therapy: Some principles and strategies for treatment. In D. F. Johns (Ed.), *Clinical management of neurogenic communicative disorders* (pp. 179–241). Boston: Little Brown.

Law, M. (2000). Strategies for implementing evidence-based practice in early intervention. *Infants and Young Children*, *13*, 32–40.

Law, J., Garrett, Z., & Nye, C. (2004). The efficacy of treatment for children with developmental speech and language delay/disorder: A meta-analysis. *Journal of Speech, Language, and Hearing Research*, *47*, 924–943.

Lenth, R. V. (2001). Some practical guidelines for effective sample-size determination. *The American Statistician*, *55*, 187–193.

Leonard, L. B. (1979). Language impairment in children. *Merrill-Palmer Quarterly*, *25*, 205–232.

Leonard, L. B., & Finneran, D. (2003). Grammatical morphemes effects on MLU: "The same can be less" revisited. *Journal of Speech-Language-Hearing Research*, *46*, 878–888.

Levant, R. F. (2005, July 1). *Report of the 2005 presidential task force on evidence-based practice*. Retrieved June 9, 2008, from http://www.apa.org/practice/ebpreport.pdf

Levin, J. R., & Wampold, B. E. (1999). Generalized single-case randomization tests: Flexible analyses for a variety of situations. *School Psychology Quarterly*, *14*, 59–93.

Leydon, C., Fisher, K. V., & Lodewyck-Falciglia, D. (2008, September 19). The cystic fibrosis transmembrane conductance regulator (CFTR) and chloride-dependent ion fluxes of ovine vocal fold epithelium [Electronic version]. *Journal of Speech, Language, and Hearing Research*. Retrieved December 10, 2008, from doi:10.1044/1092- 4388(2008/07-0192)

Likert, R. (1932). *A technique for the measurement of attitudes*. New York: Archives of Psychology.

Lincoln, Y. S., & Guba, E. G. (1985). *Naturalistic inquiry*. New York: Sage.

Locke, L., Silverman, S., & Spirduso, W. (1998). *Reading and understanding research*. Thousand Oaks, CA: Sage.

Lipsey, M. W. (1990). *Design sensitivity: Statistical power for experimental research*. Newbury Park, CA: Sage.

Lipsey, M. W. (2000). Statistical conclusion validity for intervention research. In L. Bickman (Ed.), *Validity and social experimentation* (pp. 101–119). Thousand Oaks, CA: Sage.

Lipsey, M. W., & Wilson, D. B. (1993). The efficacy of psychological, educational, and behavioral treatment: Confirmation from meta-analysis. *American Psychologist, 12*, 1181–1209.

Locke, L. F., Silverman, S. J., & Spirduso, W. W. (2004). *Reading and understanding research*. Thousand Oaks, CA: Sage.

Loewy, E. H. (2007). Ethics and evidence-based medicine: Is there a conflict? *Medscape General Medicine, 9*, 30–39.

Lof, G. L. (2006, November). *Logic, theory and evidence against the use of non-speech oral motor exercises to change speech sound productions*. Paper presented at the annual meeting of the American Speech-Language-Hearing Association, Miami Beach, FL.

Lof, G. L. (2007, November). *Reasons why non-speech oral motor exercises should not be used for speech sound disorders*. Presentation at the annual convention of the American Speech-Language-Hearing Association, Boston, MA.

Lof, G. L., & Watson, M. M. (2008). A nationwide survey of nonspeech oral motor exercise use: Implications for evidence-based practice. *Language, Speech, and Hearing Services in Schools, 39*, 392–407.

Logemann, J. A. (1987). Criteria for studies of treatment for oral-pharyngeal dysphagia. *Dysphagia, 1*, 193–199.

Logemann, J. A., & O'Toole, T. J. (2000). Identification and management of dysphagia in the public schools. *Language, Speech, and Hearing Services in Schools, 31*, 26–27.

Long, S. (2009). Computerized profiling. Retrieved April 17, 2009, from http://www.computerizedprofiling.org/

Louis, T. A., Lavori, P. W., Bailar III, J. C., & Polansky, M. (1984). Crossover and self-controlled designs in clinical research. *The New England Journal of Medicine, 310*, 24–31.

Lovelace, S., & Stewart, S. R. (2007). Increasing print awareness in preschoolers with language impairment using non-evocative print referencing. *Language, Speech, and Hearing Services in Schools, 38*, 16–30.

Lowry, R. (n.d.). *VassarStats: Website for statistical computation*. Retrieved April 18, 2009, from http://faculty.vassar.edu/lowry/VassarStats.html

Lyons, L. C. (2004). *The meta-analysis page*. Retrieved August 26, 2004, from http://www/lyonsmorris.com/MetaA/index.htm

Mastergeorge, A. M. (1999). Revelations of family perceptions of diagnosis and disorder through metaphor. In D. Kovarsky, J. Duchan, & M. Maxwell (Eds.), *Constructing (in)competence: Disabling evaluations in clinical and social interactions* (pp. 245–256). Mahwah, NJ: Erlbaum.

Max, L., & Onghena, P. (1999). Some issues in the statistical analysis of completely randomized and repeated measures designs for speech, language, and hearing research. *Journal of Speech-Language-Hearing Research, 42*, 261–270.

McAllister, L. (1998). What constitutes good qualitative research writing—in theses and papers? In J. Higgs (Ed.), *Writing qualitative research* (pp. 217–232). Sydney, Australia: Hampden Press.

McGregor, K. K., Newman, R. M., Reilly, R. M., & Capone, N. C. (2002). Semantic representation and naming in children with specific language impairment. *Journal of Speech-Language-Hearing Research*, *45*, 998–1014.

McGue, M. (2000). Authorship and intellectual property. In B. D. Sales & S. Folkman (Eds.), *Ethics in research with human* participants (pp. 75–95). Washington, DC: American Psychological Association.

McHenry, M. A. (2003). The effect of pacing strategies on the variability of speech movement sequences in dysarthria. *Journal of Speech-Language-Hearing Research*, *46*, 702–710.

Mechling, L. C., Gast, D. L., & Cronin, B. A. (2006). The effects of presenting high-preference items, paired with choice, via computer-based video programming on task completion of students with autism. *Focus on Autism and Other Developmental Disabilities*, *21*, 7–13.

Meline, T. (2003). Problems in synthesis (meta-analytic) studies: An example from the communication disorders literature. *Perceptual and Motor Skills*, *97*, 1085–1088.

Meline, T. (2006a) Evidence-based speech language pathology (practice): What's new? *Perspectives on Language Learning and Education*, *13*, 2–5.

Meline, T. (2006b). Selecting studies for systematic review: Inclusion and exclusion criteria. *Contemporary Issues in Communication Science and Disorders*, *33*, 21–27.

Meline, T. (2007a, April). *10 Steps to evidence-based practice*. Paper Presented at the annual Gruber Symposium, Lamar University, TX.

Meline, T. (2007b). Troubled waters? The evidence in evidence- based practice. *TEJAS*, *37*, 5–7.

Meline, T., Florez-Sabo, B., Hinojosa, V., & Gonzalez, E. (2004, November). *Effects of paired reading practice on children's reading fluency*. Presentation at the convention of the American Speech-Hearing-Language Association, Philadelphia, PA.

Meline, T., Gonzalez, E., Florez-Sabo, B., & Hinojosa, V. (2004, November). *Effects of paired reading practice on children's reading fluency*. Poster session presented at the annual meeting of the American Speech-Language-Hearing Association, Philadelphia, PA.

Meline, T., & Harn, W. E. (2008a). Comments on Bothe, Davidow, Bramlett, Franic, and Ingham (2006). *American Journal of Speech-Language Pathology*, *17*, 93–97.

Meline, T., & Harn, W. E. (2008b, November). *Assessing the quality of randomized controlled trials in communication disorders*. Seminar presented at the annual meeting of the American Speech-Language-Hearing Association, Chicago, IL.

Meline, T., & Mata-Pistokache, T. (2003). The perils of Pauline's e-mail: Professional issues for audiologists and speech-language pathologists. *Contemporary Issues in Communication Science and Disorders*, *30*, 118–123.

Meline, T., & Paradiso, T. (2003). Evidence-based practice in schools: Evaluating research and reducing barriers. *Language, Speech, and Hearing Services in Schools*, *34*, 273–283.

Meline, T., & Schmitt, J. F. (1997). Case studies for evaluating statistical significance in group designs. *American Journal of Speech-Language Pathology*, *6*, 33–41.

Meline, T., & Wang, B. (2004). Effect-size reporting practices in *AJSLP* and other ASHA journals: 1999–2003. *American Journal of Speech-Language Pathology*, *13*, 202–207.

Mendes, A. P. (2000). *Informed consent form: Effects of vocal training on respiration, phonation and articulation*. Indiana University of Pennsylvania School of Graduate Studies and Research (model protocols). Retrieved August 26, 2004, from http://www.iup.edu/graduate/irb/models.shtm

Menzel, O. J. (1995). Letter to the editor. *American Journal of Audiology*, *4*, 87–88.

Merton, R. K., Riske, M., & Kendall, P. L. (1956). *The focused interview. A manual* of problems and procedures. Glencoe: The Free Press.

Metz, D. E., & Folkins, J. W. (1985). Protection of human subjects in speech and hearing research. *Asha, 27*, 25–29.

Minitab. (1998). *Minitab statistical software release 12*. State College, PA: Author.

Mirrett, P. L., Roberts, J. E., & Price, J. (2003). Early intervention practices and communication intervention strategies for young males with Fragile X syndrome. *Language, Speech, and Hearing Services in Schools, 14*, 320–331.

Mizuko, M., & Reichle, J. (1989). Transparency and recall of symbols among intellectually handicapped adults. *Journal of Speech and Hearing Disorders, 54*, 627–633.

Moeschberger, M. L., Williams, J. A., & Brown, C. G. (1985). Methods of randomization in controlled clinical trials. *American Journal of Emergency Medicine, 3*, 467–473.

Moher, D., Tetzlaff, J., Tricco, A. C., Sampson, M., & Altman, D. G. (2007). Epidemiology and reporting characteristics of systematic reviews. *PLoS Medicine, 4*, 0447–0455.

Morrow, K. L., & Fridriksson, J. (2006). Comparing fixed- and randomized-interval spaced retrieval in anomia treatment. *Journal of Communication Disorders, 39*, 2–11.

Mueller, P. B., & Lisko, D. (2003). Undergraduate research in CSD programs: A solution to the PhD shortage? *Contemporary Issues in Communication Science and Disorders, 30*, 123–126.

Muma, J. (1993). The need for replication. *Journal of Speech and Hearing Research, 36*, 927–930.

Nail-Chiwetalu, B., & Bernstein Ratner, N. (2003). *Fostering information literacy competency*. Proceedings of the Council on Academic Programs in Communication Sciences and Disorders Conference. Retrieved August 26, 2004, from http://www.capcsd.org/proceedings/2003/talks/chiwetalu2003.pdf

Nathan, L., Stackhouse, J., Goulandris, N., & Snowling, M. J. (2004). The development of early listening skills among children with speech difficulties: A test of the "critical age hypothesis." *Journal of Speech-Language-Hearing Research, 47*, 377–391.

National Institute on Deafness and Other Communication Disorders. (2004). *Guidelines on communicating informed consent for individuals who are deaf or hard-of-hearing and scientists*. Retrieved August 27, 2004, from http://www.nidcd.nih.gov/news/releases/99/inform/xviii.asp

National Institutes of Health. (1979). *Regulation and ethical guidelines*. Retrieved April 11, 2009, from http://ohsr.od.nih.gov/guidelines/belmont.html

National Library of Medicine. (2004a). *MeSH*. Retrieved August 26, 2004, from http://www/ncbi.nlm.nih.gov

National Library of Medicine. (2004b). *National Information Center on Health Services Research and Health Care Technology*. Retrieved August 27, 2004, from http://www.nlm.nih.gov/nichsr/nichsr.html

National Student Speech Language Hearing Association. (2008). *Publications main page*. Retrieved June 9, 2008, from http://www.nsslha.org/NSSLHA/publications

Newman, C. W., Weinstein, B.E., Jacobson, G.P., Hug, G.A. (1990). *The Hearing Handicap Inventory for Adults*: Psychometric adequacy and audiometric correlates. *Ear and Hearing, 11*, 430–433.

NIH Office of Extramural Research. (2000). NIH *guidelines on the inclusion of women and minorities as subjects in clinical research (updated)*. Retrieved August 29, 2004, from http://grants.nih.gov/grants/funding/women_min/guidelines_update.htm

Norman, G. R., Sloan, J. A., & Wyrwich, K. W. (2003). Interpretation of changes in health-related quality of life: The remarkable university of half a standard deviation. *Medical Care, 41*, 582–592.

North Carolina Association for Biomedical Research. (2007). *NCABR.ORG: About biomedical research: FAQ*. Retrieved December 23, 2007, from http://www.ncabr.org

Norušis, M. J. (1988). *The SPSS guide to data analysis for SPSS/PC+*. Chicago: SPSS.

The Nuremberg Code. (1947). In *Trials of war criminals before the Nuremberg military tribunals under control council law no. 10* (1949), *2*, 181–182. Washington, DC: U.S. Government Printing Office (1949).

Nye, C., & Harvey, J. (2006). Interpreting and maintaining the evidence. *Contemporary Issues in Communication Science and Disorders, 33*, 56–60.

OBSSR. (n.d.). *Qualitative methods in health research: Opportunities and considerations in application and review.* Retrieved April 17, 2009, from http://obssr.od.nih.gov/pdf/Qualitative.pdf

Oelschlaeger, M., & Damico, J. S. (2000). Partnership in conversation: A study of word search strategies. *Journal of Communication Disorders, 33*, 205–225.

Office of Behavioral and Social Sciences Research, National Institutes of Health. (2004). *Qualitative methods in health research: Opportunities and considerations in applications and reviews.* Retrieved August 26, 2004, from http://obssr.od.nih.gov/Publications/Qualitative.PDF

Office of Human Subjects Research. (2004). *Research involving cognitively impaired subjects: A review of some ethical considerations (OHSR information sheet 7).* Retrieved August 27, 2004, from http://www.nihtraining.com/ohsrsite/info/info.html

Office of Laboratory Animal Welfare. (1984). *Public health service policy on humane care and use of laboratory animals.* Retrieved April 11, 2009, from http://grants.nih.gov/grants/olaw/references/phspol.htm

Ohio Board of Speech-Language Pathology and Audiology. (2004). *Ohio law and administrative rules governing the practice of speech-language pathology and audiology.* Retrieved August 27, 2004, from http://slpaud.ohio.gov/lawsandrules.htm

Olswang, L. B. (1990). Treatment efficacy research: A path to quality assurance. *Asha, 32*, 45–47.

O'Neil-Pirozzi, T. M. (2003). Language functioning of residents in family homeless shelters. *American Journal of Speech-Language Pathology, 12*, 229–242.

Orwin, R. G. (1983). A fail-safe *N* for effect size in meta-analysis. *Journal of Educational Statistics, 8*, 157–159.

Paashe-Orlow, M. K., Taylor, H. A., & Brancati, F. L. (2003). Readability standards for informed-consent forms as compared with actual readability. *The New England Journal of Medicine, 348*, 721–726.

Pannbacker, M., & Hayes, S. (2007). Controversial treatment in speech-language pathology: What are the issues? *TEJAS, 37*, 22–32.

Patten, M. L. (2004). *Understanding research methods.* Glendale, CA: Pyrczak Publishing.

Patton, M. Q. (1990). *Qualitative research & evaluation methods* (2nd ed.). Thousand Oaks, CA: Sage.

Patton, M. Q. (2002). *Qualitative research and evaluation methods* (3rd ed.). Thousand Oaks, CA: Sage.

Pawson, R., Greenhalgh, T., Harvey, G., & Walshe, K. (2005). Realist review—A new method of systematic review designed for complex policy interventions. *Journal of Health Services Research and Policy, 10*, 21–34.

Pearson, E. S., Plackett, R. L., & Barnard, G. A. (1990) *Student: A statistical biography of William Sealy Gosset.* Oxford, UK: University Press.

Plante, T. G. (1998). Teaching psychology ethics to undergraduates: An experiential model. *Teaching of Psychology, 25*, 281–285.

Preisser, D. A., Hodson, B. W., & Paden, E. P. (1988). Developmental phonology: 18–29 months. *Journal of Speech and Hearing Disorders, 53*, 125–130.

Pressman, J., & Wildavsky, A. (1973). *Implementation: How great expectations in Washington are dashed in Oakland.* Berkeley, CA: University of California Press.

Pyrczak, F., & Bruce, R. R. (2003). *Writing empirical research reports*. Los Angeles: Pyrczak Publishing.

Qualitative Interest Group. (2004). *Purpose, history and activities*. Retrieved August 26, 2004, from University of Georgia College of Education website: http://www.coe.uga.edu/quig/archives/index.html

Reid, R., Hertzog, M., & Snyder, M. (1996). Educating every teacher, every year: The public schools and parents of children with ADHD. *Seminars in Speech and Language*, *17*, 73–87.

Reilly, S., Douglas, J., & Oates, J. (Eds.). (2004). *Evidence based practice in speech pathology*. Philadelphia: Whurr.

Reynolds, M. E., Callihan, K., & Browning, E. (2003). Effect of instruction on the development of rhyming skills in young children. *Contemporary Issues in Communication Science and Disorders*, *30*, 41–46.

Robey, R. R. (1998). A meta-analysis of clinical outcomes in the treatment of aphasia. *Journal of Speech-Language-Hearing Research*, *41*, 172–187.

Robey, R. R. (2004, November). *Effect sizes in research manuscripts: Selecting, calculating, reporting, and interpreting*. Seminar presented at the annual meeting of the American Speech-Language-Hearing Association, Philadelphia.

Robey, R. R., & Dalebout, S. D. (1998). A tutorial on conducting meta-analysis of clinical outcome research. *Journal of Speech-Language-Hearing Research*, *41*, 1227–1241.

Robey, R. R., & Schultz, M. C. (1998). A model for conducting clinical-outcome research: An adaptation of the standard protocol for use in aphasiology. *Aphasiology*, *12*, 787–810.

Robey, R. R., Schultz, M. C., Crawford, A. B., & Sinner, C. A. (1999). Single-subject clinical-outcome research: Designs, data, effect sizes, and analyses. *Aphasiology*, *13*, 445–473.

Rodriguez, B. L., & Olswang, L. B. (2003). Mexican-American and Anglo-American mothers' beliefs and values about child rearing, education, and language impairment. *American Journal of Speech-Language Pathology*, *12*, 452–462.

Rogers, W. A. (2004). Evidence based medicine and justice: A framework for looking at the impact of EBM upon vulnerable or disadvantaged groups. *Journal of Medical Ethics*, *30*, 141–145.

Rosenberg, M. S., Adams, D. C., & Gurevitch, J. (2000). *MetaWin: Statistical software for meta-analysis version 2.0*. Sunderland, MA: Sinauer Associates.

Rosenfeld, R. M., & Bluestone, C. D. (Eds.). (2003). *Evidence-based otitis media* (2nd ed.). Hamilton, Ontario: BC Decker.

Rosenthal, R. (2000). Effect sizes in behavioral and biomedical research. In L. Bickman (Ed.), *Validity and social experimentation* (pp. 121–139). Thousand Oaks, CA: Sage.

Rosenthal, R., & Rosnow, R. L. (2008). Essentials of behavioral research: Methods and data analysis (3rd ed.). Boston, MA: McGraw-Hill.

Rosnow, R. L., & Rosenthal, R. (1997). *People studying people: Artifacts and ethics in behavioral research*. New York: W. H. Freeman.

Rosnow, R. L., & Rosenthal, R. (2003). Effect sizes for experimenting psychologists. *Canadian Journal of Experimental Psychology*, *57*, 221–237.

Rosnow, R. L., Rosenthal, R., & Rubin, D. B. (2000). Contrasts and correlations in effect-size estimation. *Psychological Science*, *11*, 446–453.

Rousseau, B., Hirano, S., Chan, R. W., Welham, N. V., Thibeault, S. L., Ford, C. N., & Bless, D. M. (2004). Characterization of chronic vocal fold scarring in a rabbit model. *Journal of Voice*, *18*, 116–124.

Roy, N., Weinrich, B., Gray, S. D., Tanner, K., Stemple, J. C., & Sapienza, C. M. (2003). Three treatments for teachers with voice disorders: A randomized clinical trial. *Journal of Speech-Language-Hearing Research*, *46*, 670–688.

Ryugo, D. K., Cahill, H. B., Rose, L. S., Rosenbaum, M. E., Schroeder, M. E., & Wright, A. L. (2003). Separate forms of pathology in the cochlea of congenitally deaf white cats. *Hearing Research*, *181*, 73–84.

Sacks, H., Chalmers, T. C., & Smith, H. (1982). Randomized versus historical controls for clinical trials. *The American Journal of Medicine*, *72*, 233–240.

Saghaei, M. (2008). *Random allocation software*. Retrieved June 9, 2008, from http://mahmood-saghaei.tripod.com/Softwares/randalloc.html

Sapir, S., Spielman, J., Ramig, L. O., Hinds, S., Countryman, S., Fox, C., Story, B. (2003). Effects of intensive voice treatment (the Lee Silverman Voice Treatment [LSVT]) on ataxic dysarthria: A case study. *American Journal of Speech-Language Pathology*, *12*, 387–399.

Schlosser, R. W., & Blischak, D. M. (2004). Effects of speech and print feedback on spelling by children with autism. *Journal of Speech-Language-Hearing Research*, *47*, 848–862.

Schmitt, J. F., & Meline, T. J. (1990). Subject descriptions, control groups, and research designs in published studies of language-impaired children. *Journal of Communication Disorders*, *23*, 365–382.

Schultz, K. F., Chalmers, I, Grimes, D. A., & Altman, D. G. (1994). Assessing the quality of randomization from reports of controlled trials published in obstetrics and gynecology journals. *The Journal of the American Medical Association*, *272*, 125–128.

Schwartz, H., & Drager, K. D. R. (2008). Training and knowledge in autism among speech-language pathologists: A survey. *Language, Speech, and Hearing Services in Schools*, *39*, 66–77.

Scott, N. W., McPherson, G. C., Ramsay, C. R., & Campbell, M. K. (2002). The method of minimization for allocation to clinical trials: A review. *Controlled Clinical Trials*, *23*, 662–674.

Scruggs, T. E., & Mastropieri, M. A. (2001). How to summarize single-participant research: Ideas and applications. *Exceptionality*, *9*, 227–244.

Shadish, W. R., Cook, T. D., & Campbell, D. T. (2002). *Experimental and quasi-experimental designs for generalized causal inference*. Boston: Houghton-Mifflin.

Shalala, D. (2000). Protecting research subjects—What must be done. *New England Journal of Medicine*, *343*, 808–810.

Shojania, K. G., Sampson, M., Ansari, M. T., Ji, J., Doucette, S., & Moher, D. (2007). How quickly do systematic reviews go out of date? A survival analysis. *Annals of Internal Medicine*, *147*, 224–234.

Shriberg, L. D., & Kwiatkowski, J. (1987). A retrospective study of spontaneous generalization in speech-delayed children. *Language, Speech, and Hearing Services in Schools*, *18*, 144–157.

Silliman, E. (2000). From the editor. *Language, Speech, and Hearing Services in Schools*, *31*, 211–212.

Silverman, F. H. (1988). The monster study. *Journal of Fluency Disorders*, *13*, 225–231.

Simmons-Mackie, N. N., & Damico, J. S. (2003). Contributions of qualitative research to the knowledge base of normal communication. *American Journal of Speech-Language Pathology*, *12*, 144–154.

Sininger, Y., Marsh, R., Walden, B., & Wilber, L. A. (2003). Guidelines for ethical practice in research for audiologists. *Audiology Today*, *15*, 14–17.

SISA. (2008). *SISA: Simple Interactive Statistical Analysis*. Retrieved June 9, 2008, from http://www.quantitativeskills.com/sisa/index.htm

Skarakis-Doyle, E., Dempsey, L. & Lee, C. (2008). Identifying language comprehension impairment in preschool children. *Language, Speech, and Hearing Services in Schools, 39*, 54–65.

Slavin, R. E. (1995). Best evidence synthesis: An intelligent alternative to meta-analysis. *Journal of Clinical Epidemiology, 48*, 9–18.

Smith, G. D., Egger, M., & Phillips, A. N. (1997). Meta-analysis: Beyond the grand mean? *British Medical Journal, 315*, 1600–1614.

Smith-Olinde, L., Besing, J., & Koehnke, J. (2004). Interference and enhancement effects on interaural time discrimination and level discrimination in listeners with normal hearing and those with hearing loss. *American Journal of Speech-Language Pathology, 13*, 80–95.

Southwood, F., & Russell, A. F. (2004). Comparison of conversation, freeplay, and story generation as methods of language sample elicitation. *Journal of Speech-Language-Hearing Research, 47*, 366–376.

SPSS. (2008). *SPSS statistical system*. Retrieved June 1, 2008, from http://www.spss.com/statistics

Stager, S., Calis, K., Grothe, D., Bloch, M., Berensen, N. M., Smith, P. J., & Braun, A. (2005). Treatment with medications affecting dopaminergic and serotonergic mechanisms: Effects on fluency and anxiety in persons who stutter. *Journal of Fluency Disorders, 30*, 319–335.

State of Illinois Division of Professional Regulations. (2004). *Section 1465.95 Professional Conduct Standards*. Retrieved August 26, 2004, from http://www.ildpr.com/WHO/ar/spchpath.asp

State of New Mexico, Office of the Governor (2007, May 22). *Governor Bill Richardson calls for animal-lab reforms at research universities*. Retrieved June 9, 2008, from http://www.governor.state.nm.us/press/2007/may/052207_02.pdf

Steinberg, E. P., & Luce, B. R. (2005). Evidence based? Caveat emptor! *Health Affairs, 24*, 80–92.

Sternberg, R. J. (1992). How to win acceptance by psychology journals: Twenty-one tips for better writing. *APS Observer, 12*, 13, 18.

Sternberg, R. J. (1993). *The psychologist's companion: A guide to scientific writing for students and researchers*. New York: Cambridge University Press.

Stevens, S. S. (1946). On the theory of scales of measurement. *Science, 103*, 677–680.

Stevens, S. S. (1951). Mathematics, measurement, and psychophysics. In S. S. Stevens (Ed.), *Handbook of experimental psychology* (pp. 1–49). New York: Wiley.

Stewart, M., Pankiw, R., Lehman, M. E., & Simpson, T. H. (2002). Hearing loss and hearing handicap in users of recreational firearms. *Journal of the American Academy of Audiology, 13*, 160–168.

Stillman, R., Snow, R., & Warren, K. (1999). "I used to be good with kids." Encounters between speech-language pathology students and children with pervasive developmental disorders (PDD). In D. Kovarsky, J. Duchan, & M. Maxwell (Eds.). *Constructing (in)competence: Disabling evaluations in clinical and social interaction* (pp. 29–48). Mahwah, NJ: Erlbaum.

Straus, S. E., Richardson, W. S., Glasziou, P., & Haynes, R. B. (2005). *Evidence-based medicine: How to practice and teach EBM* (3rd ed.). Edinburg, UK: Elsevier Churchill Livingstone.

Strum, J. M., & Nelson, N. W. (1997). Formal classroom lessons: New perspectives on a familiar discourse event. *Language, Speech, and Hearing Services in Schools, 28*, 255–273.

Stuart, A. (2004). An investigation of list equivalency of the Northwestern University Auditory Test No. 6 in interrupted broadband noise. *American Journal of Audiology, 13*, 23–28.

Stuart, A., Kalinowski, J., Rastatter, M., Saltuklaroglu, T., & Dayalu, V. (2004). Investigations of the impact of altered auditory feedback in-the-ear devices on the speech of people who stutter: Initial fitting and 4-month follow-up. *International Journal of Language and Communication Disorders, 39*, 93–119.

Tatano Beck, C. (1994). Achieving statistical power through research design sensitivity. *Journal of Advanced Nursing Research*, *20*, 912–916.

Taves, D. R. (1974). Minimization: A new method of assigning patients to treatment and control groups. *Clinical Pharmacology and Therapeutics*, *15*, 443–453.

ten Hallers, E. J. O., Rakhorst, G., Marres, H. A. M., Jansen, J. A., van Kooten, T. G., Schutte, H. K., et al. (2004). Animal models for tracheal research. *Biomaterials*, *25*, 1533–1543.

Tetnowski, J. A., & Franklin, T. C. (2003). Qualitative research: Implications for description and assessment. *American Journal of Speech-Language Pathology*, *12*, 155–164.

Tharpe, A. M., & Ashmead, D. H. (2001). A longitudinal investigation of infant auditory sensitivity. *American Journal of Audiology*, *10*, 1–9.

Thomas, L., & Krebs, C. J. (1997). A review of statistical power analysis software. *Bulletin of the Ecological Society of America*, *78*, 128–139.

Thompson, B. (2007). Effect sizes, confidence intervals, and confidence intervals for effect sizes. *Psychology in the Schools*, *44*, 423–432.

Timmermans, S., & Mauck, A. (2005). The promises and pitfalls of evidence-based medicine. *Health Affairs*, *24*, 18–28.

Todman, J. B., & Dugard, P. (2001). Single-case and small-n experimental designs: A practical guide to randomization tests. Mahwah, NJ: Erlbaum.

Torgerson, C. J., Brooks, G., & Hall, J. (2006). *A systematic review of the research literature on the use of phonics in the teaching of reading and spelling* (Research Report No. 71). Sheffield, UK: The University of Sheffield.

Treasure, T., & MacRae, K. D. (1998). Minimisation: The platinum standard for trials. *British Medical Journal*, *317*, 362–368.

Trochim, B. (2004). *Bill Trochim's center for social research methods*. Retrieved August 26, 2004, from http://trochim.human.cornell.edu

Trochim, W. M. (2008) *The research methods knowledge base* (2nd ed.). Retrieved June 9, 2008, from http://www.socialresearchmethods.net/kb/

Tudor, M. (1939). *An experimental study of the effect of evaluative labeling on speech fluency*. Unpublished master's thesis, University of Iowa.

Turkstra, L., Ciccia, A., & Seaton, C. (2003). Interactive behaviors in adolescent conversation dyads. *Language, Speech, and Hearing Services in Schools*, *34*, 117–127.

Tyler, A. A., Lewis, K. E., Haskill, A., & Tolbert, L. C. (2003). Outcomes of different speech and language goal attack strategies. *Journal of Speech-Language-Hearing Research*, *46*, 1077–1094.

Ukrainetz, T. A., & Fresquez, E. F. (2003). "What *isn't* language?": A qualitative study of the role of the school speech-language pathologist. *Language, Speech, and Hearing Services in Schools*, *34*, 284–298.

U.S. Department of Health and Human Services. (1990, September 28). ADAMHA/NIH policy concerning inclusion of minorities in study populations. *NIH Guide for Grants and Contracts*, *19*, 1–2.

U.S. Food and Drug Administration. (2008). *Guidance for institutional review boards, clinical investigators, and sponsors*. Retrieved June 9, 2008, from http://www.fda.gov/oc/ohrt/irbs/default.htm

Van Kleeck, A., & Beckley-McCall, A. (2002). A comparison of mothers' individual and simultaneous book sharing with preschool siblings: An exploratory study of five families. *American Journal of Speech-Language Pathology*, *11*, 175–189.

Velleman, P. F., & Wilkinson, L. (1993). Nominal, ordinal, interval, and ratio typologies are misleading. *The American Statistician*, *47*, 65–72.

Viera, A. J., & Bangdiwala, S. I. (2007). Eliminating bias in randomized controlled trials: Importance of allocation concealment and masking. *Family Medicine, 39*, 132–137.

Waddell, C. (2004). *Thesis writing*. Retrieved November 26, 2004, from http://www.rpi.edu/web/writingcenter/thesis.html

Wadsworth, B. J. (1989). *Piaget's theory of cognitive and affective development*. New York: Longman.

Walden, B. E., Surr, R. K., Cord, M. T., & Dyrlund, O. (2004). Predicting hearing aid microphone preference in everyday listening. *Journal of the American Academy of Audiology, 15*, 365–396.

Walden, T. C., & Walden, B. E. (2004). Predicting success with hearing aids in everyday living. *Journal of the American Academy of Audiology, 15*, 342–352.

Walters, D. B., & Chapman, R. S. (2000). Comprehension monitoring: A developmental effect? *American Journal of Speech-Language Pathology, 9,* 48–54.

Walton, J. H., McCardle, P., Crowe, T. A., & Wilson, B. E. (1990). Black English in a Mississippi prison population. *Journal of Speech and Hearing Disorders, 55*, 206–216.

Wambaugh, J., & Bain, B. (2002). Make research methods and integral part of your clinical practice. *ASHA Leader Online*. Retrieved August 26, 2004, from http://www.asha.org/about/publications/leader-online/archives/2002/q4/021119.htm

Watkins, M. (2008). *Marley Watkins, Ph.D., ABPP*. Retrieved April 10, 2008, from http://www.public.asu.edu/~mwwatkin/

Wegman, J. (2008). *Tips for thesis writers*. Retrieved April 18, 2009, from http://www.wesleyan.edu/writing/workshop/generalinfo/thesis.html

Wertz, R. T., LaPointe, L. L., & Rosenbeck, J. C. (1984). Apraxia of speech in adults: The disorder and its management. Needham Heights, MA: Allyn and Bacon.

White, B. (2004). Making evidence-based medicine doable in everyday practice. *Family Practice Management, 11*, 51–58.

White House Office of the Press Secretary. (1997, May 16). *Remarks by the President in apology for study done in Tuskegee*. Retrieved August 26, 2004, from http://clinton4.nara.gov/textonly/New/Remarks/Fri/19970516-898.html

Wiley, T. L., Stoppenbach, D. T., Feldhake, L. J., Moss, K. A., & Thordardottir, E. T. (1995). Audiologic practices: What is popular versus what is supported by evidence. *American Journal of Audiology, 4*, 26–34.

Williams, A. L. (2000). Multiple oppositions: Case studies of variables in phonological intervention. *American Journal of Speech-Language Pathology, 9*, 289–299.

Williams, A. L., & Elbert, M. (2003). A prospective longitudinal study of phonological development in late talkers. *Language, Speech, and Hearing Services in Schools, 34*, 138–153.

Williams, A. L., & Fagelson, M. (2003). Fostering a community of scholars in a graduate program. *ASHA Leader Online*. Retrieved August 26, 2004, from http://www.asha.org/about/publications/leader-online/archives/2003/q1/030304fa.htm

Wilson, W. J., & Mills, P. C. (2005). Brainstem auditory-evoked response in dogs. *American Journal of Veterinary Research, 66*, 2177–2187.

Yairi, E., Watkins, R., Ambrose, N., & Paden, E. (2001). What is stuttering? *Journal of Speech-Language-Hearing Research, 44*, 585–592.

Yoder, P. J. (1989). Maternal question use predicts later language development in specific-language-disordered children. *Journal of Speech and Hearing Disorders, 54*, 347–355.

SUBJECT INDEX